Pediatric Physical Examination

An Illustrated Handbook

KAREN G. DUDERSTADT, PHD, RN, CPNP, PCNS

Clinical Professor
Department of Family Health Care Nursing
School of Nursing
University of California, San Francisco
San Francisco, California;
Children's Health Center
San Francisco General Hospital
San Francisco, California

ELSEVIER

P9-BIY-713

ELSEVIER
MOSBY

3251 Riverport Lane
St. Louis, Missouri 63043

PEDIATRIC PHYSICAL EXAMINATION:
AN ILLUSTRATED HANDBOOK, SECOND EDITION

ISBN: 978-0-323-10006-9

Notices

Knowledge and best practice in this field are constantly changing. As new research and experience broaden our understanding, changes in research methods, professional practices, or medical treatment may become necessary.

Practitioners and researchers must always rely on their own experience and knowledge in evaluating and using any information, methods, compounds, or experiments described herein. In using such information or methods, they should be mindful of their own safety and the safety of others, including parties for whom they have a professional responsibility.

With respect to any drug or pharmaceutical products identified, readers are advised to check the most current information provided (i) on procedures featured or (ii) by the manufacturer of each product to be administered, to verify the recommended dose or formula, the method and duration of administration, and contraindications. It is the responsibility of practitioners, relying on their own experience and knowledge of their patients, to make diagnoses, to determine dosages and the best treatment for each individual patient, and to take all appropriate safety precautions.

To the fullest extent of the law, neither the Publisher nor the authors, contributors, or editors assume any liability for any injury and/or damage to persons or property as a matter of products liability, negligence or otherwise, or from any use or operation of any methods, products, instructions, or ideas contained in the material herein.

Library of Congress Cataloging-in-Publication Data

Duderstadt, Karen.
  Pediatric physical examination : an illustrated handbook / Karen G. Duderstadt.—2nd ed.
    p. ; cm.
  Includes bibliographical references and index.
  ISBN 978-0-323-10006-9 (pbk. : alk. paper)
  I. Title.
  [DNLM: 1. Physical Examination—Handbooks. 2. Child. WS 39]
  RJ50
  618.92'0075--dc23

2013012810

Executive Content Strategist: Lee Henderson
Content Development Specialist: Jackie Twomey
Publishing Services Manager: Jeff Patterson
Project Manager: Tracey Schriefer
Design Direction: Jessica Williams

Top cover photo: Nurse Practitioner Pat Clinton performing an ear assessment. (Photo by Tim Schoon. Copyright © University of Iowa, 2002.)

Right cover photo: Nurse Practitioner Julie Tsirambidis assessing an infant in Haiti. (Photo by Ted Stevens. Copyright © Ted Stevens, 2011.)

Printed in China

Last digit is the print number: 9 8 7 6 5 4 3 2 1

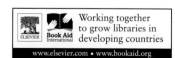

Working together
to grow libraries in
developing countries

www.elsevier.com • www.bookaid.org

To all the students who have shaped me as a teacher and a mentor;
To the children and families whom I have had the privilege of caring for and who have enriched my life; and
To Chris, my constantly patient husband, who has supported my life's work.

CONTRIBUTORS

Abbey Alkon, RN, PNP, PhD
Professor
Department of Family Health Care Nursing
School of Nursing
University of California, San Francisco
San Francisco, California
Developmental Surveillance and Screening

Patricia Jackson Allen, RN, MS, PNP-BC, FAAN
Professor, PNP Specialty Coordinator
School of Nursing
Yale University
New Haven, Connecticut
Ears
Nose, Mouth, and Throat

Angel K. Chen, RN, MSN, CPNP
Associate Clinical Professor and Vice Chair
Department of Family Health Care Nursing
School of Nursing
University of California, San Francisco
San Francisco, California;
Pediatric Urology Nurse Practitioner
Children's Health Center
San Francisco General Hospital
San Francisco, California
Male Genitalia

Karen G. Duderstadt, PhD, RN, CPNP, PCNS
Clinical Professor
Department of Family Health Care Nursing
School of Nursing
University of California, San Francisco
San Francisco, California;
Children's Health Center
San Francisco General Hospital
San Francisco, California
Approach to Care and Assessment
of Children and Adolescents
Assessment Parameters

Comprehensive Information Gathering
Environmental Health History
Head and Neck
Lymphatic System
Eyes
Musculoskeletal System
Neurological System
Charting Pediatric Comprehensive and
Symptom-Focused Health Care Visits

Victoria F. Keeton, MS, RN, CPNP, CNS
Associate Clinical Professor
Department of Family Health Care Nursing
School of Nursing
University of California, San Francisco
San Francisco, California
Abdomen and Rectum

Renee P. McLeod, PhD, APRN, CPNP, FAANP
Dean, Professor
Marybelle and S. Paul Musco School
of Nursing and Health Professions
Brandman University
Irvine, California
Skin

Erica Bisgyer Monasterio, MN, FNP-BC
Clinical Professor
Director, Family Nurse Practitioner Program
Department of Family Health Care Nursing
School of Nursing,
Clinical Professor
Division of Adolescent and Young Adult
Medicine
Department of Pediatrics
University of California, San Francisco
San Francisco, California
Male and Female Breast
Female Genitalia

Patricia O'Brien, MSN, CPNP-AC
Nurse Practitioner
Department of Nursing/Patient Services,
    Cardiovascular Program
Boston Children's Hospital
Boston, Massachusetts
Heart and Vascular System

Naomi A. Schapiro, PhD, RN, CPNP
Clinical Professor
Department of Family Health Care Nursing
School of Nursing;
Project Director
UCSF Elev8 Healthy Students & Families
University of California, San Francisco
San Francisco, California
Comprehensive Information Gathering
Musculoskeletal System
Male and Female Breast
Female Genitalia

Concettina (Tina) Tolomeo, DNP, APRN,
    FNP-BC, AE-C
Nurse Practitioner
Director of Program Development and
    Operations
Yale School of Medicine
New Haven, Connecticut
Chest and Respiratory System

Elizabeth Tong, MS, RN, PNP, FAHA, FAAN
Clinical Nurse Specialist and Research
    Coordinator (Retired)
Pediatric Cardiology;
Clinical Professor (Emeritus)
School of Nursing
University of California, San Francisco
San Francisco, California
Heart and Vascular System

Sameeya Ahmed-Winston, RN, MSN, CPNP, CPHON
Pediatric Nurse Practitioner
Children's National Medical Center
Washington, District of Columbia

Deanne Buschbach, RN, MSN, NNP, PNP
NNP and NP Team Leader for the Intensive Care Nursery
Duke University Medical Center
Durham, North Carolina

Annette Carley, RN, MS, NNP-BC, PNP-BC
Clinical Professor
School of Nursing
University of California, San Francisco
San Francisco, California

Margaret-Ann Carno, PhD, MBA, CPNP, DABSM, FAAN
Associate Professor of Clinical Nursing and Pediatrics
School of Nursing
University of Rochester
Rochester, New York

Laura Crisanti, MSN, CCRN, CPNP-PC
Pediatric Nurse Practitioner
Ann & Robert H. Lurie Children's Hospital of Chicago
Chicago, Illinois

Kari Ksar, PNP
Pediatric Nurse Practitioner
Lucile Packard Children's Hospital
Palo Alto, California

Suzanne Kujawa, MSN, RNC, CPNP-PC
Advanced Practice Nurse
Ann & Robert H. Lurie Children's Hospital of Chicago
Chicago, Illinois

Nancy McLoone, RN, MS, CPNP
Assistant Professor, Pediatric Nurse Practitioner
Mankato Clinic
Minnesota State University
Mankato, Minnesota

Jessica Pech, APN, CPNP
Ann & Robert H. Lurie Children's Hospital of Chicago
Chicago, Illinois

Susan Rice, PhD, RN, CPNP, CNS
Professor
University of Toledo
Toledo, Ohio

Caroline A. Rich, RN, MSN, CPNP, AC/PC
Pediatric Nurse Practitioner
Helen DeVos Children's Hospital
Wayne State University
Grand Rapids, Michigan

Cheryl Rodgers, PhD, RN, CPNP, CPON
Instructor, Pediatric Nurse Practitioner
Texas Children's Hospital
Baylor College of Medicine
Houston, Texas

Kerry Shields, RN, MSN, CRNP, MBE
Pediatric Critical Care Nurse Practitioner
The Children's Hospital of Philadelphia
University of Pennsylvania
Philadelphia, Pennsylvania

PREFACE

Pediatric Physical Examination: An Illustrated Handbook, second edition, is written for students, educators, and pediatric health care providers dedicated to mastering the art and technique of the comprehensive physical examination of infants, children, and adolescents. Facing increasing pressures, primary health care providers need astute assessment skills combined with quick references to assist them in caring for children and families. This second edition of *Pediatric Physical Examination: An Illustrated Handbook* will provide the novice or experienced provider with pediatric content from experts in the field, useful examination techniques from birth to adolescence, and pediatric clinical pearls not covered in other texts on health assessment across the life span. In response to suggestions by experienced clinicians who have used the text as a resource across pediatric clinical settings, the second edition features new Evidenced-Based Practice Tips, a Summary of Examination at the end of each chapter, and new Family, Cultural, Racial, and Ethnic Considerations sections. Additionally, this edition includes more than 50 new photos and drawings of important assessment findings.

The initial chapters of this handbook begin with an overview of the developmental approach to information gathering and assessment of children from birth to adolescence. Chapter 3 focuses on development surveillance and presents evidence on reliable and valid developmental and behavioral screening tools. Chapter 4 presents comprehensive information on history taking in infants, children, and adolescents, including expanded coverage of pediatric mental health assessment. Chapter 5 reviews the unique vulnerability of children to environmental hazards and focuses on the importance of the environmental health history in identifying and reducing environmental risk factors that have an impact on child health. Chapter 6 discusses inspection and palpation of the skin.

The chapters that follow are organized in the pediatric-oriented "quiet-to-active" approach to physical examination. Pediatric experts consider this to be the most effective approach to assessing young children. This format begins with the quieter parts of the exam—cardiac and respiratory—which require astute listening skills and less active participation of the young child. Then, Chapters 9 through 13, which cover assessment of the eyes, ears, nose, and throat, require more active participation from the child and are better performed after the quiet parts of the physical examination. Chapter 14 reviews abdominal assessment from birth to adolescence.

A unique feature of the text remains the developmental approach to examination of the male and female genitalia and the developing breast in males and females, presented in Chapters 15 through 17. Chapter 18 includes a comprehensive assessment of the child and adolescent athlete for sports participation, as well as the recent guidelines on assessment for concussion. Chapter 19 presents neurological assessment from a pediatric developmental perspective. Finally, Chapter 20 provides traditional charting templates for the comprehensive well-child visit and the preparticipation sports physical examination, and an example of an electronic health record commonly used in primary care clinical settings.

Working with children and families is a hopeful endeavor, and health in childhood builds the foundation for health promotion and health protection throughout life. Pediatric primary care providers have a key role in protecting and improving the health of the next generation. Through astute physical assessment, providers build trust with children and families and preserve the provider/patient relationship, ultimately improving health outcomes and decreasing health care costs. This handbook assists the pediatric health care provider with this most important undertaking: promoting the health of the next generation.

ACKNOWLEDGMENTS

The publication of the second edition would not have occurred without encouragement from my students, pediatric colleagues, family members, and the "very patient" editors at Elsevier. I would like to first acknowledge Jackie Twomey, Content Developmental Specialist, who has patiently and pleasantly mentored me through the publication of the second edition. Her attention to detail and willingness to accept my numerous edits has made this edition a wonderful resource for students and educators. Lee Henderson, Executive Content Strategist, has loyally carried my vision through to publication, including fulfilling my vision of the publication of an eBook! Tracey Schriefer, Project Manager, provided outstanding quality control for the text during the final stages of publication.

I am pleased to have several new contributors in the second edition—Abbey Alkon, Pat O'Brien, Angel Chen, Victoria Keeton, and Erica Monasterio. I am very thankful to them for bringing new pediatric and adolescent specialty expertise to this edition of the text. Their contributions were invaluable at a very busy time during the academic year. Pat Jackson Allen, my longtime mentor and friend, was willing to again support the text as a distinguished contributor, and Liz Tong, emeritus cardiac specialist, lead the revision of the cardiac chapter. Naomi Schapiro was willing to return as a contributor, all while she was completing her doctoral studies. All of these pediatric colleagues were instrumental to the second edition with their excellent contributions. Anthony Trela, PNP was my devoted research assistant and contributed the searches yielding many of the excellent references and resources used in updating the text.

Finally, I would like to acknowledge my dear husband and life companion, Christopher. Without his constant patience, love, and support, this edition would not have happened. I would also like to thank my brother, John, for his encouragement along the way! My hope is that the knowledge in this text will help to shape the next generation of pediatric health care providers who advocate for and promote optimum health for children and families.

CONTENTS

CHAPTER **1**

APPROACH TO CARE AND ASSESSMENT OF CHILDREN AND ADOLESCENTS

Karen G. Duderstadt

UNIQUE ROLE OF THE PEDIATRIC PROVIDER

Pediatric health care providers have a unique role in the development of a child's health over a lifetime. Health is an interactive process shaped by genetics, exposures, human experiences, and individual choice.[1] From a life course perspective, early experiences can "program" a child's health and development. Protective factors, such as a nurturing family and safe neighborhood, improve health and contribute to healthy development; and risk factors, such as limited access to health care and social services, impact a child's development and ability to reach his or her full developmental potential.[1]

Since physical, cognitive, and social-emotional health is established in the early years of life, a health care provider skilled in physical, behavioral, and mental health assessment can significantly promote the health and well-being of children and families. A significant body of literature indicates many chronic conditions in adulthood and disparities in adult health have their origins during childhood and increase over time.[2] Early investments in health promotion can empower individual health choices, greatly improve child health outcomes, alter the life course, and decrease the cost of health care services.

ESTABLISHING A CARING RELATIONSHIP

Children have unique needs because of their long period of dependency and development, and this presents a unique challenge to the pediatric health care provider. Children's health and well-being depend greatly on the care received from their family units and the surrounding environment in which they live. Addressing the needs of the parent while caring for the child and fostering a healthy relationship between the parent and child are the most important and challenging tasks in pediatrics.

Care is best provided in a *pediatric health care home* or *medical home,* which promotes holistic care of the child and family by partnering with a primary pediatric health care provider.[3] This model of care allows the provider to create a partnership to empower and support the family. Children, adolescents, and families benefit from motivational and anticipatory guidance in health promotion, which is particularly effective in the context of a pediatric health care home.[4] The caring relationship established by the primary care provider reinforces positive parenting and provides behavioral consultation to the family at critical periods of child development.

A caring relationship includes a patient-provider relationship without bias in regard to

1

racial, ethnic, and socioeconomic difference. Provider bias has been shown to contribute to disparities in health care and health outcomes.[5] Cultural biases may affect clinical decision making, and the perception of bias in clinical encounters undermines the caring relationship. Health care providers must make conscious efforts to overcome bias in their actions.[5] Educating providers on racial, cultural, and socioeconomic biases, self-regulating behavior, and developing new mental habits can provide the highest quality care to all children and families.[5]

PARENT AND CHILD INTERACTION

One of the most important aspects of the health interview is eliciting and observing interactions between the parent and child or adolescent. Analyzing verbal responses and interactions during the encounter gives the health care provider an idea of how the parental relationship fosters child development and child self-esteem. It also gives the health care provider a window into the child's world. Interactions between the parent or caregiver, the family members, and the health care provider reveal family dynamics, family connectedness, family authority, and the approach to problem solving.

Nonverbal cues provide the most revealing picture of the child's demeanor and of the parent/child relationship. Stop and observe these cues, and verbalize your concerns to the parent and child: "You look sad today. Can you tell me what that is about?" Ask yourself the following: Is the parent or caregiver disengaged with the child or infant during the encounter? Does the parent appear depressed or angry? Do the data from the health interview fit with the demeanor of the child during the encounter? The child or adolescent's nonverbal cues give the health care provider additional understanding of the context in which the child lives.

A child who is withdrawn, refusing to make eye contact, or who is consistently stressed when communicating with a parent is exhibiting signs of strain in her/his environment. This should alert the health care provider to communicate her/his concern to the family and provide support, counseling, and referral when indicated. Children often mirror the emotions of the adults around them. Families involved in conflict or who are under stress often cannot see their own interactions clearly or the impact their interactions have on the child. Early intervention by the health care provider in harmful or ineffective family communications is critical to the healthy psychosocial development of the child.

A large part of social and emotional development for children and adolescents is now occurring while the child or adolescent is on the Internet or on a cell phone.[6] Children's and adolescents' online lives constitute a large part of their social interactions, and there are potential risks to their privacy and safety.[6] It is important for parents and caregivers to monitor children's social media, Web, and cell phone activities for potential impact on their emotional health. Health care providers are in a unique position to urge parents to communicate with their children and educate them about the social anxiety, bullying, and risk taking that can occur with peer-to-peer communications online.[6] The American Academy of Pediatrics (AAP) provides resources for parents at http://safetynet.aap.org to assist them with safeguarding children and promoting healthy online behavior.

A CHILD'S PERSPECTIVE

The United Nations Convention on the Rights of the Child (1989) asserts that children have the right to self-determination, dignity, respect, noninterference, and to make informed decisions. Health care providers have a responsibility to ensure children's rights, and the child is encouraged or enabled to make their perspective known on issues that affect their health and well-being.[7] This perspective does present inherent conflicts for health care professionals in ensuring children's right to participate in health care decisions as well as their need for protection. Health professionals are aware of the importance of consulting with children during the health care visit, but they do not always wholly seek or acknowledge the child's or adolescent's view.[7] The view of the parent or caregiver and the view of the child may differ quite remarkably, and this difference can often impact health care decisions and treatment outcomes. Promoting opportunities for children and adolescents to contribute to health care decisions with families and caregivers creates a child-centered approach to care that empowers and enables the child or adolescent.

Shier proposed a model to facilitate children's participation in the health history.[8] The model provides a framework for communication that is attentive, sensitive, and supportive of a child's perspective while capturing the shared responsibility of families, health care professionals, and health care organizations. The model proposes the following:

- Irrespective of age the child is listened to.
- The child is supported in expressing his/her views.
- The child's views are taken into account.
- The child is involved in the decision-making process.
- The child can share power and responsibility in the decision making.

The last point is not to leave the responsibility to the child but to value the child's perspective while considering the needs and views of the family.[8] This framework provides pediatric health care providers with a child-centered approach to health care within the context of the family.

FAMILY, CULTURAL, RACIAL, AND ETHNIC CONSIDERATIONS

It is essential that health care professionals are committed to knowing the rationale and conceptual model for delivering family-centered, culturally, and linguistically competent care to provide a pediatric health care home or medical home.[9] The increasing global immigration of populations will continue to provide challenges to health care professionals working with diverse populations. Providers will be required to assess the extent to which culture plays a role in health care decisions in the family and impacts treatment plans and adherence to these plans.

There are significant disparities in pediatric health care, and children from economically disadvantaged and racially and ethnically diverse backgrounds are most affected. Recent studies have shown children with special health care needs are more racially and ethnically diverse than the general pediatric population, have less access to a pediatric health care home, and require special consideration.[9]

Cultural beliefs also impact care-seeking behavior and affect the delivery of clinical care by health care providers. Effective models of care incorporate sensitivity to cultural differences and enhance the protective factors of cultural practices within families. Studies demonstrate differences within ethnic groups are as great as the cultural differences between groups; therefore, no valid assumptions can be made in health care on the basis of physical appearance or surname. It is important for providers to acknowledge cultural differences, understand their own culture and how that influences the care they deliver, engage in self-assessment, acquire cultural knowledge and skills consistent with the practice setting, and value diversity within the health care team.[9]

Ideally, delivery of health care services should occur in the first language of the client. When this is not possible, a model framework for the encounter between the health care provider, child, and family includes the following:

- Recognizing language barriers and effectively using interpreters
- Exploring parental beliefs and their impact on the child
- Building on family strengths
- Recognizing and exploring the use of folk beliefs and alternative therapies, how they influence child health, and the impact on clinical care
- Understanding, as the health care provider, how your personal values and beliefs

influence care delivery and impact health outcomes
- Altering care practices to eliminate disparities in health care delivery related to race/ethnicity and economic status

Cultural competence is an essential component of responsible health care services for multicultural populations. Incorporating sensitive cultural understanding into the health care encounter will build honesty and trust in the caring relationship. Throughout the text, attention is given to how culture and ethnicity influence the assessment process in child health.

EFFECTIVE COMMUNICATION

Children are accepting of many different styles of interaction and will adapt to the health care provider who is at ease and competently engages the child. The skilled pediatric health care provider learns to make eye contact when a child is interested and to avoid eye contact when a child is fearful. Initially directing attention to the parent or caretaker allows the infant or young child time to adjust to the environment.

Children are comfortable when they know what to expect in an environment. Explaining clearly to the young child or adolescent exactly what you are going to assess during the physical exam will decrease anxiety and build trust. With each part of the exam, explain or "talk through" the assessment and the findings. Reassure the child or adolescent of your findings when normal and explain abnormal findings as appropriate for the child's age. Talking through every step of the encounter decreases anxiety in the child and adolescent. Even busy practitioners in time-pressured environments will find the child or adolescent to be a more willing participant when adding this *talk-through* format to the health care encounter.

INTERVIEWING CHILDREN

Engaging children in the interview process can reveal their understanding of health, allow participation in the health care encounter, and provide insight into their social-emotional world. Eye-level encounters are the most effective with young children and make the health care provider appear more approachable.

Many young children are effective communicators and can respond to questions about their dietary habits, daily activities, school or childcare, and relationships with school friends. It is important to engage children early in health information gathering. Health education can easily follow when this interview technique is used, and the child's responses create a dialogue that establishes a supportive provider-patient relationship.

Children 6 to 12 years old can be directly interviewed and can be participants in their health care. Health care providers can be role models for parents as they engage the child in the health interview and teach aspects of health and safety education. This approach teaches children from a young age to understand and care about their health and establishes the importance of building healthy habits for life.

Adolescents should always be interviewed separately from the parent. It is important to prepare the parent for this transition to a more independent role for the adolescent during the health care encounter. Allowing time to engage the adolescent independently will provide the best opening for discussion of personal or sensitive concerns that need to be voiced, and for discussion of any conflicts in the home or school environment that are impacting the adolescent's well-being.

Using the following clear communication techniques when interviewing will build a caring, trusting relationship with children/adolescents and their families.
- **Question indirectly** to encourage children and adolescents who are reluctant to discuss feelings. Engage the young child with, "I am going to tell you a story about a 5-year-old who lost his favorite pet. How do you think he feels?" or the adolescent with, "Some 15-year-olds have used marijuana. Do you have any friends who smoke marijuana?"
- **Pose scenarios** to the child or adolescent. "What would you do if . . . ?" is appropriate

for the young child, in contrast to, "How would you feel if . . . ?" which is appropriate for the older school-age child and adolescent.

- **Begin with less threatening topics** and move slowly to topics more sensitive to the child or adolescent. "Tell me how things are going at school this year," in contrast to, "Has anyone ever hurt you?" or directed to the adolescent, "Has anyone forced you to have sex against your will?"
- **State your expectations clearly.** Say to the child, "I need for you to be very quiet now so I can listen to . . . " or to the adolescent, "To take care of you, I need for you to tell me . . . "
- **Do not offer a choice** to the child or adolescent when in reality there is no choice.
- **Use "I"** when speaking to the child or adolescent. "I need to ask you this question because I want to help you . . . " in contrast to, "You need to tell me what is going on." Avoid using the word "you," which creates a defensive atmosphere when interviewing children or adolescents. This will provide positive role modeling for parents and also build the caring relationship between the health care provider, the child, and the parent.
- **Ask the young child to draw a picture.** This captures the child's attention and establishes your interest in their abilities. Children often reveal feelings or communicate important family issues through their art.[10]

THE IMPORTANCE OF PHYSICAL EXAMINATION

As health care providers increasingly rely on imaging and technology, the practice of diagnosing a health condition or disease from a physical examination has taken a backseat. The physical exam may be a ritual, but it is an important diagnostic tool when applied by skilled hands and can yield important diagnostic information and decrease the cost of health care.[11] The physical exam helps providers ask better questions of the diagnostic tests they

order.[12] Further, performing the physical examination provides important psychosocial benefits to the patient and can relieve stress and provide reassurance. Diagnostic evidence is important, but it is most valuable when decisions about diagnostic testing are made after completing a thorough health history and performing a thorough physical examination.

Besides the importance of focusing the diagnostic testing, what is also lost in eliminating the physical examination is the meaningful encounter between the patient and provider.[12] Recent studies have indicated the trusting relationship between the provider and the family is the most influential factor in assisting families in making sound decisions about the care of their child. This provider-patient relationship creates an important part of the therapeutic effect when working with families. It is crucial for pediatric health care providers to master the skills of history taking and physical examination in order to decrease or prevent medical errors and to increase the efficiency in ordering diagnostic testing and treating patients and families.

"QUIET TO ACTIVE" APPROACH TO THE PHYSICAL EXAMINATION

"Quiet to active" is an important mantra that should be adopted by the health care provider who will be caring for infants and young children. It refers to the approach of beginning with the parts of the physical examination that require the child to be quiet or silent in order for the health care provider to differentiate physical findings. The "quiet" parts of the physical examination in infants and young children include pulse and respiratory rate, auscultation of cardiac sounds and respiratory sounds, and auscultation and assessment of the abdomen. Respiratory and cardiac sounds are subtle, and accurate assessment requires a relatively cooperative child. Therefore, approaching these areas first during the physical examination produces the best results. The assessment of the genitalia and cranial nerves in the infant and young child can also be completed before the more invasive examination of the ears and mouth, and before measuring height, weight, temperature, and blood pressure when indicated. Varying the sequence of the physical examination to fit the temperament and activity level of the child is an essential part of pediatrics, but omitting an aspect of the physical exam does not serve the health care needs of the child and risks a diagnosis made on an incomplete assessment.

DEVELOPMENTAL APPROACH TO ASSESSMENT

Preterm Infants and Newborns

In the clinical setting, it is important to begin the physical assessment with the infant initially swaddled in the parent's arms or on the examining table to maintain body temperature. In this manner, auscultation of the cardiac and respiratory sounds can be accomplished before disturbing a sleeping infant or cooling the infant significantly. After the "quiet" parts of the examination are completed, transfer the infant to the examining table and begin a complete assessment with the infant wearing only a diaper. Observing the movements of the newborn for symmetry, strength, and coordination must be accomplished with the infant undressed. Assessment of overall appearance, skin color, breathing pattern, and degree of alertness or responsiveness should be noted. The health care provider should remain flexible in regard to the order of the exam throughout the encounter, because often the physical examination is performed between the eating and sleep cycles of the newborn.

Infants up to 6 Months of Age

Until 6 months of age, infants are most effectively assessed on the examination table. It provides a firm surface to support the infant's head during the physical exam and also provides a stable surface for the examination techniques required during a complete physical assessment. A calm, gentle approach works

well and avoids possibly frightening the infant. The "quiet" parts of the exam may be accomplished with the infant in the parent's arms, but other parts of the physical exam are difficult to accomplish effectively in that position. Remember never to leave the examining table at any point when evaluating a young infant.

Children 6 Months to 2 Years of Age

Inspection of infants and young children necessitates using a completely different social approach than with any other age groups. When establishing a therapeutic relationship with an adult, etiquette requires immediate eye contact. With infants 7 to 9 months of age, a progressive approach to eye contact is required because of the developmental phenomenon of stranger anxiety. First, observe the infant or young child covertly while speaking with the parent or caretaker to allow the child to adjust to your presence in the environment. If the young child is looking at you and listening, then make a glancing eye contact. If you are not rejected, then speak to the young child and, finally, reach out to touch the child. This approach will produce the best results when establishing the caring relationship. Offering puppets or washable, small toys to the child or using dolls to demonstrate parts of the physical examination for the young child also often provides a calming effect at the beginning of the encounter.

Once the infant is able to sit stably, normally around 6 to 8 months of age, the examination can proceed with the child in the parent's lap to decrease fear and stranger anxiety. Clothing should be removed gradually as the physical exam progresses from "quiet" to "active." Optimum examination of the abdomen and genitalia occurs with the child on the examining table, but in the fearful child, the exam may proceed with the child still in the parent's lap and with the examiner seated at the same level as the parent in a knee-to-knee position to create a surface for the child to lie on. With the young child's head and shoulder cradled on the parent or caretaker's lap, the examiner proceeds with assessment of the abdomen, genitalia, and hips, thereby avoiding the child's anxiety of being on the exam table. When the infant is old enough to begin walking, it is important to observe the infant toddling in only a diaper to evaluate gait and musculoskeletal coordination.

Young Children

By 3 years of age, most children, though still apprehensive, are able to make eye contact and separate briefly from the parent. Observe their ability to be comforted, evaluate their response to the environment, their level of social interaction, and their relationships with parents or caretakers and siblings, if present. How appropriate is their behavior in the setting? What is the quality and variety of their verbal responses? What is their level of activity and attention span? Young children, in general, respond best to a slow, even, steady voice. Give the young child time to warm to the situation before undressing. The confident young child should be able to be examined sitting on the examining table. The "quiet" to "active" approach is advisable with this age group also, that is, beginning with the cardiac and respiratory examination. Give children 3 to 5 years of age clear directions, allow them to respond, and recognize success. Young children particularly enjoy games, drawing, and role-playing the physical examination with dolls or stuffed animals (Figure 1-1). Modesty sets in during the preschool years, and health care providers need to be respectful and mindful of this developmental stage.

Children 6 to 12 Years of Age

Children 6 to 12 years old benefit most from the talk-through approach to the physical exam. They are interested in learning about their bodies and are forming a body image of themselves. They are becoming more independent from their parents. School-age children gain the most from education about good health habits. Learning more about their bodies helps them connect their health with their health habits. Allow the child to participate in

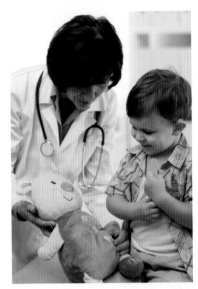

FIGURE 1-1 Use of play to decrease anxiety in a young child. (© StockLite, 2013. Used under license from Shutterstock.com.)

all aspects of the physical exam and respect their modesty. A "head-to-toe" assessment with the child on the examining table is most effective during the school-age years.

Adolescents

The approach used with the adolescent during the health care encounter should be based on the developmental stage rather than the age of the client. This is true for all children, but particularly those in adolescence. Development during early, middle, and late adolescence proceeds unevenly and can vary widely among 12- to 18-year-olds. Respect and confidentiality are essential components of developing a trusting relationship with the adolescent. Parental input is important during the health encounter, but adolescents should be interviewed and examined separately from the parent or peers. Avoid power struggles and give the adolescent control whenever possible. Involve adolescents in planning their health care and in establishing realistic goals and health habits. Chapter 4 further discusses evidence-based practice of the adolescent health visit.

REFERENCES

1. Fine A, Kotelchuck M: *Rethinking MCH: The Life Course Model as an organizing framework*, Washington DC, 2010, USDHHS.
2. Halfon N, DuPlessis H, Inkelas M: Transforming the U.S. child health system, *Health Aff (Millwood)* 26(2):315–330, 2007.
3. Duderstadt K: Medical home: Nurse practitioners role in delivery of care to vulnerable populations, *J Pediatr Health Care* 22(6):269–271, 2008.
4. Lindeke LL, Anderson SE, Chesncy ML, et al: Family-centered health care/medical home: APN roles in shaping new care models, *J Pediatr Health Care* 24(6):413–416, 2010.
5. Dovidio JF, Fiske ST: Under the radar: how unexamined biases in decision-making processes in clinical interactions can contribute to health care disparities, *Am J Public Health* 102(5):945–952, 2012.
6. Schrugin O'Keeffe G, Clarke-Pearson K: The impact of social media on children, adolescents, and families. AAP Council on Communications and Media. *Pediatrics* 127(4):800–804, 2011.
7. Soderback M, Coyne I, Harder M: The importance of including both a child perspective and the child's perspective within health care settings to provide truly child-centered care, *J Child Health Care* 15(2):99–106, 2011.
8. Shier H: Pathways to participation: Openings, opportunities and obligation. A new model for enhancing children's participation in decision making, in line with Article 12.1 of the United Nations Convention on the Rights of the Child, *Children & Society* 15: 107–117, 2001.
9. Goode TD, Haywood SH, Wells N, et al: Family-centered, culturally, and linguistically competent care: essential components of the medical home, *Pediatr Ann* 38(9):505–512, 2009.
10. Davies D: *Child development: a practitioner's guide*, ed 3, New York, 2011, The Guilford Press.
11. Verghese A, Brady E, Kapur CC, et al: The bedside evaluation: ritual and reason, *Ann Intern Med* 155(8):550–553, 2011.
12. Verghese A, Horwitz RI: In praise of the physical examination, *BMJ* 339:b5448, 2009.

CHAPTER 2

ASSESSMENT PARAMETERS

Karen G. Duderstadt

GESTATIONAL AGE IN THE NEWBORN

Obtaining an accurate assessment of gestational age begins with the prenatal history and birth history and can assist the health care provider in anticipating conditions associated with preterm birth. The prenatal assessment includes a maternal history of the last menstrual period, history of prenatal care, maternal weight gain and general health during pregnancy, maternal infections, hypertension, history of toxemia or other complications of pregnancy, and history of substance abuse or physical abuse. The birth history includes history of the onset and length of labor and the progression and method of delivery (see Chapter 4).

The *New Ballard Score (NBS)* (Figure 2-1) is the tool most often used to evaluate the gestational age of newborn infants. The NBS is a valid tool and accurately assesses gestational age for extremely low birth weight infants ≤1000 g or extremely premature infants from 20 weeks to term infants from 40 to 44 weeks of gestation.[1] The NBS is a revision of the original *Dubowitz scale,* which was used to determine gestational age of infants 35 to 42 weeks of age. The NBS consists of six physical and six neuromuscular criteria for assessing maturity. The criteria for extremely preterm infants correlates with 1 and 0 on the scale. Gestational age must be determined within 48 hours after birth except in the case of the extremely preterm infant or extremely low birth weight infant whose age should be determined within 12 hours after birth. Assessment of neuromuscular maturity score should be repeated within 48 hours after birth if neonatal asphyxia or maternal anesthesia may have affected initial assessments (Box 2-1).

The *Apgar scoring system* (Table 2-1) reflects the transition of the neonate to extrauterine life. The Apgar assessment performed at 1 minute and again at 5 minutes after birth reflects the heart rate, observation of respiratory effort, muscle tone, reflex irritability, and color of the newborn (Table 2-2). The Apgar score is not predictive of long-term perinatal outcomes or neurological status, but remains the standard for assessing viability of the newborn immediately after birth. The *Physiscore* is a physiological assessment score for preterm infants based on electronic non-invasive measurements monitored in the first 3 hours of life. It may provide higher accuracy of morbidity than the Apgar score.[2]

Term Infants

Term infants are born between the 38th and 41st weeks of gestation and normally lose about 5% to 10% of their birth weight in the first 72 hours after birth. The average weight loss is 5% to 7% over 3 to 4 days. Postterm infants are born at 42 weeks of gestation and represent about 10% of the newborn population. Postterm infants have an increased incidence of fetal distress and perinatal asphyxia, often due to increased weight gain before delivery. In term infants, a weight loss of >10% may indicate a poor feeding pattern or a more serious postnatal condition and requires thorough investigation and close follow-up. For the infant who is breastfed, observation of feeding and latch to the nipple is particularly important for the breastfed infant with a >7% to >10% weight loss. By 2 weeks of age, term infants have normally regained their birth weight.

ESTIMATION OF GESTATIONAL AGE BY MATURITY RATING

Neuromuscular Maturity

	−1	0	1	2	3	4	5
Posture							
Square Window (wrist)	> 90°	90°	60°	45°	30°	0°	
Arm Recoil		180°	140° - 180°	110° 140°	90° - 110°	< 90°	
Popliteal Angle	180°	160°	140°	120°	100°	90°	< 90°
Scarf Sign							
Heel to Ear							

Physical Maturity

								Maturity Rating	
Skin	sticky friable transparent	gelatinous red, translucent	smooth pink, visible veins	superficial peeling &/or rash, few veins	cracking pale areas rare veins	parchment deep cracking no vessels	leathery cracked wrinkled	**score**	**weeks**
								-10	20
Lanugo	none	sparse	abundant	thinning	bald areas	mostly bald		-5	22
								0	24
Plantar Surface	heel-toe 40-50 mm: -1 <40 mm: -2	>50 mm no crease	faint red marks	anterior transverse crease only	creases ant. 2/3	creases over entire sole		5	26
								10	28
Breast	imperceptible	barely perceptible	flat areola no bud	stippled areola 1-2 mm bud	raised areola 3-4 mm bud	full areola 5-10 mm bud		15	30
								20	32
Eye/Ear	lids fused loosely: -1 tightly: -2	lids open pinna flat stays folded	sl. curved pinna; soft; slow recoil	well-curved pinna; soft but ready recoil	formed & firm instant recoil	thick cartilage, ear stiff		25	34
								30	36
Genitals (male)	scrotum flat, smooth	scrotum empty faint rugae	testes in upper canal rare rugae	testes descending few rugae	testes down good rugae	testes pendulous, deep rugae		35	38
								40	40
Genitals (female)	clitoris prominent labia flat	prominent clitoris, small labia minora	prominent clitoris enlarging minora	majora & minora equally prominent	majora large minora small	majora cover clitoris & minora		45	42
								50	44

FIGURE 2-1 New Ballard Score. (From Ballard JL, Khoury JC, Wedig K et al: New Ballard Score, expanded to include extremely premature infants, *J Pediatr* 119(3):418, 1991.)

EVIDENCE-BASED PRACTICE TIP

The maximum point of weight loss can occur any day during the first week postpartum. Weight loss of greater than 10% should be evaluated and the infant should be monitored for intake.[3]

Preterm Infants

An infant is considered preterm when born before the end of the 37th week. The weight and gestational age of the infant together predict the relative risk of mortality. During the first year of life, premature infants tend to grow more slowly than term infants even when using the

| BOX 2-1 | TESTS FOR ASSESSING NEUROMUSCULAR MATURITY IN THE NEWBORN |

Posture. With infant quiet and in supine position, observe degree of flexion in arms, legs. Muscle tone and degree of flexion increase with maturity. Full flexion of the arms, legs = 4.

Square window. With thumb supporting back of arm below wrist, apply gentle pressure with index and third fingers on dorsum of hand without rotating infant's wrist. Measure angle between base of thumb and forearm. Full flexion (hand lies flat on ventral surface of forearm) = 4.

Arm recoil. With infant supine, fully flex forearms on upper arms, hold for 5 seconds; pull down on hands to fully extend and rapidly release arms. Observe rapidity and intensity of recoil to state of flexion. A brisk return to full flexion = 4.

Popliteal angle. With infant supine and pelvis flat on firm surface, flex lower leg on thigh, then flex thigh on abdomen. While holding knee with thumb and index finger, extend lower leg with index finger of other hand. Measure degree of angle behind knee (popliteal angle). Angle of <90 degrees = 5.

Scarf sign. With infant supine, support head in midline with one hand; use other hand to pull infant's arm across shoulder so that infant's hand touches shoulder. Determine location of elbow in relation to midline. Elbow does not reach midline = 4.

Heel to ear. With infant supine and pelvis flat on firm surface, pull foot as far as possible toward ear on same side. Measure distance of foot from ear and degree of knee flexion (same as popliteal angle). Knees flexed with popliteal angle of <90 degrees = 4.

Data from Hockenberry MJ, Wilson D: *Wong's essentials of pediatric nursing*, ed 8, St. Louis, 2009, Mosby.

TABLE 2-1 APGAR SCORING SYSTEM

Sign	0	1	2
Heart rate	Absent	Slow <100	>100
Respiratory rate	Absent	Irregular, slow, weak cry	Good, strong cry
Muscle tone	Limp	Some flexion of extremities	Well flexed
Reflex irritability	No response	Grimace	Cry, sneeze
Color	Blue, pale	Body pink, extremities blue	Completely pink

Data from Apgar V: Evaluation of the newborn infant, second report, *JAMA* 168(15):1985-1988, 1958.

TABLE 2-2 INTERPRETATION OF APGAR SCORES

Total Score	Assessment
0-2	Severe asphyxia
3-4	Moderate asphyxia
5-7	Mild asphyxia
8-10	No asphyxia

growth curve standard for corrected age (see Appendix A). Health care providers should use the adjusted age standard when plotting the growth of the preterm infant until the infant is 2½ years old. At this point, the difference is no longer statistically significant.

Low Birth Weight Infants

Low birth weight (LBW) infants are those infants born weighing <2500 g. Very low birth weight (VLBW) infants are those infants who weigh <1500 g at birth, and infants weighing

≤1000 g are considered extremely low birth weight (ELBW). There has been an increase in the number of VLBW infants due mainly to the increase in prematurely born multiple gestations. However, race and ethnicity, maternal age, maternal health and nutrition, substance abuse during pregnancy, environmental toxins, and access to prenatal care all contribute to the risk of LBW infants. In 2010, the prevalence of LBW infants in the United States was 8.2%, with the highest prevalence among African-Americans.[4] Box 2-2 presents maternal risk factors for LBW and VLBW infants.

Small for Gestational Age

Infants weighing <2500 g at birth or infants with weight below the 10th percentile for age are considered small for gestational age (SGA). The head may be *microcephalic,* or small in proportion to the body, and *head circumference* may be below the 5th percentile for age. With adequate nutrition, SGA infants experience overall catch-up growth. Intrauterine growth retardation (IUGR) may contribute to the reduction in growth in SGA infants, but maternal, fetal, and placental factors all affect pregnancy outcomes. *Head circumference* is normally the first growth parameter to show catch-up growth, followed by weight, and then length. Fifty percent of SGA infants remain below average weight at 3 years of age.[5] The mortality rate for the SGA infant is almost five times that of term infants.[6]

Large for Gestational Age

Large for gestational age (LGA) is defined as birth weight >2 standard deviations (SD) above the mean for gestational age or weight above the 90th percentile for age. The increased weight may result from fetal factors, which include genetic and chromosomal disorders, or from maternal factors, such as obesity or diabetes. *Maternal hyperglycemia* exposes the fetus to increased levels of glucose, which increases fetal insulin secretion.[5] Increased insulin levels increase fat deposits in the fetus and often result in LGA infants. Diabetic mothers who are insulin-dependent and in poor control during the early trimesters of pregnancy have characteristically large infants. LGA infants are at risk for birth trauma, neonatal asphyxia, hypoglycemia, polycythemia, and hyperbilirubinemia.

NORMAL GROWTH

Growth is the most dynamic aspect of childhood. In the early years, the measurements of height and weight are key indicators of health. Abnormal progression of growth and maturation is often the first indicator to the health care provider of abnormalities in the growth pattern. Normal growth proceeds in a predictable pattern during childhood from *cephalocaudal* (head to tail) and from *proximodistal*

BOX 2-2	MATERNAL RISK FACTORS FOR LOW BIRTH WEIGHT AND VERY LOW BIRTH WEIGHT INFANTS

Maternal Risks
- Maternal age
- Race and ethnicity
- Maternal health and nutrition
- Environmental toxins or occupational chemical toxins
- Access to prenatal care

Maternal Substance Abuse
- Alcoholism
- Tobacco use
- Illicit drug use
- Over-the-counter drug use

Data from Malloy MH: Size for gestational age at birth: Impact on risk for sudden infant death and other causes of death, USA 2002, *Arch Dis Child Fetal Neonatal Ed,* 92(6):F473-478, 2007.

(near to far). Plotting serial measurements regularly on a standardized growth curve for age and gender is a reliable method of monitoring growth and is an essential component of comprehensive well-child care (see Appendix A). Accurate assessment of growth begins in the newborn period by evaluating progress on the growth curve and continues throughout childhood and adolescence by evaluating growth in relation to age (see the inside back cover). Using the correct technique when gathering measurements is one of the significant challenges in pediatrics.

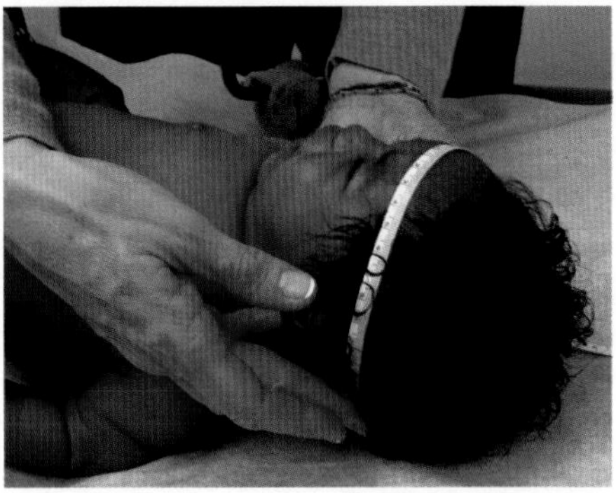

FIGURE 2-2 Accurate measurement of head circumference.

MEASUREMENT

Head Circumference

Measurement of *head circumference* is a routine part of growth assessment in the first 2 years of life. Accurate measurement of the head is taken with the measuring tape around the head placed at the point of greatest circumference from the occipital protuberance above the base of the skull to the midforehead or point of greatest bossing of the frontal bone (Figure 2-2). The head circumference measurement is then plotted on the growth curve specific for sex and age at each well-child visit to determine if the growth pattern is normal. If the initial head measurement is plotted on the growth chart and indicates a concerning pattern of growth, it is important to remeasure the head to ensure accuracy of head size. A *head circumference* that plots 1 to 2 SD above height and weight on the growth curve or >95th percentile or <5th percentile for age should be evaluated. *Microcephaly* may be indicative of an SGA infant, IUGR, or premature closure of the cranial sutures, termed *craniosynostosis*, which requires immediate referral. *Macrocephaly,* a large head in proportion to the body, may indicate increased intracranial pressure or may be a familial variant. Consistent and accurate assessment of the *head circumference* is a critical part of the assessment of normal growth and development.

Chest Circumference

Chest circumference is smaller at birth than *head circumference. Chest circumference* is measured at the nipple line. The head circumference is normally 2 cm greater than the chest circumference in the first 6 months of life. Molding of the head in the term newborn may make it appear as though the measurements are equal. By 1 year of age, the *chest circumference* should closely equal the head circumference. With the progression of growth, the *chest circumference* becomes larger than the head circumference at about 2 years of age and continues to grow more rapidly during childhood. Chest measurements are not routinely taken unless an infant has abnormal physical findings at birth or demonstrates abnormal growth.

Height

Height is the most stable measurement of growth and maturation in childhood. Linear growth is genetically predetermined, and therefore adult height generally occurs within a predictable range if accurate family history is available. Linear growth often occurs in spurts followed by long quiescent periods in which no growth occurs. Infants and young children may demonstrate an increase in appetite before a growth spurt, followed by an increased need for sleep.

For the infant or toddler, *recumbent* height is required for accurate measurement of linear growth. Place the infant supine on a flat surface or examination table equipped with a measuring device. Accurate measurement requires the infant's legs to be flat against the examination table and the foot in the level position. Term newborns vary in height between 18 and 22 inches (45 to 55 cm) at birth, and height increases by approximately 1 inch per month over the first few months of life. Although less accurate than the measuring device, infant measurement can be taken on the examination table by marking the position of the top of the head and the bottom of the foot on table paper and then determining length with a measuring tape. Term infants generally increase in length by 50% in the first year. The increase is primarily in truncal growth. Doubling the height at 2 years of age can give an estimate of adult height. Obese children are taller than children of average weight, often 1 SD above their counterparts for age (Box 2-3).

After 2 years of age, transition to standing height is appropriate, although recumbent height is often easier to obtain in the first part of the second year if the child is fearful. The increase in height averages 3 inches (7.5 cm) over the second and third years. Measurement is recorded to the nearest 0.1 cm or 0.25 inch without shoes. Standing height should be taken without shoes using a wall-mounted or portable *stadiometer* for accuracy. Accurate measurement requires a cooperative child to stand erect with head level, feet flat, and heels against the measuring surface (Figure 2-3). From the end of the third year until the onset of puberty, the increase in height averages 2 inches (9.5 cm) per year. In adolescence, girls' height potential is generally realized by

---

BOX 2-3	ACCURATE MEASUREMENT OF HEIGHT AND WEIGHT

Height

Birth to 24 months
- Infant's head must be held firm on flat surface against top of measuring bar.
- Push knees gently toward table while leg is extended. Bottom of foot is placed directly against footboard of measuring device.

24 to 36 months
- Toddlers are best measured lying on a flat surface or examination table equipped with a measuring device as described above.

36 months through school age
- For accurate height in the young child, maintain head erect by placing slight upward pressure under chin.
- Child should be standing erect with buttocks and back against stadiometer or wall.

Weight

Birth to 12 months
- Infant should be undressed (without diaper) or weighed consistently with clean, dry diaper.

- *Safety* is of primary concern. Examiner cannot leave infant unattended at any time.

12 to 24 months
- Before 2 years of age, weight is measured most accurately on infant balance scale with dry diaper. *Exceptions:* when child is very large or more cooperative/stable on standing scale.

2 to 6 years of age
- At 2 years, weight can be measured accurately on standing balance scale when child is cooperative.
- Weight should be measured with child in underwear consistently when using standing balance scale until 3 years of age.
- From 3 to 6 years children can be weighed in clothing without shoes.

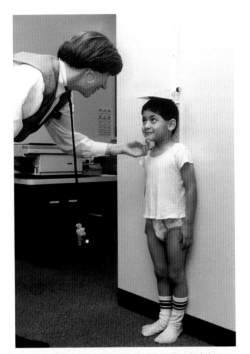

FIGURE 2-3 Measuring standing height.

16 years of age, and boys' growth potential continues until 18 to 21 years of age. Linear growth ceases when the maturation of the skeleton is complete (see Chapters 15 and 16 for discussion of growth and sexual maturity rating).

Familial *short stature* is often not recognized as the most likely assessment for slow linear growth when parents are anxious for their child to achieve a socially acceptable height. *Short stature* also may be a key indicator in children with poor nutritional status or indicative of chronic conditions including cardiac and renal disease, fetal alcohol syndrome, methadone exposure, growth hormone deficiency, or congenital syndromes.[5]

PEDIATRIC PEARLS

Height at 2 years of age is approximately 50% of adult height. To estimate adult height, double the height at 2 years of age.

Arm Span

An adolescent male or female of tall stature with a disproportionate arm length should be evaluated for arm span measurement. An *arm span* measurement should be taken with the arms outstretched. Measure the distance from the tip of the middle finger across the crest of the shoulders to the other middle fingertip. The arm span measurement should equal the height. In *Marfan syndrome,* the arm span measurement exceeds the height and is associated with a disproportionate appearance.

Weight

The average birth weight in term infants is 7 to 7.5 pounds (3175 to 3400 g). The average range of weight in a healthy term newborn is from 5 pounds 8 ounces to 8 pounds 13 ounces (2500 to 4000 g) (see the inside back cover). Poor weight gain in early infancy is indicative of *failure to thrive* and may be caused by poor feeding patterns, malnutrition, neglect, cardiac or renal disease, chronic infection, or congenital anomalies.

Infants can be accurately weighed lying on an infant balance scale while wearing a dry diaper. Infants should be weighed in the sitting position only with extreme caution and only after they are able to sit without support. Weight is recorded to the nearest 0.5 ounce or 0.01 kg (10 g). After 2 years of age, standing weight should be recorded to the nearest 0.25 pound or 0.1 kg (100 g) (see Box 2-3). If a young child is very fearful or irritable, parent and child can be weighed together on standing scale; then parental weight is subtracted from total weight to obtain an *estimate* of child's weight. For children with special health care needs or disabilities, accommodations for wheelchair scales or special purpose scales should be made in the clinical setting.

From infancy through adolescence, more children are becoming overweight. The overall prevalence of obesity in children 2 to 5 years of age is 12.1%, and the trend of overweight and obesity in this age group has been increasing.[7] For children 6 to 11 years old, the overall prevalence of obesity is 18%, but the rate is 29.7% in black, non-Hispanic males and 27.9% in black, non-Hispanic females. The overall prevalence of obesity in adolescence is 18.4%.[7] Obesity has its origins in early life and routine serial measurements of height and weight in the growing infant and child are most important in evaluating trends in weight gain early and communicating this information to families. Rapid weight gain in early infancy, early adiposity rebound in childhood, and early pubertal development all influence the risk of becoming overweight and have been implicated in the development of obesity.[8]

Adiposity

Adipose tissue is a unique form of connective tissue with cells that maintain a large intracellular space. These *adipocytes,* or fat cells, store large quantities of triglycerides and are a repository of energy in the body. More than 90% of the body's energy is stored in the adipose tissue, and lipids are the main source for stored fuel in the body.[5] Although *adipocytes* do not reproduce, they do have a long life span, and infants born with a large numbers of fat cells are at risk for obesity. Adiposity typically declines in later infancy and early childhood, then rebounds, as shown by the upturn in the childhood growth charts and the body mass index (BMI) curve. This upturn in the growth curve is known as *adiposity rebound* and is expected at about 5 to 7 years of age.[9] Large weight gains during the preschool years alter the normal pattern of growth. Thus early adiposity rebound is associated with increased depositions of fat in middle childhood, and risks associated with early adiposity rebound persist at least until early adulthood.[9] Gestation, early infancy, middle childhood, and adolescence are critical periods for the development of adiposity.[8]

Body Mass Index for Age in Children

Body mass index (BMI) provides a guideline for health care providers to determine the healthy weight of a child beginning at 2 years

of age based on height. The formula for determining BMI is weight in kilograms divided by height in meters squared (BMI = weight [kg]/height squared [m²]). Calculating and plotting BMI during the routine health visit and discussing this information with families is an important part of providing comprehensive well-child care. The BMI growth curve may be easier to use than the standard weight-for-height growth charts to point out weight trends to parents (see Appendix B). BMI is used to determine whether a child or adolescent is overweight or underweight, and interpretation of the BMI in children depends on age. Children with a BMI greater than the 95th percentile for age and sex or a BMI greater than or equal to 30 are considered obese, and children with a BMI between the 85th percentile and 94th percentile for age and sex are considered overweight (Table 2-3).[10]

As children grow, their composition of body fat changes over time, and the amount of body fat compared to height differs between boys and girls during maturation. BMI normally decreases during the preschool years, increases during the prepubertal years, and continues to increase into early and middle adolescence. Preadolescent girls often experience their peak weight gain before beginning peak increase in height. Children with BMIs that do not follow this pattern or who demonstrate an earlier increase in body fat or adiposity rebound are more likely to have an increased BMI as an adult.

TABLE 2-3	INTERPRETATION OF BMI STANDARDS	
Weight	BMI for Age and Sex (Percentile)
Underweight	<5th percentile
Overweight	85th to 94th percentile
Obese	≥95th percentile or BMI ≥30

Data from Barlow SE, Expert Committee: Expert Committee recommendations regarding the prevention, assessment, and treatment of child and adolescent overweight and obesity, *Pediatrics* 120(Supp14):S164-S192, 2007.

The categories of BMI percentiles may not adequately define risk of obesity-related comorbid conditions in children such as diabetes and hyperlipidemia.[11] Overweight children have different body fatness and risk factor levels. Recent trends in childhood obesity have shown a marked increase in the number of children with a high *waist-to-height* ratio—a 65% increase in waist circumference among boys and a 69% increase among girls.[12] Abdominal obesity is identified as an important factor in the adverse health effects of childhood obesity. A high waist-to-height ratio has been associated with *metabolic syndrome* and *type II diabetes* in adolescents. Among overweight children, high *waist-to-height* ratio is more strongly associated with adverse risk factors than a high BMI for age or skinfold thickness.[11] Overweight children with a high waist-to-height ratio are two to three times more likely to have adverse levels of most risk factors than are those with a low waist-to-height ratio.[11]

There are no BMI parameters for children under 2 years of age. Children younger than 2 years who have a weight-to-height ratio on the standard growth curves of ≥95th percentile for age and sex are considered overweight.

FAMILY, CULTURAL, RACIAL, AND ETHNIC CONSIDERATIONS IN HEIGHT AND WEIGHT

The incidence of LBW and ELBW is higher in African-American infants. Birth weight averages 180 to 240 g lower in African-Americans than in other racial and ethnic groups. Native American newborns have the largest average birth weight of over 4000 g, reflecting a higher incidence of gestational diabetes during pregnancy.

Asian children may be at risk for comorbidities due to obesity at lower BMI thresholds than for other ethnic groups.[13] Ethnicity-specific BMI cut points may be needed; however, it is increasingly difficult to assign ethnicity to some individuals in a global population.

DEVELOPMENTAL CONSIDERATIONS

Temperament

Assessment of *temperament* is a key part of comprehensive health assessment in infants, children, and adolescents. Temperament is the inborn tendency to react to one's environment in certain ways and is thought to be generally constant and at least partially genetically determined. The personality of an individual child reflects the interaction between the child's temperament and environment. Temperament can be assessed by report, clinical observation, or by a formal assessment tool. The term *"goodness of fit"* describes the concept of how well the child's temperament meets the expectations of his or her parents and caregivers. *Goodness of fit* promotes healthy development in the family unit through adaptation to the infant's personality, and it has a critical influence on a child's emotional well-being and behavior. Table 2-4 identifies the nine characteristics of temperament. Certain temperament characteristics may be associated with resiliency in children or signal emotional difficulties. Characteristics of frustration tolerance and intensity may be specific indicators of emotional dysregulation in some children and may indicate an underlying dysfunction in affective processes that significantly increase risk for mood disorders in later childhood or in adulthood.[14] An easy temperament with strong characteristics of regularity and adaptability acts as a protective factor for social-emotional development and could be related to resilience in children living in an adverse social environment.[15]

Understanding temperament characteristics removes judgment and blame and assists parents in recognizing that some rules do not work equally well with all children. Setting limits and time out is more difficult with some children, and some children are more difficult to discipline and require more parental ingenuity. Temperament theory objectifies these differences. A comprehensive approach to assessing

TABLE 2-4	TEMPERAMENT CHARACTERISTICS
Characteristics	**Description**
Activity	Amount of motor activity and proportion of active to inactive periods
Intensity	Amount of emotional energy released with responses
Sensitivity	Amount of sensory stimuli required to produce response
Approach/ withdrawal	Nature of initial response to new stimuli
Adaptability	Ease of accepting new situation after initial response
Frustration tolerance	Length of time activity is pursued
Mood	Amount of pleasant versus unpleasant behavior child exhibits
Distractibility	Effectiveness of extraneous stimuli in altering direction of ongoing behavior
Regularity	Predictability of physiological functions such as hunger, sleep, elimination

development includes assessing and understanding temperament and sharing this information with parents and caregivers. A temperament assessment tool for parents may be accessed online at http://www.preventiveoz.org.

VITAL SIGNS

Temperature

Measurement of temperature continues to be a dynamic process in the infant and young child. Much discussion has occurred on the accuracy of temperature measurement and the ideal instrument to use. Currently there is a range of methods for measuring temperature in the infant and young child.

Temporal artery thermometers have been studied for accuracy in children from birth to 18 years of age in relation to standard rectal thermometers. The sensitivity and specificity of the temporal artery thermometer for detecting fever has been reported at 67.9% and 98.3%, respectively.[16] The diagnostic accuracy of the temporal artery thermometer in detecting fever in children of all ages is low. Therefore current practice does not support the use of the temporal artery thermometers for infants and young children to accurately measure fever.

Non-contact infrared thermometers are gaining in popularity in pediatric settings as a noninvasive method for measuring temperature for infants and young children with less discomfort. However, recent research comparing the accuracy of the non-contact infrared thermometers with non-mercury liquid-in-glass thermometers has been inconclusive. Infrared thermometry tended to overestimate the temperature of afebrile children and underestimate the temperature of febrile patients ($P < .01$).[17] Temperatures measured with non-contact infrared thermometers in comparison to rectal temperatures varied significantly and did not reliably predict fever in infants and young children.[18] The digital thermometer provides the best agreement with the mercury thermometer in detecting fever in infants and young children.[19]

Axillary temperature measurement is the most favored method for the healthy newborn. Place the non-mercury liquid-in-glass thermometer under the arm at the base of the axilla for 3 to 5 minutes and hold the arm firmly against the side of the body with swaddling. Research has shown parental report of axillary temperature measurement can be considered reliable and has shown a high correlation with measurement by trained, experienced staff.[20]

Rectal temperature remains the most reliable method for detecting core body temperature in infants and young children. In early infancy to 8 to 9 months, rectal temperature is most accurately measured with the infant placed in the supine position on the examining table with knees flexed toward the abdomen.

The infant can see the practitioner and be secured more easily in this position. Proper positioning prevents injury. In males, stimulation often elicits urination so the penis should be covered. A child from 9 months to 2 years of age can be placed in the parent's arms or laid supine on the parent's lap. Insert the lubricated tip of thermometer into the anal opening of the rectum a distance of 0.5 to 1 inch. Rectal measurement of temperature remains the recommended standard in clinical practice for infants under 1 month of age to determine fever when considering further diagnostic evaluation. Oral measurement is the preferred method for cooperative children over 4 years of age.

Pulse

Pulses should be assessed for the quality of rate, rhythm, and volume or strength. Children under 2 years of age require apical pulse (AP) measurements. Readings should be taken when the child is quiet. AP measurements are taken with the stethoscope placed over the heart below the nipple at the apex. For children over 2 years of age, the radial pulse is a satisfactory measurement. In infants and young children, the pulse should be counted for a full minute to account for irregularities in rhythm. Figure 2-4 illustrates the location of the pulses. Although pulse is most often monitored electronically, it is important to detect any differences in pulse between the upper and lower extremities. The radial and femoral pulses should be evaluated and compared for strength and quality. Detecting the femoral pulse in newborn and young infants requires focus and concentration by the examiner. The femoral pulse is located in the mid-inguinal area over the head of the femur. In children who are overweight and obese, locating the femoral pulse is challenging and requires palpating through adipose tissue to determine presence and strength of the pulse. An absent or weak pulse in the lower extremities compared to the upper extremities is diagnostic of *coarctation of the aorta*. Table 2-5 presents the grading of pulses used to evaluate strength and quality.

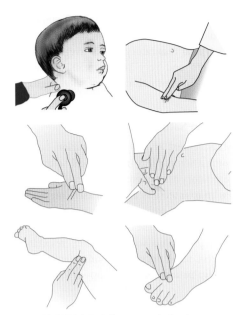

FIGURE 2-4 Assessment of pulses.

TABLE 2-5	STRENGTH AND QUALITY OF PULSES	
Strength	Quality
0	Not palpable
1+	Difficult to palpate, thready, obliterated by pressure
2+	Weak, difficult to palpate, may obliterate with pressure
3+	Palpable, normal strength
4+	Strong, bounding, not affected by pressure

Respirations

Respirations should be assessed for rate and pattern. Respirations should be taken when the child is quiet to accurately assess the rate and quality of breathing. In infants and young children, observe the abdominal movements when evaluating respiratory rate. An infant's breathing is primarily diaphragmatic. Also evaluate the use of any accessory muscles in the upper chest or difficulty breathing. Respirations should be assessed for a full minute because the typical respiratory rate is irregular in the newborn and very young infant. Table 2-6 shows the normal range of vital signs in children.

Oxygen Saturation

Measurement of *oxygen saturation* has become a standard in most clinical settings for respiratory assessment in the pediatric patient. *Pulse oximetry* is a noninvasive method of determining oxygen saturation (Spo_2) and should be part of the criteria for evaluating any child presenting with wheezing, respiratory distress, respiratory compromise, or preoperative evaluation. A normal Spo_2 of 95% to 96%

is adequate, and 97% is generally considered to be normal. An Spo_2 of $\leq$92% is considered *hypoxemic*. Spo_2 assists the practitioner in clinical decision making when determining the need for prolonged observation or hospital admission. *Pulse oximetry* alone may detect cyanotic heart disease in the asymptomatic newborn, preventing morbidity and delayed diagnosis of cardiac disease.[5]

Blood Pressure

Blood pressure should be assessed at all routine well-child visits beginning at 3 years of age. In infants and children younger than 3 years of age, blood pressure should be evaluated in children who are at risk or who have chronic conditions. The size of the blood pressure cuff is

TABLE 2-6 EXPECTED RANGE OF VITAL SIGNS

	Temperature	Respirations	Heart Rate*	Blood Pressure
Newborn	36.5° C-37° C, clothed and swaddled	30-60 without signs of respiratory distress (grunting, flaring, retracting, stridor)	80-160 AP (range 80 when sleeping to 220 when active/crying)	65/41 mean 75/49 90th percentile 78/52 95th percentile
1 week to 3 months	37° C-37.5° C average	30-50	100-220 AP (range 100 when sleeping to 220 with fever/crying)	87/52 mean 104/64 90th percentile 106/68 95th percentile
3 months to 2 years	37.4° C-37.7° C	24-38	80-150 AP	95/58 mean 106/68 90th percentile 110/71 95th percentile
2 to 6 years	37° C-37.2° C	20-28	75-120	101/57 mean 112/66 90th percentile 115/68 95th percentile
6 to 12 years	36.8° C-37° C	16-22	70-110	112/73 mean 115/75 90th percentile 120/80 95th percentile
12 years to adult	36.6° C-36.7° C	12-20	50-105	119/78 mean 132/85 90th percentile 138/87 95th percentile

AP, Apical pulse.
*Apical pulse rate taken in children younger than 2 years of age.

critical to obtaining an accurate measurement. The blood pressure cuff should cover about two thirds of the upper arm and should encircle the arm once. A cuff that is too large will result in a low blood pressure reading. If the cuff is too small, the blood pressure reading may be too high. For obese children and adolescents, an extra-large adult cuff may be needed to obtain an accurate measurement. Blood pressure readings can increase in children who are crying and in children and adolescents who are feeling anxious. Table 2-6 reviews the normal range of blood pressure at different ages. For healthy children and adolescents with a blood pressure reading above the 95th percentile for age, three independent readings should be taken to confirm the diagnosis of *hypertension*.

Pain

An accurate assessment of pain response in infants and young children requires strategies specific to the developmental level of the child. The use of the pain scale in children 3 years of age and older has greatly improved the ability of the health care practitioner to accurately assess and treat pain in the pediatric patient. Figure 2-5 presents the FACES pain rating scale used across most pediatric clinical settings.[21]

For nonverbal children, cognitively impaired children or children with special health care needs, the revised Face, Legs, Activity, Cry, Consolability (FLACC) Behavioral Scale has been validated for evaluating postoperative pain in the acute care setting and for pain secondary to trauma or other chronic conditions.[22] Zero to two points is assigned to each of the five categories on the scale, and total score from 0 to 10 reflects no pain to severe pain. Table 2-7 presents the FLACC Behavioral Scale.

PHYSICAL ASSESSMENT TECHNIQUES

Inspection

Inspection is about *looking. Inspection* is a skill acquired by developing detailed and meticulous observation of children and learning to see the whole as well as the parts. It involves not only the sense of sight but also the senses of hearing and smell. Inspection requires good room lighting and complete visibility of the body part to be examined to accurately assess symmetry, shape, color, and odor. It is an essential skill for the pediatric health care provider, particularly when interacting with the nonverbal child, the young pediatric patient, or a child who is ill.

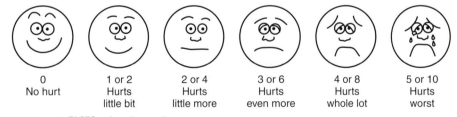

0	1 or 2	2 or 4	3 or 6	4 or 8	5 or 10
No hurt	Hurts little bit	Hurts little more	Hurts even more	Hurts whole lot	Hurts worst

FIGURE 2-5 FACES pain rating scale.
Brief word instructions: Point to each face using the words to describe the pain intensity. Ask the child to choose the face that best describes own pain, and record the appropriate number. NOTE: Use of these instructions is recommended. Rating scale can be used with people 3 years and older.
Original instructions: Explain to the person that each face is for a person who feels happy because he has no pain (hurt) or sad because he has some or a lot of pain. **FACE 0** is very happy because he doesn't hurt at all. **FACE 1** hurts just a little bit. **FACE 2** hurts a little more. **FACE 3** hurts even more. **FACE 4** hurts a whole lot. **FACE 5** hurts as much as you can imagine, although you don't have to be crying to feel this bad. Ask the person to choose face that best describes how much hurt he has. Record the number under the chosen face on the pain assessment record. (From Hockenberry MJ, Wilson D: *Wong's nursing of infants and children,* ed 9, St. Louis, 2011, Copyrighted by Mosby. Reprinted by permission.)

TABLE 2-7	FACE, LEGS, ACTIVITY, CRY, CONSOLABILITY (FLACC) BEHAVIORAL SCALE

	Scoring		
Categories	0	1	2
Face	No particular expression or smile	Occasional grimace or frown, withdrawn or disinterested	Frequent to constant frown, clenched jaw, quivering chin
Legs	Normal position or relaxed	Uneasy, restless, or tense	Kicking, or legs drawn up
Activity	Lying quietly, normal position, moves easily	Squirming, shifting back and forth, or tense	Arched, rigid or jerking
Cry	No cry	Moans, whimpers, or occasional complaint	Crying steadily, screams or sobs, frequent complaints
Consolability	Content, relaxed	Reassured by occasional touching, hugging, or being talked to; distractable	Difficult to console or comfort

From Merkel SI, Voepel-Lewis T, Shayevitz JR, Malviya S: The FLACC: a behavioral scale for scoring postoperative pain in young children, *Pediatr Nurs* 23:293-297, 1997.

Palpation

Palpation is about *touching* and *feeling,* a skill used to detect temperature, vibration, position, and mobility of body organs and glands. *Palpation* appreciates shape, pulsation, texture, and hydration of the skin and tenderness. *Palpation* detects masses and differences in size and shape of glands, organs, muscles, and bones in all parts of the body. The fingertips are most sensitive to tactile differences, the backs of the fingers are most sensitive to temperature, and flattened fingers and palm on the chest detect vibrations when palpating. The examiner's hands should move smoothly over the body without hesitation, first using light palpation, then followed by deep, firm pressure with palpation. It is important to know the distinction between palpation and massage. Massage incorporates *rubbing* in contrast to the technique of *palpation,* which is the movement of the fingers over an area using light to firm pressure for the purpose of identifying size, location, mobility, sensitivity, and temperature of lymph nodes, muscles, tissues, and body organs.

Percussion

Percussion is a helpful skill for mapping out the borders of the organs or sternum and for determining the presence of solid tumors. *Percussion* requires using the examiner's fingers and hands to produce sounds on the area of the body being examined. The density of the body parts is determined by the sounds emitted when the examiner's finger strikes the middle finger of the opposite hand. The fingers produce sounds ranging from the least dense sound, *tympany* or *resonance,* as heard over the stomach or intestines, to the most dense sound, *dullness* or *flatness,* produced by striking over bone. This technique can be useful when examining the abdomen to detect the size of an organ prior to diagnostic imaging.

Auscultation

Auscultation is listening to body sounds transmitted through the stethoscope. With infants and small children, low-pitched cardiac sounds are heard best with the bell-shaped side of the stethoscope, and high-pitched lung and bowel sounds are best heard with the diaphragm, or flat portion, of the stethoscope. The bell shape is effective in isolating cardiac sounds from stomach sounds in the young infant. For best results during the physical examination of a child, it is essential to match the size of the stethoscope head to the size of the child proportionately or the pressure on the head of a dynamic stethoscope. It is important to develop the skill to screen out adventitious sounds that occur in infants and children when listening to lungs and heart. The close proximity of the organs requires the practitioner to screen out stomach and abdominal sounds when listening to the heart and the respirations in the lung.

REFERENCES

1. Ballard J, Khoury J, Wedig K, et al: New Ballard score, expanded to include extremely premature infants, *J Pediatr* 119(3):417-423, 1991.
2. Saria S, Rajani AK, Gould J, et al: Integration of early physiological responses predicts later illness severity in preterm infants, *Sci Transl Med* 2(48):48-65, 2010.
3. Grossman X, Chaudhuri JH, Feldman-Winter L, et al: Neonatal weight loss at a U.S. Baby-Friendly Hospital, *J Acad Nutr Diet* 112(3):410-413, 2012.
4. National Center for Health Statistics, Centers for Disease Control and Prevention: Births and natality, FastStats, 2010. Available from http://www.cdc.gov/nchs/fastats/births.htm.
5. Porth CM, Matfin G: *Pathophysiology: concepts of altered health status*, ed 8, Philadelphia, 2010, Lippincott.
6. Malloy MH: Size for gestational age at birth: impact on risk for sudden infant death and other causes of death, USA 2002, *Arch Dis Child Fetal Neonatal Ed* 92(6):F473-478, 2007.
7. Ogden C, Carroll M, Kit B, et al: Prevalence of obesity in the United States, 2009-2010, *NCHS Data Brief* 82:1-8, 2012.
8. Adair LS: Child and adolescent obesity: epidemiology and developmental perspectives, *Physiol Behav* 94(1):8-16, 2008.
9. Williams SM, Goulding A: Patterns of growth associated with the timing of adiposity rebound. *Obesity (Silver Spring, Md)* 17(2):335-341, 2009.
10. Barlow SE, Expert Committee: Expert Committee recommendations regarding the prevention, assessment, and treatment of child and adolescent overweight and obesity, *Pediatrics* 120(Supp 14): S164-S192, 2007.
11. Freedman DS, Dietz WH, Srinivasan SR, et al: Risk factors and adult body mass index among overweight children: the Bogalusa Heart Study, *Pediatrics* 123(3):750-757, 2009.
12. Li C, Ford ES, Mokdad AH, et al: Recent trends in waist circumference and waist-height ratio among U.S. children and adolescents, *Pediatrics* 118(5): e1390-e1398, 2008.
13. Daniels SR: The use of BMI in the clinical setting, *Pediatrics* 124 Suppl 1:S35-41, 2009.
14. West AE, Schenkel LS, Pavuluri MN: Early childhood temperament in pediatric bipolar disorder and attention deficit hyperactivity disorder, *J Clin Psychol* 64(4):402-421, 2008.
15. Derauf D, LaGlasse L, Smith L, et al: Infant temperament and high-risk environment relate to behavior problems and language in toddlers, *J Dev Behav Pediatr* 32(2):125-135, 2011.
16. Penning C, van der Linden JH, Tibboel D, et al: Is the temporal artery thermometer a reliable instrument for detecting fever in children?, *J Clin Nurs* 20(11-12):1632-1639, 2011.
17. Fortuna EL, Carney MM, Macy M, et al: Accuracy of non-contact infrared thermometry versus rectal thermometry in young children evaluated in the emergency department for fever, *J Emerg Nurs* 36(2):101-104, 2010.
18. Paes BF, Vermeulen K, Brohet RM, et al: Accuracy of tympanic and infrared skin thermometers in children, *Arch Dis Child* 95(12):974-978, 2010.
19. Fadzil FM, Choon D, Arumugam K: A comparative study on the accuracy of noninvasive thermometers, *Aust Fam Physician* 39(4):237-239, 2010.
20. Klein M, DeWitt TG: Reliability of parent-measured axillary temperatures, *Clin Pediatr (Phila)* 49(3): 271-273, 2010.
21. Hockenberry MJ, Wilson D: *Wong's essentials of pediatric nursing*, ed 8, St. Louis, 2009, Mosby.
22. Voepel-Lewis T, Zanotti J, Dammeyer JA, et al: Reliability and validity of the face, legs, activity, cry, consolability behavioral tool in assessing acute pain in crtically ill patients, *Am J Crit Care* 19(1):55-61, 2010.

CHAPTER 3

DEVELOPMENTAL SURVEILLANCE AND SCREENING

Abbey Alkon

Each child achieves developmental milestones at his or her own pace, although the sequence of developmental milestones is generally incremental and stepwise in all children. Screening children for developmental delay and emotional and behavioral difficulties is one of the most challenging aspects of well-child care. Screening is an important step toward referral for evaluation and diagnosis of developmental delay and emotional and behavioral problems, and health care professionals are mandated by the Individuals with Disabilities Education Act (IDEA) and Title V of the Social Security Act to provide screening, early identification, and intervention for children with developmental delays and disabilities.[1]

In the United States, 12% to 16% of children have at least one developmental delay.[2] The most common childhood developmental and behavioral problems identified are speech and language delay, hearing loss, emotional and behavioral concerns, learning disabilities, delay in developmental milestones, and mental retardation.[3] Health care providers can identify young children with developmental and mental health problems early in life by providing surveillance at every well-child visit and implementing standardized developmental screening tests at the 9-month, 18-month, and 24- or 30-month well-child visit.[1] Timely identification of developmental and behavioral problems and prompt referral for early intervention can lead to interventions that resolve or lessen the impact of a delay or disability on the functioning of the child and family. Effective interventions in early childhood increase a child's readiness for school entry and for optimum learning in the classroom.

PEDIATRIC PEARLS

The care environment vastly impacts the development of a child's full potential.

DEVELOPMENTAL SURVEILLANCE IN EARLY CHILDHOOD

The first component of a developmental screening program is developmental surveillance. Developmental surveillance includes eliciting parental concerns, collecting and documenting a developmental history, and identifying risks and protective factors for developmental delay or emotional and behavioral problems in the child's environment. Observations of the child's development include speech and language skills, communication and social skills, activity level, and parent/child relationship. It is important to identify strengths in the parent and caregiver that are protective factors in the child's developmental progress. The primary care provider must include input from parents, other caregivers, and teachers in childcare and school settings to make informed observations of the child's developmental progress and accurately document the ongoing developmental surveillance in the health record.

Surveillance for vision and hearing includes asking parents about any concerns they may have about their infant or young child's developing vision or response to voices or sounds in the environment. Observable normal visual behaviors include fixing on and following near faces at 6 to 8 weeks of age; visually tracking at 4 months of age, including seeing the parent or caregiver at a distance of 5 feet; and visually fixating at 5 months on a 1-inch cube or small object at

12 inches.[4] Health care providers should ask parents about their child's ability to hear quiet sounds and turn and locate voices. All children referred for emotional and behavioral concerns should also have formal vision and hearing screening tests conducted to identify deficits or delays. Reviews of screening practices for vision and hearing are presented in Chapters 11 and 12, respectively.

Speech refers to the mechanics of oral communication, and language encompasses the understanding, processing, and production of communication during the early developmental years and throughout childhood. Surveillance of speech and language skills in childhood in-

cludes eliciting any parental concerns about communication problems, dysfluency, stuttering, articulation disorders, or an unusual voice quality.[5] Approximately 10% to 15% of children 2 years of age have language delays, and 4% to 5% remain language delayed after 3 years of age.[6] Early referral and intervention is key to optimizing speech and language development in early childhood. Health care providers need to conduct ongoing surveillance at each health encounter and identify children with parental concerns about speech and language development. Table 3-1 presents normal developmental speech and language patterns in infancy and early childhood.

TABLE 3-1 NORMAL RANGE OF DEVELOPMENTAL SPEECH AND LANGUAGE PATTERNS IN INFANCY AND EARLY CHILDHOOD

Age	Preverbal Communication to Developing Language and Attention to Speech Sounds
8 weeks	Grunting, crying, cooing
4 months	Squeals, yells, repeating vowel sounds or sounds in repeated patterns Turns head to look at the speaker by 4 months
6 months	More complex consonant-vowel combinations ("da," "ba") Vocal play with parent or caregiver repeating sounds Responding to own and family names by 6 months
8 to 10 months	Multisyllable babble (vowel-consonant combinations) Appears to listen to conversation of others by 8 months Looks at or gives common objects used at home by 8 months Wordlike sounds with intonation by 9 months Jargon Waves bye-bye and/or plays pat-a-cake by 10 months
10 to 12 months	Infant learned favored sounds of parent's and caregiver's language
12 to 13 months	Emergence of first word ranges from 8 to 18 months (mean 13 months) Consonant-vowel word by 12 months Single words, other than mama/dada, with consistent meaning by 12-13 months Infant communicates actively by pointing
13 to 15 months	Follows familiar requests by 12 to 15 months
18 to 20 months	Understands about 50 words Speaks about 20 words
24 months	Median speaking vocabulary 300 words 10th percentile speaking 60 words 90th percentile speaking 500 words

Data from Sharma A: Developmental examination: birth to 5 years, *Arch Dis Child Educ Pract Ed* 96:162-175, 2011; Davies D: *Child development: a practitioner's guide*, ed 3, New York, 2011, Guildford Press.

As a component of developmental surveillance for language deficits, pediatric health care providers can promote literacy by adopting the *Reach Out and Read* (ROR) program. ROR was designed to target children in early childhood who are at risk for poor early school performance and to provide families with books and anticipatory guidance about the importance of reading to young children. Several studies have shown that ROR can significantly enhance a young child's early literacy environment by increasing the frequency of parent-child book-sharing activities and facilitating language development.[7] Pediatric health care settings interested in establishing a pediatric literacy promotion program may contact the national Reach Out and Read program at http://www.reachoutandread.org.

The clinical assessment or surveillance of development without using standardized developmental screening tests identifies less than 50% of children with developmental delays.[8] The ultimate goal of developmental surveillance and screening is to improve outcomes for children with developmental delays and disorders. Table 3-2 presents normal developmental milestones of communication, fine and gross motor, problem solving, and social/emotional skills from 6 months to 5 years of age in accordance with *Ages and Stages Questionnaires* (ASQ-3) (2009). Guidelines for developmental surveillance

> ### EVIDENCE-BASED PRACTICE TIP
>
> Children who participate in *Reach Out and Read* demonstrate increased receptive and expressive language in early childhood and are less likely to suffer school failure.[7]

TABLE 3-2   ASQ-3 DEVELOPMENTAL MILESTONES BY AGE

Age	Communication-Linguistic Skills	Gross Motor	Fine Motor	Problem Solving	Social-Emotional
6 months	Makes sounds like "da," "ba", makes high-pitched squeals, turns in direction of loud noise	Rolls from back to tummy, sits with support of own hands, bears weight with feet flat on surface	Grabs toy, picks up small toy with one hand, reaches for crumb with thumb or raking motion	Reaches or grasps toy using both hands, looks for fallen object, picks up toy and mouths it	Smile or coo in front of mirror; grabs own foot while lying on back; tries to get out-of-reach toy
12 months	Makes two similar sounds, such as "ba-ba," "da-da"; plays peekaboo; says three words; points to objects	Walks holding on to furniture or holding both your hands, stands alone	Picks up string, uses pincer grasp, throws ball with forward arm motion, turns pages of book	Claps two toys together, looks for hidden object (object constancy), copies scribbles on paper	Helps with dressing, rolls or throw a ball, hugs stuffed animal or doll
18 months	Points to objects and pictures in book, says eight or more words, imitates two-word sentence	Picks up object from the floor, walks, climbs, walks down stairs, kicks large ball	Throws small ball, stacks two to three blocks, marks paper, turns pages of book, uses spoon	Dumps things out of container, copies single line drawing	Gets attention by pulling on your hand or clothes, comes to you for help, drinks from a cup, copies activities

TABLE 3-2	ASQ-3 DEVELOPMENTAL MILESTONES BY AGE—CONT'D				
Age	Communication-Linguistic Skills	Gross Motor	Fine Motor	Problem Solving	Social-Emotional
2 years	Points to correct picture in book, imitates two-word sentences, follows directions, names objects	Walks down stairs holding rail, kicks large ball, runs, jumps with both feet	Uses spoon without spilling; turns pages of book, flips switches on and off, stacks seven blocks, strings beads	Copies line drawings, pretend play, puts things away, climbs on chair to reach object	Drinks from cup without spilling, copies activities such as sweeping, combs hair, pushes toys on wheels
3 years	Points to seven body parts, speaks with three- to four-word sentences, follows directions, identifies action in picture book, knows own first and last name	Kicks ball by swinging leg forward, jumps forward at least 6 inches, walks up stairs, stands on one foot for 1 second, throws ball overhand	Draws line in vertical direction and circle, strings beads, cuts paper, holds crayon between fingers and thumb	Lines up four objects in a row, repeats two numbers, makes a bridge with blocks	Pushes and steers wagon or toy on wheels, dresses self, knows sex, takes turns
4 years	Follows simple directions; Follows three directions, speaks in complete sentences	Jumps forward at least 6 inches, catches a large ball with both hands, climbs a ladder	Traces a circle, cuts paper with scissors, puts together five- to seven-piece puzzle	Repeats three numbers, identifies small versus large circle, pretend play	Dresses self with coat and shirt, takes turns, serves food to self, washes hands using soap and water
5 years	Follows three unrelated directions; uses four- to five-word sentences, uses past tense and comparison words, answers questions	Throws ball at least 6 feet away, catches large ball with both hands, stands on one foot for 5 seconds, walks on tiptoes for 15 feet, hops on one foot 4-6 feet, skips	Draws picture of person with three or more body parts, cuts with scissors, copies shapes and letters, prints first name	Identifies colors; counts up to 15, knows opposites, names three numbers and four letters	Serves food to self, washes and dries hands and face without help, knows phone number and city of residence, dresses and undresses self, uses toilet by self, takes turns and shares with others

Data from Squires J, Bricker D: *Ages and stages questionnaires*, ed 3 (ASQ-3), Baltimore, MD, 2009, Brookes Publishing.

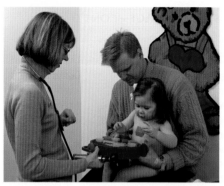

FIGURE 3-1 Developmental tasks for toddler.

and developmental screening are available at the website for the American Academy of Pediatrics (AAP) *Bright Futures: Guidelines for Health Supervision of Infants, Children, and Adolescents* (http://brightfutures. aap.org).[9]

PEDIATRIC PEARLS

Parental concern regarding delays in fine and gross motor skills, language skills, and social/emotional development are often highly accurate and should always warrant further evaluation.

DEVELOPMENTAL RISK FACTORS

Certain biological, family, and social risk factors increase the likelihood that a child will exhibit developmental delay. Biological factors that influence development include prenatal factors such as maternal substance abuse, maternal infection, maternal chronic health conditions, maternal medications, and severe toxemia. Neonatal risk factors include history of prematurity, gestational age <33 weeks, birth weight <1500 g, Apgar score <3 at 5 minutes, neonatal infections (sepsis or meningitis), and severe hyperbilirubinemia. A family history of maternal depression, low maternal education, poverty, a lack of maternal bonding, child abuse and neglect, and a lack of developmentally appropriate opportunities for learning can impact early child development. Environmental factors such as disadvantaged neighborhoods, high lead levels, exposure to environmental toxins, and limited access to health care may also contribute to developmental delays.[4]

Children at risk require especially diligent developmental surveillance, including implementing recommended use of developmental screening tools in the first 3 years of life and prompt referral for early intervention services, including a pediatric neurologist or pediatric developmental specialist when indicated. Box 3-1

BOX 3-1	DEVELOPMENTAL RED FLAGS IN EARLY CHILDHOOD INDICATING NEED FOR REFERRAL

3 Months
Persistent fisting
Failure to alert to visual/auditory stimuli
Lack of fixation

4-6 Months
Poor head control while sitting
Failure to reach for objects by 5 months
No social smile
Lack of visual tracking by 4 months
Failure to turn to sound or voice at 6 months

6-12 Months
Inability to sit by 9 months
Persistence of primitive reflexes after 6 months
No babbling by 6 months

No reciprocal vocalizations by 9 months
Inability to localize sound by 10 months

12-24 Months
No consonant production by 15 months
No word other than mama/dada by 18 months
Hand dominance before 18 months
Inability to walk independently by 18 months
Inability to walk up/down stairs by 24 months
No two-word sentences by 24 months
Echolalia beyond 24 months
Unable to follow simple command by 24 months
Does not play with toys in functional way (such as push car to make it go by 24 months)
Cannot name one picture in book by 27 months

BOX 3-1	DEVELOPMENTAL RED FLAGS IN EARLY CHILDHOOD INDICATING NEED FOR REFERRAL—CONT'D

3 Years
Speech is less than 75% intelligible
Lack of or inappropriate pronoun use
Sentences contain less than 3 to 4 words
Cannot feed independently with fork/spoon

4 Years
Speech is less than 95% intelligible
Has not achieved independent daytime toileting

Cannot separate from parent without crying
Cannot balance on one foot for 2 seconds
Cannot copy circle or use mature pencil grasp
Unable to name two to three colors
Not able to take turns and share most of
   the time

Data from Gerber R, Wilks T, Erdie-Lalena C: Developmental milestones: motor development, *Pediatr Rev* 31(7):267-277, 2010; Wilks T, Gerber R, Erdie-Lalena C: Developmental milestones: cognitive development, *Pediatr Rev* 31(9):364-367, 2010; Moses S: Developmental red flags, *Family practice notebook,* 2012, available at: www.fpnotebook.com/Peds/Neuro/DvlpmntlRdFlgs.htm.

presents red flags for developmental delay and language delay in infancy and early childhood that warrant referral for early intervention.

DEVELOPMENTAL SCREENING

Over 25% of children under 5 years of age are at risk for developmental, emotional, and behavioral problems, but fewer than one in five children receive the recommended developmental screening.[10] Many parents with children under 6 years of age are concerned about their child's development or behavior, yet only 20% of parents report that developmental screening was conducted at their child's primary care visits before entering kindergarten.[11] The AAP recommendations for developmental screening are based on evidence that indicates standardized screening tools capture up to 80% of children with early developmental delays.[12]

Developmental screening focuses on positive development and also identifies children with delays or problems early in life. It assists the health care provider with anticipatory guidance for parents and caregivers by identifying the developmental milestones met at each age as the infant grows and develops. Identification of a deficit or delay on a developmental screening test does not provide a diagnosis, but it identifies children who need

further evaluation, referral, and intervention services. Table 3-3 presents the common developmental screening tools used in the pediatric clinical setting.

STANDARDIZED DEVELOPMENTAL SCREENING TOOLS

Psychometrics

The psychometric properties of developmental screening tools are important considerations when deciding which screening tool to use in the pediatric health care setting.[1] Psychometric properties include reliability, validity, and sensitivity and specificity. Reliability is the ability of a measure to produce consistent results. The validity of a screening test is its ability to discriminate between a child with a problem and one without such a problem. Sensitivity is the accuracy of the test in identifying a problem, and specificity is the accuracy of the test in identifying individuals who do not have a problem. The sensitivity and specificity, the developmental domains measured, the number of test items, available languages, and the time to complete and score the common developmental, behavioral, and emotional screening tools are included in Tables 3-3 and 3-4. Other important considerations for pediatric developmental surveillance

TABLE 3-3   GENERAL DEVELOPMENTAL SCREENING TOOLS

Tool	Age Range	Informant and Time to Administer	Description	Access
Ages and Stages Questionnaires-3 (ASQ-3)	0-5 years	Parent, 5 minutes	10-15 items for each age range Directions are simple Screens communication, gross motor, fine motor, problem solving, and personal-social skills Available in multiple languages Sensitivity = 70%-90% Specificity = 76%-91%	Brookes Publishing www.brookespublishing. com www.agesandstages. com
Parent's Evaluation of Developmental Status (PEDS)	0-8 years	Parent, 2 minutes	10 items elicit parent's concerns for children of all ages Screens for developmental and behavioral problems Available in multiple languages Sensitivity = 75% Specificity = 74%	Ellsworth and Vandemeer Press, Ltd. www.pedstest.com
Denver II Developmental Screening Test (DDST II)	0-6 years	Provider, 20 minutes	20 items on gross motor, language, fine motor/adaptive, personal/social domains Provider elicits behavior or parent report Available in English and Spanish Sensitivity = 56%-83% Specificity= 43%-80%	Denver Developmental Materials, Inc. http://denverii.com/ denverii/
Bayley Infant Neurodevelopmental Screen (BINS)	3-24 months	Provider, 10-15 minutes	Trained examiner uses 10-13 directly elicited items to assess neurological processes, neurodevelopmental skills, and developmental achievements Sensitivity = 75% to 86% Specificity = 75% and 86%	Pearson Assessments www.pearsonassess. com

TABLE 3-4 EMOTIONAL, BEHAVIORAL, AND MENTAL HEALTH SCREENING TOOLS

Tool	Age Range	Informant and Time to Administer	Description	Access
Ages and Stages Questionnaires-SE (ASQ-SE)	3-66 months	Parent, 10-15 minutes	30 items Screens self-regulation, compliance, communication, adaptive behaviors, autonomy, affect, interaction with people Available in English and Spanish Sensitivity = 78% Specificity = 94%	Brookes Publishing www.brookespublishing.com www.agesandstages.com
Brief Infant/ Toddler Social Emotional Assessment (BITSEA)	12-36 months	Parent, 5-7 minutes	42-item report measure for identifying social emotional/behavioral problems with domains for externalizing, internalizing, dysregulation, and competence Available in different languages Sensitivity = 80%-85% Specificity= 75%-80%	Pearson Assessments www.pearsonassess.com
Modified Checklist for Autism in Toddlers (M-CHAT)	16-30 months	Parent, 5-10 minutes	23 items Identifies children at risk of autism spectrum disorders (ASD) Available in multiple languages Sensitivity = 85% Specificity= 93%	First Signs, Inc. http://www.firstsigns.org/downloads/m-chat.PDF
Pediatric Symptom Checklist (PSC35; Y-PSC)	4-16 years	Parent (PSC) or child over 11 years (Y-PSC), 5 minutes	35 items elicit parent's or teen's response on short statements about problem behaviors including conduct, depression, anxiety, adjustment Available in English, Spanish, Japanese Sensitivity = 80%-95% Specificity = 68%-100%	American Academy of Pediatrics www.brightfutures.org/mentalhealth/pdf/professionals/ped_sympton_chklst.pdf
Children's Depression Inventory 2 (CDI 2)	7-17 years	Parental report, teacher report, self-report, 5 to 10 minutes for short form	12 to 28 items Measures cognitive, affective and behavioral signs of depression	Multi-Health Systems, Inc. www.mhs.com

and screening are the costs to administer a screening tool.

The AAP strongly endorses the use of standardized, reliable (≥80%), well-validated, and accurate developmental screening tools with a sensitivity and specificity to ≥70% for the early identification of developmental-behavioral problems.[12] Screening tools should be directly administered by providers or trained staff or be parent-report questionnaires. Use of developmental screening tools with lower sensitivity and specificity may identify children without significant delays and may result in unnecessary referrals. Emotional and behavioral screening tests with low specificity may identify mental health symptoms that are below the level of a *Diagnostic and Statistical Manual of Mental Disorders* (DSM-IV-TR) diagnosis.[13] However, these children may benefit from early interventions in the home or improved developmental learning opportunities to address developing emotional and behavioral problems. Continual tracking of a child's developmental status and follow-up on referrals is critical to optimum child health and developmental outcomes.

Developmental Screening Tools for Early and Middle Childhood

The Parents' Evaluation of Developmental Status (PEDS)[14] and the Ages and Stages Questionnaires (ASQ-3)[15] use parental report as an effective screening tool for identifying children with possible developmental delays. Parent-completed developmental screening tools are found to be efficient, feasible, and cost-effective compared to provider-completed screening tools.

The Bayley Infant Neurodevelopmental Screener (BINS) is a tool designed specifically for high-risk infants and assesses cognitive, social, language, and gross and fine motor skills. It has a high sensitivity and specificity in identifying delays in preterm and low birth weight infants and is reliable as an indicator for referral for developmental

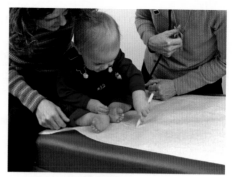

FIGURE 3-2 Scribbling to assess handedness.

delays in preterm infants at 6 months who remain delayed at 12 months of age; therefore, it is reliable as an indicator for referral.[16]

The Denver-II Developmental Screening Test (DDST-II) was previously the most widely used developmental screening tool by primary care providers but has significantly lower sensitivity and specificity than other developmental screening tools currently being used in pediatric clinical settings. The sensitivity (56% to 83%) and specificity (43% to 80%) is low to modest and has a wide range, which may result in over-referral of those infants and children who do not have a developmental delay and under-identification of those children who do not have developmental deficits.

Mental Health, Emotional, and Behavioral Screening Tools for Early and Middle Childhood and Adolescence

The Ages and Stages Questionnaire-Social/Emotional (ASQ-SE) is a parent-completed questionnaire to monitor the social and emotional development of infants and young children and screens for adaptive behaviors, communication, autonomy, affect, and interaction with adults. The Brief Infant/Toddler Social Emotional Assessment (BITSEA) is a parental report screening tool and is also a good measure of children's social, emotional, and behavioral development.[17] Both tools identify children with developing social and emotional disorders who may benefit from a more in-depth evaluation and referral.

The Modified Checklist for Autism in Toddlers (M-CHAT) is a 23-item parental-report questionnaire that can be administered to parents or caregivers to identify children at risk for autism spectrum disorders (ASD). The M-CHAT is valid and reliable in children from 16 to 30 months of age and requires about 5 to 10 minutes to complete. It has a high sensitivity and specificity for identifying as many children as possible with ASD and assists health care providers in assessing the need for referral for early intervention services. The M-CHAT is available in Appendix C.

The Pediatric Symptom Checklist (PSC) is the most commonly used mental health screening tool for children in middle childhood and adolescents in pediatric primary care settings.[18] The PSC has 35 items and screens children and adolescents from 4 years to 16 years of age. Beginning at 11 years of age, the PSC can be completed by the child or adolescent (see Appendix D). Approximately one in every four to five adolescents has one or more mental health, emotional, or behavioral problems, which may include depression, conduct disorder, or substance abuse.[19] Routine screening for mental health and emotional and behavioral disorders needs to be a primary focus for health care providers caring for adolescents. Health history screening tools for anxiety and depression in adolescence are presented in Chapter 4.

The Children's Depression Inventory 2 (CDI 2) (http://www.mhs.com) is used to screen children and adolescents from 7 years to 17 years of age for cognitive, affective, and behavioral signs of depression. It is administered as a parental report, teacher report, and/or self-report screening tool.

Other valid and reliable mental health screening tools for adolescents can be found at TeenScreen (http://www.teenscreen.org).

DEVELOPMENTAL AND BEHAVIORAL HEALTH CONDITIONS

Autism Spectrum Disorders

An autism spectrum disorder (ASD) is a complex neurodevelopmental disorder that is characterized by delays in communication and language skills, and social and behavioral development. ASDs include autism; pervasive developmental disorder, not otherwise specified (PDD-NOS); and Asperger syndrome. The onset of ASD is before 3 years of age. ASD is at least partially genetically linked, though no single gene abnormality or mode of inheritance has yet been identified.

The Centers for Disease Control and Prevention (CDC) reports the prevalence of ASD is currently 1 in 88 children, but 40% of affected children do not get a diagnosis until after 4 years of age.[3,20] The ratio of ASD is 5:1, male to female.[20] Autism screening is recommended for all children before 24 months of age.[21,22] Screening for ASD should be completed at the 18- and/or 24-month well-child visit. Early identification and intervention has been shown to be highly effective in helping children with ASD gain social and emotional skills. Some of the concerning behaviors identified by 18 months of age are not smiling in response to parent's face, not responding to his/her name, not using an index finger to point to objects, not taking an interest in other children, not playing peekaboo or hide-and-seek, wandering or staring without a purpose, and making unusual finger movements near his/her face.

The M-CHAT is the recommended screening tool to identify children at risk for ASD. Questions include: "Does your child take an interest in other children?" "Does your child ever use his/her index finger to point, to indicate interest in something?" "Does your child ever bring objects to you (parent) to show you something?" "If you point at a toy across the room, does your child look at it?" "Does your child imitate you? (e.g., if you make a face, will your child imitate it?)". If a child fails on 3 out of the 23 items or 2 critical domain items, the child should be referred for a diagnostic evaluation. Children at risk for other developmental disorders or delays may also be identified with the M-CHAT screening tool.

Learning Disorders

Learning disorders may result from neurodevelopmental or genetic causes or occur as comorbidities with other physical or mental disabilities. *Learning disability* refers to difficulty in acquiring and using basic reading and writing skills, reading comprehension, oral expression, listening comprehension, mathematical reasoning, and mathematical comprehension that occurs without an environmental precipitant in otherwise normally intelligent children. Learning disorders are neurologically based and persist into adulthood. The incidence of learning disorders is 10% to 15% of the population.[23] Pediatric primary care providers assist with the diagnosis of learning disabilities by performing an initial thorough history and physical examination including a complete neurological examination and an evaluation of school performance. Confirmation of learning disabilities includes referral for neuropsychometric testing and evaluation by a licensed psychologist.

Attention-Deficit/Hyperactivity Disorder

Attention-deficit/hyperactivity disorder (ADHD) occurs in 4% to 12% of the pediatric population in the community, with males outnumbering females 3:1 to 6:1.[24] The diagnosis of ADHD is based on a characteristic clinical presentation and observable behaviors. The problematic behaviors include inattention, hyperactivity, and impulsivity. The practitioner must rule out the possibility that such behaviors merely represent variations in normal development or temperament, and that they are not attributable to environmental factors such as a poor fit with the teacher and/or classroom. Furthermore, ADHD may coexist with other disorders or conditions that must be addressed before an appropriate diagnosis can be given. Between 10% and 40% of children with ADHD have learning disabilities. Schools are federally mandated to perform appropriate evaluations if a child is suspected of having a disability such as ADHD. Parents should be assisted in requesting evaluations for ADHD, which include a comprehensive history, with careful attention given to developmental level; complete physical examination, including neurological exam; vision and hearing screening; lead and hematocrit levels in preschool children; input elicited from teachers; initiation of an individual education plan coordinated with the child's school; and referral to a developmental-behavioral specialist, pediatric neurologist, or mental health professional.

CHARTING

Documentation of developmental surveillance and screening also provides a record of the child's neuromaturational progress over time.

Charting

A Healthy 9-Month-Old Infant

Mother without concerns regarding child's development or behavior, states she reads to child daily. Infant initially exhibits stranger anxiety, consolable by mother. Creeps, pulls to stand, claps, has thumb-finger grasp, plays peekaboo. Plays pat-a-cake per parental report. Passed ASQ-3.

REFERENCES

1. Council on Children With Disabilities, Section on Developmental Behavioral Pediatrics, Bright Futures Steering Committee, Medical Home Initiatives for Children With Special Needs Project Advisory Committee: Identifying infants and young children with developmental disorders in the medical home: an algorithm for developmental surveillance and screening, *Pediatrics* 118(1):405-420, 2006.

2. Mackrides PS, Ryherd SJ: Screening for developmental delay, *Am Fam Physician* 84(5):544-549, 2011.

3. Slomski A: Chronic mental health issues in children now loom larger than physical problems, *JAMA* 308(3):223-225, 2012.

4. Sharma A: Developmental examination: birth to 5 years, *Arch Dis Child Educ Pract Ed.* 96:162-175, 2011.

5. US Preventive Services Task Force: Screening for speech and language delay in preschool children: recommendation statement, *Pediatrics* 117(2): 497-501, 2006.

6. Stein MT, Parker S, Coplan J, et al: Expressive language delay in a toddler, *J Dev Behav Pediatr* 22:S99, 2001.

7. Willis E, Kabler-Babbitt C, Zuckerman B: Early literacy interventions: reach out and read, *Pediatr Clin North Am* 54(3):625-642, viii, 2007.

8. Aylward G: Developmental screening and assessment: what are we thinking? *J Dev Behav Pediatr* 30(2): 169-173, 2009.

9. Hagan JF, Shaw JS, Duncan PM: *Bright Futures: Guidelines for health supervision of infants, childrens, and adolescents*, ed 3, Elk Grove Village, Ill., 2008, American Academy of Pediatrics.

10. U.S. Department of Health and Human Services, Maternal and Child Health Bureau: *National survey of children's health 2007*. Available at http://www.cdc.gov/nchs/slaits/nsch.htm#2007nsch.

11. Bethell C, Reuland C, Schor E, et al: Rates of parent-centers developmental screening: disparities and links to services access, *Pediatrics* 128(1):146-155, 2011.

12. Marks KP, LaRosa AC: Understanding developmental-behavioral screening measures, *Pediatr Rev* 30(10): 448-458, 2012.

13. American Psychiatric Association Task Force on DSM-IV: *Diagnostic and statistical manual of mental disorders: DSM-IV-TR*, ed 4, Washington D.C., 2000, American Psychiatric Association.

14. Glascoe FP: *Parents' evaluation of developmental status (PEDS)*, Nashville, Tenn., 2006, Ellsworth & Vandermeer Press, LLC.

15. Squires J, Bricker D: *Ages and Stages Questionnaires*, ed 3, Baltimore, 2009, Brookes Publishing.

16. Leonard CH, Piecuch RE, Cooper BA: Use of Bayley Infant Neurodevelopmental Screener with low birth weight infants, *J Pediatr Psychol* 26(1):33-40, 2001.

17. Briggs-Gowan M, Carter A, Irwin J, et al: The Brief Infant-Toddler Social and Emotional Assessment: screening for social-emotional problems and delays in competence, *J Pediatr Psychol* 29(2):143-155, 2004.

18. Jellinek M, Murphy J, Little M, et al: Use of the Pediatric Symptom Checklist (PSC) to screen for psychosocial problems in pediatric primary care: a national feasibility study, *Arch Pediatr Adolesc Med* 153(3):254-260, 1999.

19. Merikangas K, He J, Burstein M, et al: Life-time prevalence of mental disorders in U.S. adolescents: results from the National Co-morbidity Survey Replication-Adolescent Supplement, *J Am Acad Child Adolesc Psychiatry* 49(10):980-989, 2010.

20. Autism and Developmental Disabilities Monitoring Network Surveillance 2008 Principal Investigators, Centers for Disease Control and Prevention: Prevalence of autism spectrum disorders—Autism and Developmental Disabilities Monitoring Network, 14 sites, United States, 2008. *MMWR Surveill Summ* 61(3):1-19, 2012.

21. Johnson CP, Meyers SM: Identification and evaluation of children with autism spectrum disorders, *Pediatrics* 120:1183-1215, 2007.

22. Robins DL: Screening for autism spectrum disorders in primary care settings, *Autism* 12(5):537-556, 2008.

23. Wolraich ML, American Academy of Pediatrics: *Caring for children with ADHD: A resource toolkit for clinicians*, ed 2, Elk Grove Village, Ill., 2011, American Academy of Pediatrics.

24. Leslie L, Weckerly J, Plemmons D, et al: Implementing the American Academy of Pediatrics attention-deficit/hyperactivity disorder diagnostic guidelines in primary care settings, *Pediatrics* 114(1):129-140, 2004.

CHAPTER 4

COMPREHENSIVE INFORMATION GATHERING

Karen G. Duderstadt; Naomi A. Schapiro

The skill of obtaining a comprehensive, holistic health history remains the most important clinical tool for pediatrics. Despite the technological advances in health care and electronic medical records, expert assessment is most influenced by observing, listening, and thinking critically in a clinical setting. Recognizing patterns of health and illness in infants, children, and adolescents requires obtaining relevant pieces of data from the health history, thinking about their meaning, and explaining them logically. Taking a comprehensive history with families not only develops a profile to guide physical assessment, diagnosis, and treatment, but also contributes to the development of a continuity relationship between the family and health care provider.

Information gathered from the family history is also key to identifying genetic patterns of inheritance in health conditions and is a guide to health education and promoting responsible health behaviors in the child and adolescent.[1] Identifying and counseling children and adolescents at risk for chronic health conditions such as diabetes, hypertension, and cardiovascular disease begins with gathering a comprehensive family history.[1]

Identifying and counseling for childhood overweight and obesity remains a top priority in pediatrics. Identifying early childhood factors in the comprehensive history that are significant predictors of obesity in adulthood is an important role for pediatric health care providers in prevention and anticipatory guidance. Probable early markers of obesity include maternal body mass index; childhood growth patterns, particularly early rapid growth and early adiposity rebound; childhood obesity; and parental employment, a marker for socioeconomic status of the family.[2] When gathering the health history, it is important to talk to children and adolescents about the importance of physical activity and their dietary routines to establish early positive health habits.

The comprehensive health history in children and adolescents also includes psychosocial screening. In child health, the top five chronic health conditions in pediatrics currently are speech and language delays, learning disabilities, attention-deficit/hyperactivity disorders, developmental disabilities, and emotional, behavioral, and mental health problems.[3] These findings indicate the importance of psychosocial screening during every well-child and adolescent encounter in a clinical setting.

Another important component of comprehensive information gathering is oral health. Tooth decay continues to be the single most common chronic health condition in pediatrics. Tooth decay affects more than one fourth of U.S. children from 2 to 5 years of age and half of adolescents 12 to 15 years of age.[4] Globally, 60% to 90% of school children have dental caries.[5] Assessing children's oral health and access to dental health services is key to establishing positive dental health behaviors early in life.

THE GENETIC FAMILY HISTORY

Genetics has transformed the use of family history information and has led to the reemergence of the detailed *genetic family history*. The increased use of genetic screening is creating a paradigm shift in medical treatment by emphasizing primary prevention and early

TABLE 4-1 THE SCREEN MNEMONIC FOR FAMILY HISTORY COLLECTION

SC	Some concerns	"Do you have any (some) concerns about diseases or conditions that run in the family?"
R	Reproduction	"Have there been any problems with pregnancy, infertility, or birth defects in your family?"
E	Early disease, death, or disability	"Have any members of your family died or become sick at an early age?"
E	Ethnicity	"How would you describe your ethnicity?" or "Where were your parents born?"
N	Nongenetic	"Are there any other risk factors or nonmedical conditions that run in your family?"

From Trotter TL, Martin HM: Family history in pediatric primary care, *Pediatrics* 120(Suppl 2):S60-65, 2007.

intervention for families with hereditarily linked health conditions.[6] Gathering of the comprehensive family history is necessary to make this link and advance the health of children and families. It is important to be aware of the emotional and ethical issues that may arise when taking a genetic family history, such as the hereditary link between breast cancer in female relatives and familial gene testing. Pediatric health care providers are well placed to provide this support to individuals and families.[7] Also, pediatric providers are particularly well positioned to use this knowledge as they provide primary care for children from birth to young adults, the period during which many genetic disorders emerge.[1]

The genetic family history establishes a family pedigree. The *family pedigree* or *genogram* is a visual way to enhance recognition of patterns of inheritance. This approach leads to insights in patterns of inheritance across generations, and gives health care providers an opportunity to counsel families on prevention and offer referrals for further genetic testing. Knowledge of the genetic family history can aid in the diagnosis of rare single-gene disorders such as cystic fibrosis, fragile X syndrome, Huntington disease, or familial hypercholesterolemia.

An accurate genetic family history requires the availability of a reliable family source and the knowledge of a three-generation family history. The challenge is to gather a family and genetic history within the brief time available in the clinical setting. Table 4-1 presents the SCREEN mnemonic for an initial genetic family history.[8] The SCREEN mnemonic represents an initial series of questions used to quickly identify potential genetically influenced health conditions in the family that require further intervention, counseling, referral, or screening by a geneticist. Figure 4-1 is

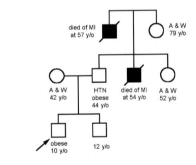

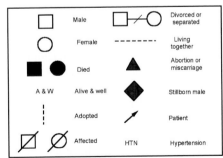

FIGURE 4-1 Family pedigree with a multigenerational inheritance of cardiovascular disease. (From Bennett RL: *The practical guide to the genetic family history,* New York, 1999, Wiley-Liss, Inc.)

an example of a family pedigree with a multigenerational inheritance of cardiovascular disease.

FAMILY-CENTERED HISTORY

The following key strategies are involved in developing a successful family-centered relationship with children and families in the pediatric setting:

- Listen actively to the concerns of the family. A caring relationship is established by developing an understanding of the feelings and values within the family context.
- Understand the family expectations for the encounter. To successfully establish a caring relationship, the parent's agenda must be identified and addressed during the encounter.
- Ask open-ended questions, thereby allowing relevant data to unfold.
- Personalize your care. Ask about the health and well-being of other family members and extended family members to personalize your care and demonstrate your connectedness with the family unit. Taking the time to obtain and integrate this relevant personal data on the child and family will assist in building the family profile and family-centered relationship.
- Learn and understand the role and importance of cultural influences in the family and the primary language spoken in the home. The health interview should be conducted in the family's primary language if possible to promote family engagement.

- Identify protective factors in the family that create a positive environment for the child. Social supports for the parents, involvement of relatives or extended family, and shared family interest in activities such as sports, cultural events, or religious services often help to form a supportive and protective community for children and adolescents.
- Build a sense of confidence in parents by confirming and complimenting their strengths in caring for their child. This approach also builds a trusting relationship between the family and health care provider.
- Time management is key. With the increased workload in health care settings and the implementation of electronic health records, being present when talking with children and families becomes more challenging. Remember to sit rather than stand, maintain eye contact with the child and family in between screen time, and share screen health information such as growth chart and lab results to engage with families.

Pediatric health care providers are uniquely suited to assess children from a family-centered perspective. Box 4-1 approaches the family-centered interview from three levels to assess family strengths, stressors, and threats to the family unit. Families hold trust in the pediatric provider, and their relationship is based on the knowledge, understanding, respect, and care the pediatric provider demonstrates during the encounter with their child.

BOX 4-1 THREE LEVELS OF FAMILY-CENTERED ASSESSMENT

Level 1: Micro Level
The child, parent or parents, partner, caregiver, other adults or children in household
- *Consider* intersecting characteristics and temperament of the individuals in the family unit, style of parenting, relationship between parents, and impact of family dynamics on physical, developmental, behavioral, and emotional health of child.

Level 2: Mezzo Level
The extended family, family supports and resources, community-based systems
- *Consider* housing, school, childcare, parental work and income, health care access, church and religious community, safety of community, immigration status, and impact on child well-being.

Level 3: Macro Level
The social context of child and family
- *Consider* impact of the community, cultural influences, economic status, environmental health, political climate, and impact on physical and mental health of child.

FAMILY, CULTURAL, RACIAL, AND ETHNIC CONSIDERATIONS

A *cultural assessment* should be included in every comprehensive family health history, and gathering information on family culture begins with the interview questions. The cultural assessment should include the family's beliefs about the origin of wellness or illness and their perceptions of the child's health. Cultural values and beliefs strongly influence a family's perception of cause and effect of common and chronic health conditions. Establishing positive health behaviors within the family may hinge upon a family's understanding of the cause of an illness and their beliefs about the impact of therapies on the illness. Integrating respect for culture is a continual process in the provider/family relationship.

The following questions should be included in a *family cultural assessment* with the goal of developing an understanding of culture within the context of the family:

- Where was the child born? *If an immigrant:* How long has the child lived in this country? What is the family's cultural identity?
- *If multiracial family:* What culture(s)/race(s) does the family identify with most closely? *If interviewing an adolescent:* What culture(s)/race(s) do you identify with most closely?
- What are the child's primary and secondary languages? What is the family's speaking and reading ability of the primary language (languages) in the home?
- What is the family's religion, and do they practice their religion daily or weekly?
- Are the family's food preferences linked to cultural or religious preferences?
- Are there beliefs about health or illness related to the family's culture?
- *If interviewing an adolescent:* Are there conflicts with parents or peers concerning cultural norms or customs? Have you experienced discrimination?

COMPONENTS OF INFORMATION GATHERING

The information gathered during an encounter reflects the parent's or caretaker's opinions and experience and therefore needs to be viewed as *subjective* information. The subjective information guides the *objective* findings of the physical examination and assists the health care provider in evaluating the family functioning, the family's approach to health and illness, and the reliability of the historian—parent, partner of the biological parent, guardian, or grandparent.

The type of health history gathered during an encounter depends on whether the child and family are presenting for a *comprehensive well-child visit, acute care visit, symptom-focused visit,* or a *preparticipation sports physical examination* (see Chapter 18). Examples of medical charting and electronic medical record (EMR) templates for different types of health visits for different pediatric age groups are presented in Chapter 20.

INFORMATION GATHERING OF SUBJECTIVE DATA

Child Profile

The demographic and biographical information for a child and family should be gathered at the initial health visit and verified at each health encounter. In an initial visit, the child profile should include information on the previous health care provider, date of the child's or adolescent's last health care visit, and contact information on parents or stepparent, partner of biological parent, caregiver, guardian, or grandparent. Family units change and this information should be updated at each health encounter.

The Open-Ended Question

Begin the interview with an open-ended question such as, "What brings you here today?" This allows the family to tell their story in their own words and centers the health visit around the family concerns and establishes the basis of the *family-centered interview.* Clarifying the expectations of the child and family for the health visit and negotiating a time frame and plan for care are important to establishing trust in a provider/parent relationship.

Present Concern

After summarizing the family concerns gathered in the initial interview, transition to the *provider-centered interview* to complete gathering information on the present health history and past medical history. If this is a symptom-focused or acute care visit, begin gathering information in the following areas to clarify information the family has not already addressed:

- When did you first notice the symptoms? Or date/time child was last well?
- Character of symptoms (time of day, location, intensity, duration, quality)?
- Progression of symptoms (How is child doing now? Symptoms getting better or worse?)

- Associated symptoms (vomiting, fever, rash, cough etc.)? Anything else bothering child?
- Exposure to household member, classmates, or others who have been ill? Pets in home?
- Any recent travel?
- Changes in appetite or activity level (eating regularly, school/daycare attendance, sleeping pattern)?
- Medications taken (dosage, time, date)? Did the medication help or relieve the symptoms?
- Home management (What has the family tried? What has helped?) Use of alternative therapies or healing practices?
- Pertinent family medical history? (Is anyone in the family immunosuppressed or does anyone have a chronic illness?)
- What changes have occurred in the family as a result of this illness (effects or secondary gain)?
- Has the family seen other health care providers for the concern?

For a symptom-focused or acute care visit, the health care provider should include only pertinent parts of the comprehensive history presented in the following sections.

Prenatal and Birth History

The initial history of the child is important in relation to the first 2 years of life and particularly relevant for infants and children with developmental delays, abnormal neurological findings, or congenital syndromes.

Prenatal History

- GTPAL (Gravidity, number of pregnancies; Term deliveries; Premature deliveries; Abortions, spontaneous or induced; Living children)
- Maternal and paternal age, month prenatal care started, planned pregnancy?
- Length of pregnancy, weight gain, history of fetal movement/activity
- Maternal health before and during pregnancy—overweight or obese; hypertension; gestational diabetes; infectious diseases,

including TB and HIV status; asthma or other chronic health conditions; hospitalizations

- Maternal substance use or abuse; tobacco use; prescription drug use; over-the-counter drug use or abuse; intimate partner violence or exposure to abuse or family violence
- History of maternal depression or anxiety disorders

Birth and Neonatal History

- Length of labor, location of birth, cesarean or vaginal delivery, epidural/anesthesia? Vacuum-assisted vaginal birth? Breech or shoulder presentation?
- Infant born on or near expected due date? Born preterm or post term? *If preterm*: Was infant in intensive care? Intubated?
- Birth weight and length? Gestational age?
- Apgar score, if known? Breathing problems after birth?
- Who was present at delivery, how soon after birth did mother or parent(s) touch or hold baby?
- Difficulties in feeding or stooling? Irritability or jitteriness? Jaundice?
- Length of hospitalization? Was infant discharged with mother?

Past Medical History

A comprehensive health history includes a review of the *past medical history* from birth to adolescence. For symptom-focused or acute care visits, past medical history information is often focused on system-specific symptoms, which are presented in the chapters that follow. The following are components of the past medical history:

- **Childhood conditions:** Frequent upper respiratory infections (URIs) or viral infections, history of ear infections—how often? Sore throats; streptococcal or bacterial infections? Eczema or frequent skin rashes? Dental caries?
- **Chronic conditions:** Seasonal or household allergies, wheezing or asthma; recurrent bronchitis; frequent ear infections or fluid in ears; hearing problems; overweight or obesity; diabetes; bed-wetting; dental decay or poor oral health? HIV or immunodeficiency? Onset of chronic condition?
- **Hospitalizations:** Date and reason for hospitalization, history of surgery, length of stay, complications after hospitalization?
- **Unintentional injuries:** Falls, nature of injury, age of child when injury occurred, problems after injury? Motor vehicle, bicycle, scooter/skateboard, or pedestrian-related injuries?
- **Intentional injuries:** History of family violence, physical abuse, or intimate partner violence? Child interview should include the following questions: Has anyone hurt you? Have you felt afraid someone would harm you? Is there any bullying or verbal abuse from family members or during school, after-school programs, or childcare?
- **Immunization:** Review immunization dates and current status including status of annual flu vaccine; ask parent/caregiver about reactions to vaccines; date of last TB skin testing and result? If under-immunized, reasons for withholding vaccines or parental concerns about vaccine safety?
- **Allergies:** Allergic to prescription medications or antibiotics; reaction to over-the-counter (OTC) medications? Any food allergies noted? What type of reaction occurred? Severity of the reaction? Was an epinephrine pen (EpiPen) recommended? Reaction to insect bites or bee stings? Pets in home? Environmental triggers?
- **Medications:** Is child taking vitamins, fluoride, or medications regularly? Type of medication? Use of OTC medications? Use of herbs or natural or homeopathic medicines? Cultural healing practices?
- **Laboratory tests:** Review of newborn screening results? Result of newborn hearing screening? Hemoglobin or hematocrit screening for anemia? Lead screening? Tuberculin purified protein derivative (PPD) screening?

Activities of Daily Living

Nutrition and Feeding

- Obtain a history of the infant feeding pattern. Exclusively breastfeeding? Formula feeding? Feeding both breast milk and formula? How often and quantity of formula daily?
- Obtain a 24-hour dietary recall during every early childhood, middle childhood, and adolescent encounter. (See later on age-specific content on nutrition and feeding.)
- Is there a usual time daily when the family has a common meal? Are there usual family eating patterns? How often does the family eat together at a meal? Who does the food shopping? How often are meals prepared at home? Daily or number of times per week? Number of fast food meals per week?
- Vegetarian or vegan diet in family? Are there any special cultural or religious food preferences?
- Does the family participate in any supplemental food programs? WIC (Special Supplemental Nutrition Program for Women, Infants, and Children) or SNAP (Supplemental Nutrition Assistance Program)?

Stooling and Elimination Patterns

- **Infancy:** Stooling pattern, frequency, and consistency?
- **Early childhood (1 year to 4 years of age):** Stooling pattern and frequency, plans for toilet training; resistance to toilet training, difficulties with bowel or bladder control; age bowel and bladder control attained?
- **Middle childhood (5 to 10 years of age):** Daytime or nighttime wetting? Soiling or difficulty with bowel control? Parental attitudes toward wetting incidents? History of encopresis or enuresis? History of constipation or diarrhea?

Sleep

- Sleep patterns and amount of sleep day and night for infants and young children? Bedtime routines? Regular bedtime? Hours of sleep nightly? Where does the child sleep? Co-sleeping until what age? Always sleeps in same household? Concerns about nightmares, night terrors, night waking, somnambulism (sleepwalking)?

Oral Health and Dentition

- Number of teeth? Use of night bottle or frequent breastfeeding? Weaning occurred at what age? Use of sugary foods/sodas/juices? Snacks and snack frequency? Has child seen dentist? Does child have a dental home? Last dental appointment? Tooth loss pattern? History of dental caries?

School/After-School Programs/Childcare

- **Infancy (birth to 11 months):** Who is primary caregiver for infant? If infant is in childcare: Is infant in home daycare or in a childcare center? Number of children in home daycare?
- **Early childhood (1 year to 4 years of age):** Where does the child spend the day? Who is primary caregiver? What is your child's school experience? Daycare, preschool, or prekindergarten experience? How well did your child adjust to school entry?
- **Middle childhood (5 years to 10 years of age):** School performance? Likes school? What are child's strengths? Number of missed school days? Reason for school absence? Teacher has concerns about learning? Attends special education classes? Any history of bullying in the classroom or during school hours?

EVIDENCE-BASED PRACTICE TIP

Children as young as 3 years of age can effectively participate in the health interview. Involving children at this age establishes the health care provider as an advocate for the child and gives voice to the concerns of the child in an objective manner. Eighty-four percent of pediatric providers obtain part of the health history from preschool children.[10]

Interests/Hobbies/Sports

- Screen time? Number of hours daily of TV, video gaming, cell phone use, computer use, and computer gaming?
- After-school activities? At school or in the community?
- Interested in sports? Participates in after-school sports programs?
- Daily amount of physical activity?

Safety[11]

- **Infancy:** *Car seat:* Rear-facing car seat in back seat of car? Any concern about installation of car seat? Safely installed? If preterm infant or infant with special health care needs, is infant using supports in car seat or car bed for safe transport?[12] *Household:* Is household water temperature set at ≤120° F? Choking hazards? Is infant in smoke-free environment? Avoid parental tobacco use or counsel on smoking cessation.
- **Early childhood (1 year to 4 years of age):** *Car seat:* Rear-facing car seat in back seat of car until age 2 years? Child meets manufacturer's weight/height for front-facing infant car seat? Any concern about installation of car seat? Safely installed? *Household:* Child-proofing of household? Preventing burns and falls? Number for poison control? Choking hazards? Tobacco use in home? Presence of gun in home, loaded/unloaded, how stored? Stranger safety taught? Teaching pet safety? Drowning risks? Home or community pool? Empty cleaning buckets? Sunscreen use?
- **Middle childhood (5 years to 10 years of age):** *Car safety:* Transition to booster seat at what age? Belt-positioning booster seat required until 4 feet 9 inches or until child is at least 8 years of age. Seat belt used regularly? Riding in backseat of motor vehicle? Pedestrian safety? *Household:* Bicycle safety? Helmet use? Sports safety equipment used? Swimming safety? Sunscreen use? Stranger safety taught? Supervision with friends/peers? Presence of gun in home? Loaded/unloaded, how stored? Fire safety? Smoke detectors? Monitoring of screen time and content (TV, computer, and cell phone)? Discussion about tobacco, alcohol, and drug use risks with child?
- **Adolescence (11 years to 21 years of age):** See later section on adolescent history.

Developmental History

The timing of developmental markers and normal developmental progress is critical during infancy and early childhood. Parental concerns about delayed physical growth or delayed psychomotor or cognitive development is of primary importance in the health history interview. Parental expectations of developmental markers vary widely in families, so it is important to elicit in the history not only what the infant or child is doing, but also what the family expects and allows.[11] Note the ages at which the child attained key developmental markers.

Infancy

- **Gross motor skills:** Holds head up while prone; supervised tummy time? Rolls over; sits without support; crawling/cruising? Pulls to standing? Starting to stand and walk?
- **Fine motor skills:** Hand-eye coordination; reaching and grasping? Beginning to feed self finger foods? Scribbling by 1 year of age? Pointing?
- **Communication:** Is infant hearing? First word? How many words by 1 year of age?
- **Social/emotional:** Smiles, socially engaged with family? Points? Stranger anxiety?
- **Sexual development:** Normal self-pleasure exploration in infant?

Early Childhood (1 Year to 4 Years of Age)

The health care provider should explore parental concerns about the child's temperament and behavior and about temper tantrums and parental reaction. Breath-holding spells can occur during early childhood, and discussions about establishing discipline and parental response to child's increasing demands are important during this period. Habits such as thumb-sucking are common with this age group and should be reviewed.

- **Gross and fine motor skills:** Manual dexterity, handedness, uses utensils/self-feeding, tying shoes, drawing, writing, coordination when walking and running?
- **Communication:** Do you have any concerns about your child's speech? Do you understand your child's speech? Do others? Does child follow directions? Does child combine words? Does child get confused, stutter, repeat words?
- **Social/emotional:** Dresses without help, separates from mother or parent? Names friend, peer interaction?
- **Temperament/personality:** Activity level, attention span, consolability?
- **Discipline:** What type of discipline do you use when your child misbehaves? When do you use it? Is discipline effective?
- **Sexual development:** Normal self-pleasure exploration and masturbation in preschooler, parental attitude towards normal self-pleasure exploration? Parental comfort with answering child's questions?

Middle Childhood (5 Years to 10 Years of Age)

The health care provider should explore developing interests with the school-age child and parent and encourage participation in physical activity. Exploring the quality of the child's friendships and the school performance and experience (current grades, relationship with teacher) gives a view into the child's world. Children who are bullying, being bullied, or both should be counseled and considered for possible referral. Habits such as nail biting and tics should be explored.

- **Gross and fine motors skills:** Physical balance and coordination? Participating in sports? Handwriting ability?
- **Communication:** Readiness to learn? Speech or language delays? Communication patterns with peers and adults?
- **Social/emotional:** Increasing independence? Self-esteem? Relationships with parents, siblings? Peer relationships and best friend?

Experienced bullying in school or from family members? Mood or symptoms of depression? History of suicidal ideation?

- **Temperament/personality:** Congenial with peers? Self-image? Ability to adapt to change?
- **Discipline:** What type of discipline do you use when your child misbehaves? When do you use it? Is discipline effective? Consistent parenting styles? Does child live at more than one home? Behavior issues at home or at school?
- **Sexual development:** Gender identity, comfort with biological sex, child or family concerns about gender expression; sex education provided in the home and school?

Adolescence (11 Years to 21 Years of Age)

See adolescent-specific content later in the chapter.

Family History

- **Family health history:** Hypertension, heart disease, diabetes, stroke, cancer, asthma, nasal allergy, eczema, mental health problems, history of substance abuse or alcoholism, sexually transmitted infections (STIs) or HIV+, family history of headaches or migraine, congenital anomalies or mental retardation, sickle cell trait or disease, kidney disease, learning problems, death in first year of life, early death from heart attack or any cause, epilepsy, or treatment for tuberculosis. (Information can be incorporated in genogram and genetic family history.)
- **Socioeconomic history:** Employment status, parental occupations, parental or caregiver work schedules, parental education and parental literacy level, access to health insurance, medical or health care home, uninsured or underinsured. (See Family, Cultural, Racial, and Ethnic Considerations section.)
- **Home and housing situation:** Who lives in the household? Number of adults and children living in home? Type of home, apartment, or housing situation? Living with extended family members or relatives? Is

housing secure or temporary? Housing problems? Is the neighborhood and community safe? Sleeping arrangements?

- **Support systems:** With whom do you talk when you have a problem? Family support or extended family living near or in home? Help with childcare? Supportive or close friends?
- **Family violence or intimate partner violence:** Do you feel safe in the home? Is there a history of family violence or intimate partner violence in home?

Review of Systems

The *review of systems* is often included in the comprehensive health history for children and adolescents, particularly those with chronic health conditions impacting multiple systems in the body. Table 4-2 presents a guide for the information gathered in a review of systems.

TABLE 4-2	REVIEW OF SYSTEMS FOR MIDDLE CHILDHOOD AND ADOLESCENCE
General	General health/well-being, weight gain/loss, fevers, appetite, sleep, malaise, fatigue
Skin	Rashes, eruptions, skin infections, pigmentations, growths/lumps, easy bruising
Eyes	Itching, redness, dryness, mucous discharge, tearing, rubbing eyes frequently, vision problems, squinting, trouble reading and/or sitting close to TV, has glasses or wears glasses, vision screening results
Ears	History of frequent infections, earaches, pulling at ears, ear drainage, wax impaction, trouble hearing, newborn hearing screening results, history of failed audiogram
Nose	Frequent runny nose or nasal allergy, frequent upper respiratory infection, nose bleeds
Mouth/Throat	Frequent sore throats, large tonsils, mouth breathing, speech difficulties, number of teeth, signs of teething, most recent dental visit, thumb-sucking
Neck/Lymphatic	Pain or stiffness in neck, swollen or tender lymph nodes or glands, any lumps or bumps noted
Chest	For females over 9 years of age: breast development For males over 9 years of age: breast swelling or gynecomastia
Respiratory	Frequent cough, nighttime cough, shortness of breath when exercising, respiratory distress, nasal flaring, retractions, rate, wheezing, cyanosis, pain, tuberculosis exposure and testing, previous chest x-rays (CXR), history of asthma, sleep apnea, snoring, secondhand smoke exposure
Cardiovascular	Shortness of breath, tire easily with exercise, history of heart murmur, any chest pain, hypertension, history of anemia
Gastrointestinal	Appetite, weight gain/loss, food intolerance, frequent abdominal pain or stomachaches, history of colic, lactose intolerance, frequent loose stool or diarrhea, constipation, vomiting (description), anal itching, blood or mucus in stool
Genitourinary	Frequency of urination, blood in urine, burning/dysuria, urgency, hesitancy, enuresis, history of urinary tract infections (UTI)
Gynecological	Females: age of puberty, age of first menses, frequency of periods, duration of periods, pain with menses, vaginal discharge, vaginal itching Females/Males: sexual debut, sexual history, questions about sex Males: wet dreams, testicular pain

Continued

TABLE 4-2	REVIEW OF SYSTEMS FOR MIDDLE CHILDHOOD AND ADOLESCENCE—CONT'D
Musculoskeletal	Pain, redness, or swelling around joints; sprains or strains; history of injuries; recent change in gait; hip or feet deformities; weakness; awkwardness; or clumsiness
Neurological	Headaches, dizziness, fainting, tremors, tics, breathholding spells, night terrors, sleepwalking, history of head trauma, convulsions or seizures, concussions, unconsciousness, falls
Endocrine	Polyuria, polydipsia, polyphagia, any hair/skin changes (including acne, skin pigmentations, extra body hair), parental or child concerns about rate of growth, early or late puberty, elevated blood glucose
Hematological	History of anemia, blood transfusions, any problems with bleeding, frequent bruising, sickle cell trait or disease
Psychosocial and behavioral	Behavioral problems, concerns about unusual behavior, difficulty focusing, learning problems, anxiety, nervousness, extreme shyness, fearful, depressed

Experienced providers will incorporate the *review of systems* questions into the physical examination to prompt families to remember areas of past medical history that may have been overlooked in the initial interview. Interview questions for the *review of systems* are also found in the system-specific chapters that follow.

CHILDREN WITH SPECIAL HEALTH CARE NEEDS

Children with special health care needs (CSHCN) require special consideration when gathering information on health history, family cohesion, and family functioning. Children with special health care needs are those who have a chronic physical, developmental, behavioral, or emotional condition and who also require health and related services of a type or amount beyond that required by children generally.[13] Assessing the level of care management required for a child with special health care needs is important to assist families in optimizing daily functioning of the child and in order to provide a framework for continuity of care in a medical home or health care home setting. The CSHCN Screener is a five-item survey-based tool completed by the parent and is an efficient and flexible standardized method of identifying children across the range and diversity of chronic health conditions and special needs.[14] See Appendix E for the CSHCN Screener tool and the scoring for a child to meet the criteria for a chronic health condition or a special health care need. Implementing the CSHCN Screener can be an effective part of the comprehensive health history and child and family assessment.

AGE-SPECIFIC NUTRITIONAL INFORMATION GATHERING

Infancy

Adequate nutrition in the first 2 years of life is critical for the period of rapid growth and brain development. A thorough dietary history in the infant recognizes problems early and allows the health care provider to counsel families for developing issues of overweight, underweight, or failure to thrive. Dietary history for the first year of life includes the following:

- **Breastfeeding:** Frequency and duration of infant feeds; use of supplemental formula feedings or water; difficulties with nippling or feeding patterns? Concern about infant weight gain? Any vomiting after feeds? Mother's diet or dietary restrictions? Father's participation in feeding routines? Mother receiving adequate rest? Experiencing nipple soreness? Plans for return to work? Plan for expression of breast milk or weaning?

- **Formula feeding:** Type of infant formula, how is formula stored and prepared? Powdered formula or concentrated formula? Amount and frequency of feeds? Concern about infant weight gain? Bottle-feeding at night? How often? Difficulty feeding or slow feeder? Plans for bottle weaning and transition to cup?
- **Fluids:** Drinking juice and/or water daily? Type of juice? Drinking juice in cup or bottle? Amount of juice and/or water daily?
- **Solid foods:** Age at introduction of solid foods? Portion size/amount of baby foods? Introduction of table foods and finger foods? Regular meal pattern? Introduction of cup?

Early Childhood (1 Year to 4 Years of Age)

During the toddler years, it is particularly important to establish weaning. Persistent bottle-feeding or breastfeeding may be associated with iron deficiency anemia and early childhood caries; therefore reducing milk intake during this period is key to understanding overall healthy nutrition patterns and protecting oral health. Eating habits are established during the early years and a balanced diet is important to maintain a healthy weight and for optimum growth and development. Dietary history for early childhood includes the following:

- Obtain a 24-hour dietary history.
- Document servings of fruits and vegetables, sources of protein, iron, vitamin C, and calcium (Ca^{++}).
- Food likes and dislikes?

- Snacking and meal pattern? Frequency of juice and soda?
- Any parental concerns about the child's appetite or overeating?

Parental concerns and attitudes about the child's eating should be addressed. Review the importance of introducing a variety of foods often. Portion size should be reviewed. Food may be used for discipline or reward and this may establish an early unhealthy relationship with food. It is also important to discuss avoidance of foods commonly associated with choking or inhalation—round slices of hot dogs/sausage, popcorn, peanuts, chips, grapes, chewing gum, hardy candy, gummy candies, and carrot sticks. Feeding a child while driving should be avoided to prevent choking incidents. In early childhood, only 100% juice is recommended and should be limited to 4 to 6 ounces daily. Soda and carbonated beverages should be discouraged. Caffeinated drinks should not be consumed.

Middle Childhood (5 Years to 10 Years of Age)

In middle childhood, the prevalence of overweight is higher in boys than girls; 20.1% of boys and 15.7% of girls 6 to 11 years old are overweight.[15] Overweight children and adolescents have a 70% chance of becoming overweight or obese adults. Therefore during the health history interview with the school-age child and parent, it is important to discuss the importance of healthy eating habits. Determine whether the parent uses food as a reward or punishment and what the parental attitude is toward the weight of the child. Review gender and age-specific growth charts and body mass index (BMI) at every health encounter during middle childhood.

Dietary history for middle childhood should include the following:

- Obtain a 24-hour dietary history. Begin with the child's recall of dietary intake and then elicit dietary information from parent or caregiver.

- Document servings of fruits and vegetables, sources of protein, iron, vitamin C, and calcium (Ca^{++}).
- Review daily meal pattern and snacking habits, amount of soda and fast foods weekly, daily quantity of juice and water, consumption of sports drinks or caffeinated drinks daily or weekly? (Consumption of large amounts of juice, soda and carbonated beverages, and sports drinks suggests inadequate intake of Ca^{++} and other nutrients.[11])
- Review amount of high-fat, salty, and sugary foods in the diet.
- How many meals does child eat away from home daily or weekly? Does child contribute to preparation or planning of family meals at home? Does the child have any interest in cooking?
- Any parental concerns about appetite or overeating? Any parental struggles around food and weight gain or weight loss?

Adolescence (11 Years to 21 Years of Age)

"Disordered eating" is unfortunately the norm for many adolescents who do not necessarily have an eating disorder. According to the 2011 National Youth Risk Behavior Surveillance System, 5.7% of adolescents reported no vegetable intake, 17.3% reported drinking no milk, 13.1% reported no breakfast intake in the 7 days before the survey, 12.2% had fasted for 24 hours, 5.1% had taken diet pills or powders without medical advice, and 4.3% had vomited or taken laxatives to control their weight within the 30 days before the survey.[16] Teens may skip breakfast, either because of lack of time, lack of available food, or the misconception that skipping breakfast will aid in weight loss. Although a vegetarian diet is often a healthy choice for adults or for children who have been raised as vegetarians, in teens a sudden switch to a vegetarian diet may actually be a red flag for a developing eating disorder.[17] Even though eating disorders are more common among adolescent girls, boys are also at risk. A 24- or 48-hour diet recall can be helpful in evaluating nutrition status. While an assessment of the context of nutrition and activity can take longer than a traditional diet recall (e.g., "Tell me how eating and activity fit into your day yesterday."), this contextual information can be very useful in client-centered counseling techniques, such as motivational interviewing, for improved nutritional and dietary habits.

When asking adolescents about body image, the provider should avoid the assumptions that an adolescent with a low BMI for age is satisfied with his or her weight, or that an adolescent with a high BMI wants to lose weight (Box 4-2). See Table 4-3 for a screening tool for evaluating adolescents for eating disorders.

BOX 4-2   BODY IMAGE AND DIETING BEHAVIOR IN THE ADOLESCENT

Ask the following questions to gather nutritional information when assessing an adolescent.

Satisfaction with Weight
- Is adolescent happy with weight?
- What has he or she done to gain/lose weight?
- Exercise history?

Diet and Dieting History
- Number of diets in past year? Does adolescent feel he or she should be dieting? Dissatisfaction with body size?
- Is adolescent eating in secret? Using supplements, laxatives, or diuretics?

Self Image
- How much does weight affect how adolescent feels about herself or himself?
- Has a specific binge/purge cycle been established?

Data from Anstine D, Grinenko D: Rapid screening for disordered eating in college-aged females in the primary care setting, *J Adolesc Health* 26(5): 338-342, 2000.

TABLE 4-3	SCOFF SCREENING TOOL FOR EATING DISORDERS
S	Do you make yourself **S**ick (vomit) because you feel uncomfortably full?
C	Do you worry you have lost **C**ontrol over how much you eat?
O	Have you recently lost more than **O**ne stone (15 pounds) in a 3-month period?
F	Do you believe yourself to be **F**at when others say you are thin?
F	Would you say that **F**ood dominates your life?

From Morgan JF, Reid F, Lacey JH: The SCOFF questionnaire: assessment of a new screening tool for eating disorders, *BMJ* 319:1467, 1999.

ADOLESCENT PSYCHOSOCIAL HISTORY AND CONFIDENTIALITY

The most important caveat of the adolescent psychosocial history is that it should be conducted without the parent or guardian in the room. A review of studies on adolescent access to health care services shows that a perceived lack of confidentiality is a barrier to care and discussing sensitive topics improves the adolescent's satisfaction with care, yet only a minority of adolescents have ever discussed the importance of the confidentiality of the health visit with a health care provider.[18,19]

All 50 states have laws allowing adolescents to consent to STI testing and treatment; however confidential access to contraception, prenatal care, abortion, adoption, medical care of the minor's child, and mental health services vary from state to state, as do laws restricting or requiring disclosure of confidential care to a parent.[20] In all 50 states, there are some limitations to confidentiality. Providers are generally required to notify parents and/or police or child protective services if an adolescent under 18 years of age expresses a desire to harm himself or herself or others, or if an adolescent has been abused or neglected. In addition, some states have mandatory reporting laws about consensual sexual activity, depending on the age and age discrepancy of the teen and the sexual partner; other states encourage reporting but give the provider some discretion. It is crucial for the provider to become familiar with the specific state laws pertaining to adolescent consent, confidentiality, privacy, child abuse reporting, and the amount of control the adolescent has over the release of medical records related to confidential services. Federal regulations under the Health Insurance Portability and Accountability Act (HIPAA), as well as the adoption of electronic health records, affect the control and privacy of medical records for services the adolescent may have accessed confidentially.[21]

Adolescent Psychosocial Screen: from HEADSSS to SSHADESS

The SSHADESS psychosocial history (Box 4-3) is a key part of a comprehensive adolescent health history and assessment.[22] The SSHADESS psychosocial history is currently used over the more familiar HEADSSS mnemonic, which covers similar health history.[23] The SSHADESS offers the advantages of a strength-based approach and a more holistic exploration of the adolescent's emotional states.[22] The order of questioning, in general, proceeds from less private and sensitive questions to more sensitive, giving the provider and adolescent an opportunity to establish some rapport. The SSHADESS can be tailored to early, middle, or late adolescents by modifying the questions. Remember early adolescents and occasionally middle adolescents can have concrete thinking[24] and may wonder why the provider is asking such unusual questions. It is important to explain to early adolescents that you ask all teens the same questions and you start the health history interview by asking questions about the activities of peers before asking about the teen directly. Avoid medical jargon and try to use the teen's own terminology without sounding as though you are trying to talk like a teen. Remember that adolescents tend to be

BOX 4-3 SSHADESS ADOLESCENT HISTORY

Strengths
- What are some of your strengths that help you cope with stress?
- How would your friends describe you?
- If you were applying for a job, how would you describe yourself to encourage someone to hire you?

School
- Are you in school? (Regular or continuation? English learner/bilingual? Special education/504 plan?) Attend regularly? Suspensions?
- Favorite/most difficult subjects?
- What are your grades/GPA?
  - Low: Recent if changes in GPA? Is work too difficult? Not doing homework?
  - High: Any stress about college goals or grades?
- Plans after high school graduation? (Realistic? Is teen taking right courses/activities? Taking SATs, sending college applications on time? Taking vocational training?)
  - If no specific plans, end of high school can be a difficult, vulnerable time.

Home
- Who lives with you? (One or both parents, grandparents, aunts/uncles, adult siblings, group home, foster care?) Do you live with boyfriend/girlfriend and family?
  - Immigrant teens may live with adult siblings/extended family while parents live in home country.
- Have you lived with . . . your whole life? Changes because of divorce or death of parent? Separation/reunification with parents resulting from immigration? Conflict with parents/guardians? Illness, incarceration, homelessness of family members?
- How do you get along with . . . ? How are conflicts handled at home?

Activities
- How do you spend free time? What do you do for fun? Sports/other extracurricular activities? Exercise? Hobbies? Church or community activities?
  - Responses reflect a measure of connection to school, extra motivation for attendance/grades

- Jobs? (Number of hours/week, schedule, location, hazards)
- Names of friends, best friend?

Drugs/Alcohol/Tobacco
Introduce the subject gently, especially with young teens; can be more direct with older teens
- Does anyone at your school . . . ? Do any of your friends . . . ? Then, have you . . . ?
- If yes, use CRAFFT questions (see Box 4-4).
- Attempts to quit?
- Family members using drugs/alcohol/tobacco?

Emotions
- How would you describe your moods? (Elicits rich information if teen given time to elaborate)
- Depression/anger: Changes in energy, appetite, weight? Sleep disturbances, difficulty concentrating? Irritability is hallmark of depression in teens. Difficulty with homework, school? How teen copes with anger?
- Present/past suicidal ideation, attempts? Suicide gesture versus self-cutting without suicidal intent?
  - Suicidal gestures/attempts may be impulsive acts after disagreement with parents, peers; teen may not self-identify as depressed.
- Warn parent/guardian if teen contemplating suicide, even if not at immediate risk.

Sexuality and Sexual Abuse
Warn the teen of limits of confidentiality in your setting or state.
- "Have you ever had sex or ever come close to having sex?"
  - "Come close to" covers a broad range, includes oral/anal sex, which teens often do not define as sex. For teens with the intention to initiate sexual activity, it is important to explore choice and decisions about sex in relationship. It is important to elicit history before discussing safer sex, contraception, and need for pelvic exam.
- "Are your partners girls, boys, or both?" or "Are you attracted to girls, boys, or both?"
  - Ask of everyone. Be sensitive to teens engaging in same-sex activities.
- Condom/barrier (if appropriate): "At what point in the sexual encounter do you use

---

BOX 4-3   SSHADESS ADOLESCENT HISTORY—CONT'D

condoms?" ("late use" problem). Condom education in school? Knowledge of other barriers (gloves, dental dams)? Difficulties in negotiating condom use with partner?

- Teens with less formal education may lack awareness of anatomy/physiology of genitals and reproductive organs.
- Are you doing anything to prevent pregnancy (if indicated)? Are you experiencing any pressure from partners or family to not use birth control or interference with condom or birth control use?
- "Has anyone ever touched you sexually without permission or tried to force you to have sex?" *If yes*, history of childhood sexual abuse? Acquaintance or date rape? Stranger assault?
- "Has anyone you were seeing ever put you down or made you feel ashamed? Pressured you to go the next step when you are not ready? Grabbed your arm, yelled at you, or pushed you when they were angry or

frustrated? Treated you badly when you were alone but acted differently in front of friends and family? Pushed you to have sex or do sexual things when you didn't want to?"

Safety Issues
- Do you have to do anything special to be safe in your home, at school, or in your neighborhood (e.g., positive climates, presence of gangs, etc.)?
- Guns or other weapons in home or school?
- Physical fighting/abuse in home (between siblings, parents, parent-child)?
- Teen involved in physical fights at home, neighborhood, school?
- Adolescent relationship abuse? (See previous questions under Sexuality.)
- Friends in gangs? Have you ever been a gang member or do you wear a color/insignia? Teen, peers, siblings/cousins involved in gangs?
  - Be sensitive to potential reluctance to disclose.

Data from Ginsburg KR, Carlson EC: Resilience in action: an evidence-informed, theoretically driven approach to building strengths in an office-based setting, *Adolesc Med State Art Rev* 22(3):458-481, 2011; Griswold KS, Aronoff H, Kernan JB, Kahn LS: Adolescent substance use and abuse: recognition and management, *Am Fam Physician* 77(3):331-336, 2008; Miller E, Levenson R: *Hanging out or hooking up: clinical guidelines on responding to adolescent relationship abuse, an integrated approach to prevention and intervention*, San Francisco, 2012, Futures Without Violence.

BOX 4-4   CRAFFT SUBSTANCE ABUSE SCREENING TEST

The **CRAFFT** test is intended specifically for adolescents. It draws upon adult screening instruments, covers alcohol and other drugs, and calls upon situations that are suited to adolescents.

CRAFFT Substance Abuse Screening Test	Yes	No
C—Have you ever ridden in a **C**ar driven by someone (including yourself) who was high or had been using alcohol or drugs?		
R—Do you ever use alcohol or drugs to **R**elax, feel better about yourself, or fit in?		
A—Do you ever use alcohol or drugs while you are **A**lone?		
F—Do you ever **F**orget things you did while using alcohol or drugs?		
F—Do your **F**amily or **F**riends ever tell you that you should cut down on your drinking or drug use?		
T—Have you ever gotten into **T**rouble while you were using alcohol or drugs?		

Scoring: Two or more positive items indicate the need for further assessment and consideration for referral for counseling.

oriented in the here and now. A "long time ago" may refer to years or months ago or as little as a few weeks ago.

Begin the interview with an opening such as "I'm going to ask you questions about sex, drugs, and feelings. What you tell me is private, unless you tell me that you have been hurt by someone else, you are thinking of hurting someone else, or you are thinking of hurting yourself." Questions are asked in as neutral and nonjudgmental manner as possible to avoid making assumptions about the family structure, kinds of sexual activity, or sexual orientation of the adolescent. Asking open-ended questions such as, "How are things at home?" sets a neutral tone.

SSHADESS Assessment for Adolescence[22]

(S) Strengths: Personal characteristics that help youth cope and succeed

(S) School: Connection to, disconnection from school

(H) Home: Family structure and living arrangement, supports, and any problems at home

(A) Activities: Sports, school activities (school connection), hobbies, church involvement, youth groups, jobs, and hours per week for each

(D) Drugs: Drug, alcohol, tobacco experimentation and abuse

(E) Emotions/eating/depression: Positive and negative emotional states, including potential depression and suicidal ideation, healthy and unhealthy eating habits

(S) Sexuality: Sexual attractions, sexual activity or intentions, and any history of coercion or sexual abuse

(S) Safety issues: Protective factors (seat belts, helmets, problem-solving skills) and risk factors (guns in home, engaging in fights, gang activity), home and neighborhood safety

Health History for Sexually Active Male and Female Teens

- Sexually active? Gender of partner(s)—male, female, both, other?

- Type of activity (oral, vaginal, anal), number of sexual partners, change of recent partners, any coercion

- History of gonorrhea/chlamydia screen (urine or genital probe), other STI screens (syphilis, HIV, hepatitis, HPV, herpes simplex)?

Sexually Active Female

- Age at menarche, last menstrual period, regularity of menses, days of menstrual flow, pain during menstruation?

- In addition to other STI screening (described previously), screening for trichomoniasis, bacterial vaginosis, candida?

- If history of pregnancy: GTPAL (Gravidity [number of pregnancies], Term deliveries, Premature deliveries, Abortions [spontaneous or induced], Living children)

See Chapter 17 for detailed information on female health history.

Adolescent Depression and Anxiety

Approximately 11% of adolescents suffer from a serious mental health disorder and about 70% of adolescent mental health disorders are unrecognized and untreated.[25,26] Anxiety and depression place affected adolescents at greater risk for poor developmental and health outcomes such as life-long anxiety and depression, ADHD, conduct disorders, and substance abuse.[27] Adolescents who suffer from anxiety and depression also have difficulty forming important peer relationships, tend to suffer from low self-esteem, and lack self-advocacy skills due to their developmental stage.[28] Anxiety and depression can lead to school absenteeism, poor performance, and underachievement.[27] Screening for these conditions in primary care has become an important part of routine adolescent health care. Table 4-4 provides information on the Patient Health Questionnaire Screening for Depression-9 (PHQ-9), Screen for Child Anxiety Related Disorders (SCARED), and Generalized Anxiety Disorder 7-Item Scale (GAD-7), frequently used screening tools for adolescent psychosocial screening for anxiety and depression across clinical settings.[17,19,29]

TABLE 4-4	SCREENING TOOLS FOR DEPRESSION AND ANXIETY IN ADOLESCENTS	
Ages	**Completed by**	**Tool Available**
13 yr and up	Adolescent	Generalized Anxiety Disorder 7-Item Scale (GAD-7) (available at http://www.phqscreeners.com/overview.aspx?Screener=03_GAD-7)
13 yr and up	Parent, adolescent	Patient Health Questionnaire Screening for Depression-9 (PHQ-9) (available at http://www.phqscreeners.com/overview.aspx?Screener=02_PHQ-9)
8 yr and up	Parent, child, adolescent	Screen for Child Anxiety Related Disorders (SCARED) (available at http://psychiatry.pitt.edu/research/tools-research/assessment-instruments)
All ages	Parent, child, adolescent	Mental Health Screening Tools for Children and Adolescents (available at http://www2.massgeneral.org/schoolpsychiatry/screeningtools_table.asp.)

REFERENCES

1. Trotter TL, Martin HM: Family history in pediatric primary care, *Pediatrics* 120 Suppl 2:S60-65, 2007.
2. Brisbois TD, Farmer AP, McCargar LJ: Early markers of adult obesity: a review, *Obes Rev* 13(4): 347-367, 2012.
3. Slomski A: Chronic mental health issues in children now loom larger than physical problems, *JAMA* 308(3):223-225, 2012.
4. Centers for Disease Control and Prevention: Oral health: Preventing cavities, gum disease, tooth loss, and oral cancers, 2011. Available at http://www.cdc.gov/chronicdisease/resources/publications/aag/doh.htm.
5. World Health Organization: Oral health: Fact sheet No. 318, 2012.
6. Hinton RB, Jr: The family history: reemergence of an established tool, *Crit Care Nurs Clin North Am* 20(2):149-158, v, 2008.
7. Bishop M, Newton R, Farndon P: Genetics in family health care: putting it into action, *J Fam Health Care* 20(5):155-157, 2010.
8. Rich EC: Reconsidering the family history in primary care, *J Gen Intern Med* 19(3):273-280, 2004.
9. Swaydena KJ, Anderson KK, Connelly LM, et al: Effect of sitting vs. standing on perception of provider time at bedside: a pilot study, *Patient Educ Couns* 86(2):166-171, 2012.
10. Mendelsohn JS, Quinn MT, McNabb WL: Interview strategies commonly used by pediatricians, *Arch Pediatr Adolesc Med* 153(2):154-157, 1999.
11. Hagan JF, Duncan PM: *Bright Futures: Guidelines for health supervision of infants, children, and adolescents,* ed 3, Elk Grove Village, Ill., 2008, American Academy of Pediatrics.
12. Bull MJ, Engle WA: Safe transportation of preterm and LBW infant, *Pediatrics* 123(5):1425-1429, 2009.
13. McPherson M, Arango P, Fox H, et al: A new definition of children with special health care needs, *Pediatrics* 102(1 Pt 1):137-140, 1998.
14. Bethell CD, Read D, Stein REK, et al: Identifying children with special health care needs: development and evaluation of a short screening instrument, *Ambul Pediatr* 2(1):38-47, 2002.
15. Ogden C, Carroll M, Kit B, et al: Prevalence of obesity in the United States, 2009-2010, *NCHS Data Brief* 82:1-8, 2012.
16. Eaton DK, Kann L, Kinchen S, et al: Youth risk behavior surveillance - United States, 2011, *MMWR Surveill Summ* 61(4):1-162, 2012.
17. Robinson-O'Brien R, Perry CL, Wall MM, et al: Adolescent and young adult vegetarianism: better dietary intake and weight outcomes but increased risk of disordered eating behaviors, *J Am Diet Assoc* 109(4):648-655, 2009.
18. Brown JD, Wissow LS: Discussion of sensitive health topics with youth during primary care visits: relationship to youth perceptions of care, *J Adolesc Health* 44(1):48-54, 2009.
19. Jones RK, Boonstra H: Confidential reproductive health care for adolescents, *Curr Opin Obstet Gynecol* 17(5):456-460, 2005.
20. Guttmacher Institute: *An overview of minors' consent law* (website). www.guttmacher.org/statecenter/spibs/spib_OMCL.pdf. Accessed December 18, 2012.

21. Berlan ED, Bravender T: Confidentiality, consent, and caring for the adolescent patient, *Curr Opin Pediatr* 21(4):450-456, 2009.
22. Ginsburg KR, Carlson EC: Resilience in action: an evidence-informed, theoretically driven approach to building strengths in an office-based setting, *Adolesc Med State Art Rev* 22(3):458-481, xi, 2011.
23. Goldenring J, Rosen D: Getting into adolescent heads: an essential update, *Contemporary Pediatrics* 21:64-80, 2004.
24. Radzik M, Sherer S, Neinstein LS: Psychosocial development in normal adolescents. In Neinstein LS, Gordon CM, Katzman DK, Rosen DS, Woods ER: *Adolescent health care: a practical guide,* ed 5, Philadelphia, 2008, Wolters Kluwer/Lippincott, Williams & Wilkins, pp. 27-31.
25. Knopp DM, Park MJ, Paul-Mulye T: The mental health of adolescents: a national profile 2008, San Francisco, CA, 2008, National Adolescent Health Information Center, University of California, San Francisco.
26. National Center for Mental Health Checkups at Columbia University: Teen screen primary care fact sheet: Research supporting the integration of mental health checkups into adolescent health care, New York, 2010, National Center for Mental Health Checkups at Columbia University.
27. Connolly SD, Suarez L, Sylvester C: Assessment and treatment of anxiety disorders in children and adolescents, *Curr Psychiatry Rep* 13(2):99-110, 2011.
28. Birmaher B, Brent D, Bernet W, et al: AACP Work Group on Quality Issues. Practice parameter for the assessment and treatment of children and adolescents with depressive disorders, *J Am Acad Child Adolesc Psychiatry* 46(11):1503-1526, 2007.
29. Richardson LP, McCauley E, Grossman DC, et al: Evaluation of the patient health questionnaire-9 item for detecting major depression among adolescents, *Pediatrics* 126(6):1117-1123, 2010.

CHAPTER 5

ENVIRONMENTAL HEALTH HISTORY

Karen G. Duderstadt

Environment is a key determinant of health, and children are uniquely vulnerable to environmental hazards. Children's genetic predisposition, social milieu, and nutrition play an important role in their susceptibility to environmental hazards.[1] Recent estimated costs of the burden of disease in children from environmental hazards is $76.6 billion annually.[2] The burden of disease stems primarily from exposure to toxic chemicals and air pollutants, and the related health conditions include lead poisoning, exposure to mercury pollution, childhood cancers, asthma, autism, intellectual and learning disabilities, and attention-deficit/hyperactivity disorder.[2]

Toxic substances are those chemicals in the environment capable of causing harm. *Toxicants* are environmental hazards from chemical pollutants, and *toxins* are environmental hazards from biological sources. Children have a larger ratio of surface area to body mass than adults which increases their susceptibility to pesticides and other environmental toxicants. Therefore, children absorb larger amounts of environmental toxins, kilogram (kg) for kg, than adults. Infants have three times as large a surface area and children have twice the surface area to body mass of an adult.[1] Young children breathe more air and drink more water per pound of body weight than adults. They have greater exposure to toxic chemicals and air pollutants for their body weight than adults, and they *absorb* toxic substances at a higher rate than that of adults.[3] The skin, respiratory tract, and gastrointestinal tract in children are particularly vulnerable to toxic substances and absorb them more readily and efficiently than in the adult. The high gastric pH in children facilitates absorption of environmental toxins. The developing fetus and the young child are particularly vulnerable to the neurodevelopmental effects of environmental toxins because of their rapid periods of brain growth and development in the first 2 years of life.

Children also live and play closer to environmental hazards on the ground, which increases their concentrations of inhaled toxic substances. The breathing zone of a child is lower than adults, and chemical pollutants such as lead or mercury and chemicals vaporizing from carpets, flooring or nap mats impact children at a greater rate than adults.[1] Children's metabolic pathways are immature, and they *metabolize* toxic chemicals differently than adults because they lack the enzymes to break down and remove toxic chemicals from the body.[3] Their higher metabolic rate increases their oxygen consumption and production of carbon dioxide (CO_2). The increased CO_2 requires higher minute ventilation in infants and children and increases exposure to particulate matter in the air.[1] The *dose-response* rate for exposure in children is far more rapid than in adults.

Environmental health is defined as "freedom from illness or injury related to exposure to toxic agents and other environmental conditions encountered in the home, workplace, and community environments that are potentially detrimental to human health."[4] It is critically important for pediatric health care providers

55

to understand the impact of environmental hazards and exposures on the healthy growth and development of infants, children, and adolescents. Health care providers have a professional responsibility to identify and understand the environmental health risks present in the communities they work in, to access available health risk data from community surveillance programs, and to report exposures to appropriate local and state authorities. Furthermore, providers are mandated to conduct appropriate screening tests and to educate children and families about toxic environmental health risks.

ENVIRONMENTAL RISK FACTORS

Children can encounter environmental hazards and be exposed to many different toxic substances in the home, car, school, childcare setting, play environments, and community. Young children spend 80% to 90% of their time indoors so environmental hazards in the home and childcare environments are the primary sources of exposures.[1] Environmental health hazards include physical agents; chemical agents; outdoor and indoor air contaminants; water, soil, or dust contaminants; biological irritants; allergens; toxins; and infectious agents.[5] Box 5-1 presents common indoor and outdoor air pollutants, contaminants in water and soil, food contaminants, and hazardous substances that children may be exposed to through parental or family employment or hobbies.

DEVELOPMENTAL VULNERABILITIES

Different developmental stages put children at risk for different types of exposures to

---

BOX 5-1 RISK CATEGORIES OF ENVIRONMENTAL HAZARDS

Household Exposures and Indoor Air Pollutants
- Mold spores
- Animal dander
- Carbon monoxide
- Tobacco smoke
- Mercury vapors
- Radon
- Smoke from wood-burning stoves
- Lead
- Phthalates and plasticizers
- Personal care products or cosmetics

Outdoor Air Pollutants
- Pesticides
- Air particulates
- Ozone
- Insecticides
- Herbicides

School or Daycare Exposures
- Polychlorinated biphenyls (PCBs)
- Arsenic from pesticide-treated wood
- Pesticides
- Friable asbestos

Community and Outdoor Exposures
- Insecticides
- Herbicides

Water Pollutants
- Bacteria
- Parasites

Food Contaminants
- Mercury
- Pesticides

Unintentional Ingestions or Poisonings

Family Members' Occupations/Hobbies
- Paint contractors
- Car mechanics
- Smelters
- Agricultural workers or farmworkers
- Miners
- Jewelry artist
- Stained-glass artist

Data from American Academy of Pediatrics, Etzel RA, Balk SJ: *Pediatric environmental health*, ed 3, Elk Grove Village, IL, 2011, American Academy of Pediatrics.

environmental hazards. Prenatal exposure of the fetus to maternal smoking, substance use, and chemical or biological agents increases risk of absorption of toxicants and toxins. Toxicants such as illicit drugs, alcohol, cotinine from environmental tobacco smoke, mercury, and lead, which cross the placental barrier, contribute to low birth weight, intrauterine growth retardation, cognitive and developmental delays, and congenital birth defects.[6] In the newborn, particular attention should be given to toxicants in breast milk or preparation of infant formula, dermal contacts, and parental occupations.

Infants and toddlers have expanded mobility, giving them increased exposure to their environment. They are particularly vulnerable to oral exposures because of their hand-to-mouth activity and inhaled substances within the physical zone they occupy near the ground. Preschool and school-age children become susceptible to toxicants in the school, childcare setting, or playground environments. Occupational hazards are of particular concern in adolescents and young adults, as well as harmful exposures that occur through experimentation with illicit drugs; alcohol and tobacco; intentional inhalation, known as *huffing,* of leaded gasoline, glues, and other substances; and excessive exposure to the sun and ultraviolet radiation (UVR) through tanning salons.

SOURCES OF ENVIRONMENTAL TOXINS

Children are at risk for environmental toxins in lead paint chips (pre-1970 housing); lead-contaminated soil; dust in homes from paint or soil; industrial toxicants in or near neighborhoods, landfill sites, or waste treatment sites; charcoal mills; pre-1989 plumbing suggesting presence of lead pipes or lead solder; well water or contaminated tap water; and drinking water contaminated with lead. They may also play near high-traffic areas with old deposits from leaded gasoline. Children also consume more fruits and vegetables per pound of body weight and are at increased risk for pesticide and organophosphate exposure. Children of farm workers are particularly vulnerable to pesticide exposure.

Children are at risk for indoor air pollutants such as environmental tobacco smoke, mold, pesticides in the home or school, and products containing lead, such as leaded candlewicks, pottery with lead glaze, and imported products containing lead. Hobbies of family members and household contacts, such as soldering stained glass or refinishing old painted furniture, can put children at risk. Children's exposure to toxins may also occur through contact with parent's workplace or work clothes.

Children with asthma are at higher risk from exposure to outdoor air pollutants. Increased particulate matter created by air pollution, release of known environmental toxins from industrial sources, and increased allergens due to extreme weather events exacerbate childhood asthma. Children living in low-income communities are at greater risk for exposure to outdoor air pollutants and environmental toxins. Children living in families with food insecurity are at risk for poor nutrition resulting in iron or calcium deficiency which may enhance lead toxicity in the body.

ENVIRONMENTAL HEALTH SCREENING HISTORY

All children and adolescents should have an environmental health screening history during routine primary care visits to establish risk of exposures.[7] An environmental health screening history establishes known home, school, and/or community environmental health risks and a family history of parental or sibling exposure in the workplace. Table 5-1 presents an environmental health screening history for use in establishing a risk profile for exposure to pesticides, poor indoor or outdoor air quality, contaminated drinking water, or chemical toxicants. A Pediatric Environmental History

TABLE 5-1   QUICK ENVIRONMENTAL SCREENING QUESTIONNAIRE

Source	Exposure
Where does your child spend time during the day?	
Home	
Do you have a basement where children sleep or play?	Asbestos, radon
Do you have water damage or visible mold in home?	Indoor air pollutants
Do you use pesticides in lawn/garden area or in home?	Pesticide
Do you have a gas stove or wall heater?	Carbon monoxide
Do you live near a freeway, industrial area, or polluted site?	Outdoor air/water pollutants
Smoking	
Does anyone smoke in the home environment?	Environmental tobacco smoke (ETS)
Food and Water	
Do you use tap water or well water? Do you wash fresh fruits/vegetables?	Pesticides, nitrates, lead, biological agents
Workplace	
What do family members and household contacts do for a living?	Chemical, physical, and biological agents
Is anyone in the household involved in a hobby at home?	
Sun Exposure	
Do you use sun protection for your child?	UV index

Data from American Academy of Pediatrics, Etzel RA, Balk SJ: *Pediatric environmental health*, ed 3, Elk Grove Village, IL, 2011, American Academy of Pediatrics.

form for children from birth to 18 years of age, categories and questions for children with a positive screen for environmental risks, and an Environmental History Form for Pediatric Asthma Patient are presented in the Appendix F.

The concept of *health risk communication* is particularly important to assessing environmental health in children and is part of a holistic approach to working with families in the clinical setting. *Health risk communication* requires active listening to identify parental concern and the knowledge of public health risks of exposure to indoor and outdoor hazardous substances in the surrounding community. It requires

determining the presence of an environmental hazard, assessment of the health risk, the severity of the exposure or dose, acceptability of the health risk and the impact on the health of the child or adolescent, and communicating the health risk effectively to the family.[1]

LEAD EXPOSURE

The Centers for Disease Control and Prevention (CDC) recently supported ending the use of the term "level of concern" in discussing blood lead levels (BLLs) in children, because evidence supports no level of lead is safe, and therefore all elevated levels of lead are of concern.[8] Health care providers should take the primary role in educating individual families and screening for risk of environmental exposure to lead. Lead screening in children is routinely performed in most pediatric health care settings at 1 year of age and 2 years of age. For those infants and children with BLL >97.5th percentile or >2.0 mcg/dL, health care providers should monitor the health status of children until environmental investigation and mitigation has been implemented.[9] Also, the risk of lead exposure must be relayed to families through routine health visits and culturally and linguistically appropriate health education materials.

Ongoing lead toxicity among immigrant and refugee children in the United States has been well documented.[10] Malnutrition is a known risk factor for increased BLL in immigrant and refugee children. In one study, the median age of immigrant and refugee children with elevated BLL was 4.9 years, with an age range from 14 months to 13 years.[11] Since this age range is considerably older than the ages of recommended screening for most children in the United States, it is particularly important for health care providers to screen the pediatric immigrant population for lead toxicity. The most common lead exposures identified among children with elevated BLL at repeat testing were lead-based paints and lead-contaminated soil where the children had played.[10] Infants and children can be exposed to lead contaminants from a variety of substances including household dust, household products, candies, and medications. Children living in immigrant families are particularly vulnerable to household and medicinal exposures to lead. Box 5-2 provides questions for assessing health risks for lead exposure in children and families. Table 5-2 presents common substances associated with elevated BLLs in immigrant and refugee children.

Children with excess lead levels usually show no unique features on physical examination. Environmental exposures are often insidious and affect the internal organs and brain. Children with lead toxicity may present

---

BOX 5-2 QUICK LEAD SCREENING QUESTIONNAIRE FOR CHILDREN

1. Within the last 6 months, has your child lived in or regularly visited a house, apartment, or school built before 1978 or before 1950? Are there paint surfaces that are peeling or chipped in the home or school?
2. Does your child live in or regularly visit a house or school built before 1978 or before 1950 that is undergoing renovation or has been recently renovated?
3. Have you ever seen your child eating paint chips or other nonfood substances such as paper?
4. Has your child ever taken home remedies such as *azarcon, pay-loo-ah, carol, ghasard, kohl, greta, bala goli, shurma,* or *rueda*?
5. Do you use ceramic pottery from Mexico, Central America, South America, or Asia for cooking, serving, or storing food or beverages?
6. Have you ever been told that your child has an elevated blood lead?

Data from Centers for Disease Control and Prevention: Childhood lead poisoning prevention program, 2009. Available at http://www.cdc.gov/nceh/lead/about/program.htm. Accessed January 3, 2013.

---

with one or more of the following symptoms: fatigue, malaise, abdominal pain, loss of appetite, constipation, irritability, headache, weakness, or clumsiness. Any signs of developmental delay, neurobehavioral disorders such as tics, persistent hand-to-mouth activity such as pica, unexplained seizures, anemia, chronic abdominal pain, learning difficulties, or attention deficit disorder warrant an in-depth environmental health history to relate positive exposure to environmental hazards. Figure 5-1 illustrates the primary organs and body systems affected by exposure to environmental hazards.

TABLE 5-2   EXAMPLES OF CULTURE-SPECIFIC EXPOSURES ASSOCIATED WITH
ELEVATED LEAD LEVELS IN CHILDREN

Exposure	Area of Origin	Reported Uses	Description
Pay-loo-ah	Southeast Asia	Treatment of fever and rash	Orange-red powder Administered by itself or mixed in tea
Greta	Mexico	Treatment of digestive problems	Yellow-orange powder Administered with oil, milk, sugar, or tea Sometimes added to baby bottles or tortilla dough
Azarcon	Mexico	Treatment of digestive problems	Bright orange powder Administered similarly to greta
Litargirio	Dominican Republic	Deodorant/antiperspirant; treatment of burns and fungal infections of the feet	Yellow or peach-colored powder
Surma	India	Improve eyesight	Black powder administered to inner lower eyelid
Unidentified ayurvedic	Tibet	Treatment for slow development	Small gray-brown balls administered several times a day
Lozeena	Iraq	Added to rice and meat dishes for flavor	Bright orange spice
Tamarind candies (multiple brand names)	Mexico	Lollipops, fruit rolls, candied jams	"Bolirindo" lollipops are soft and dark brown Candied jams are typically packaged in ceramic jars
Lead-glazed ceramics	Often made in Latin America	Bean pots, water jugs	
Makeup and beauty products	Multiple cultures	Decoration	Many types

Modified from Walker P, Barrett E: *Immigrant medicine*, Philadelphia, 2008, Saunders. In Centers for Disease Control and Prevention: Refugee health guidelines: lead screening, 2010. Available at http://www.cdc.gov/immigrantrefugeehealth/guidelines/lead-guidelines.html. Accessed January 3, 2013.

ENDOCRINE-DISRUPTING CHEMICALS

Endocrine disruptors are chemically manufactured substances or naturally occurring substances that interfere with the function of hormones in the body. They can mimic naturally occurring hormones such as estrogens (female sex hormones), androgens (male sex hormones), and thyroid hormones, producing overstimulation of the endocrine system.[12] Endocrine disruptors affect the normal function of tissues and organs, resulting in abnormal gonadal development, decline in the age of the onset of puberty, reduced fertility, intellectual

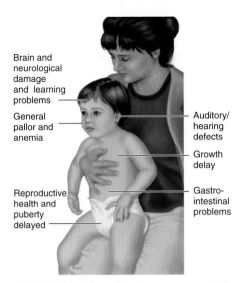

Brain and
neurological
damage
and learning
problems

General
pallor and
anemia

Auditory/
hearing
defects

Growth
delay

Reproductive
health and
puberty
delayed

Gastro-
intestinal
problems

FIGURE 5-1 Effects of lead exposure on a child's body.

disabilities, thyroid disorders, diabetes, and some childhood cancers.[6,12,13]

Endocrine disruptors are present in the environment in food, water, soil, plastics, and personal care products. Phthalates, bisphenol A (BPA), and polychlorinated biphenyls (PCBs) are three of the high volume chemicals present in the environment and are known endocrine disruptors. Phthalates and BPA are chemicals used in the production of soft plastics, polycarbonated plastics, and epoxy resins. Epoxy resins are used as coatings for liners of food and beverage cans. Phthalates are also found in personal care products. BPA is an endocrine-disrupting chemical with a wide range of health effects. PCBs are synthetic organic chemicals associated with risks for harmful effects in humans. Although PCBs are no longer manufactured in the United States, they are resistant to degradation in the environment and therefore remain hazardous to human and animal health. Phytoestrogens, which are naturally occurring substances found in soy products, also can have hormone-like activity.

EVIDENCE-BASED PRACTICE TIP

Breast milk and polycarbonate feeding bottles are the primary source of BPA exposure among infants, and canned foods are the primary source of BPA exposure in children.[14]

DIAGNOSTICS

For most environmental toxins, valid and reliable laboratory tests have not been developed.[6] Laboratory testing that is available for toxins is not performed at all laboratories. Further, there may be a lapse between exposure and testing, and the levels may not reflect the total burden of the environmental contaminant on the developing child.[6] See Table 5-3 for

TABLE 5-3 LABORATORY TESTING FOR ENVIRONMENTAL TOXINS

Environmental Hazard Exposure	Diagnostic Study
Lead	Blood lead level (BLL), free erythrocyte protoporphyrin (FEP), zinc protoporphyrin (ZPP)
Carbon monoxide	Carboxyhemoglobin
Mercury	Blood mercury level, 24-hour urine sample, hair analysis with atomic absorption spectrometry (AAS)
Pesticide metabolites and organophosphates	Plasma cholinesterase (ChE) levels
Tobacco metabolites	Urine cotinine assays
PCBs (polychlorinated biphenyls)	Gas-liquid chromatography
Heavy metals, arsenic	24-hour urine sample

Data from Burns CE, Dunn AM, Brady MA, et al: *Pediatric primary care,* ed 5, St. Louis, 2012, Elsevier.

BOX 5-3 ENVIRONMENTAL HEALTH RESOURCES

Children's Environmental Health Network
www.cehn.org
National Center for Environmental Health
www.cdc.gov/nceh
Center for Health, Environment and Justice
www.chej.org
Columbia University's Center for Children's Environmental Health
www.ccceh.org
The National Environmental Education Foundation
www.neefusa.org/
Healthy Schools Network, Inc.
www.healthyschools.org
U.S. Environmental Protection Agency: Ground Water and Drinking Water Topics
www.epa.gov/safewater/topics.html

World Health Organization: Health Impact Assessment
www.who.int/hia/en/
National Institute of Environmental Health Sciences: Endocrine Disruptors
www.niehs.nih.gov/health/topics/agents/endocrine/index.cfm
U.S. Department of Health & Human Services: Bisphenol A (BPA) Information for Parents
www.hhs.gov/safety/bpa/
Association of Occupational and Environmental Clinics
www.aoec.org/pehsu.htm

---

available laboratory tests for environmental hazards. Exposure to significant levels of toxicants should be reported to local and state authorities, and the regional Pediatric Environmental Health Specialty Units (PESHU) at http://www.aoec.org/pehsu.htm.

RESOURCES

Resources on environmental health and the impact on children and families are available to pediatric health care providers through governmental, public health, and environmental health agencies and are important in assisting with comprehensive screening for environmental hazards (Box 5-3). Having access to evidence-based research and resources on environmental health is key to responsible health risk screening and health risk communication to parents, caregivers, and families.

SUMMARY OF ENVIRONMENTAL HEALTH SCREENING

- Children are uniquely vulnerable to environmental hazards. Children have a larger surface area/body mass ratio than adults.
- The skin, respiratory tract, and gastrointestinal tract are particularly vulnerable to toxic substances and absorb substances more readily and efficiently than in the adult.
- Children live and play closer to environmental hazards on the ground, which increases their concentrations of inhaled toxic substances.
- Children's metabolic pathways are immature, and they metabolize toxic chemicals differently than adults do because they lack the enzymes to break down and remove toxic chemicals from the body.[3]
- Environmental health hazards include physical agents; chemical agents; outdoor and indoor air contaminants; water, soil or dust contaminants; biological irritants; allergens; toxins; and infectious agents.[5]
- Children are at risk for indoor air pollutants such as environmental tobacco smoke, mold, pesticides in the home or school, and products containing lead such as leaded candlewicks, pottery with lead glaze, and imported products containing lead.

- Children living in low-income communities are a greater risk for exposure to environmental toxins. Ongoing lead toxicity among immigrant and refugee children in the United States has been well documented.[10]

- An environmental health screening history establishes known home, school, and/or community environmental health risks and a family history of parental or sibling exposure in the workplace.

Charting

Environmental Exposure History on 2½-Year-Old

2½-year-old healthy-appearing female living in subsidized housing built before 1978. Mother gives history of obvious mold on the bedroom and bathroom walls. The building has water damage on the walls that has not been repaired over the past 2 years. The building overlooks a large gas station and a high-traffic area adjacent to the freeway.

Charting

Environmental Exposure History on 5-Year-Old

5-year-old healthy-appearing male who lives on a farm where pesticides are used seasonally on crops. Father works part-time as a crop duster. House built before 1950 with some restoration underway in the family living area. House is partially heated with wood stove. Parents refinish old furniture as a hobby in garage area adjacent to house. Well water is primary source of drinking water for family.

REFERENCES

1. Etzel RA, Balk SJ, eds: *Pediatric environmental health*, ed 3, Elk Grove Village, Ill., 2011, American Academy of Pediatrics.
2. Trasande L, Liu Y: Reducing the staggering costs of environmental disease in children, estimated at $76.6 billion in 2008, *Health Aff (Millwood)* 30:863-870, 2011.
3. Landrigan PJ, Goldman LR: Children's vulnerabiltiy to toxic chemicals: a challenge and opportunity to strengthen health and environmental policy, *Health Aff (Millwood)* 30:824-850, 2011.
4. Pope AM, Snyder MA, Mood LH: *Nursing, health, and the environment*, Washington, DC, 1995, Institute of Medicine.
5. Schneider D, Freeman N: *Children's environmental health: reducing risk in a dangerous world*, Washington, DC, 2000, American Public Health Association.
6. Burns CE, Dunn AM, Brady MA, et al: *Pediatric primary care*, ed 5, Philadelphia, 2012, Elsevier.
7. NEEF: *National Environmental Education Foundation* (website). www.neefusa.org/health/PEHI/HistoryForm.htm. Accessed September 1, 2012.
8. Centers for Disease Control and Prevention: *CDC response to Advisory Committee on Childhood Lead Poisoning Prevention recommendations in "Low level lead exposure harms children: a renewed call of primary prevention"*, Atlanta, GA, 2012, Center for Disease Control and Prevention.
9. Advisory Committee on Childhood Lead Poisoning Prevention: *Low level lead exposure harms children: a renewed call for primary prevention*, Atlanta, GA, 2012, US Department of Health and Human Services, CDC, Advisory Committee on Childhood Lead Poisoning Prevention. Available at http://www.cdc.gov/nceh/lead/acclpp/final_document_010412.pdf.
10. Centers for Disease Control and Prevention: *Refugee health guidelines: lead screening* (website). www.cdc.gov/immigrantrefugeehealth/guidelines/lead-guidelines.html. Accessed September 1, 2012.
11. Centers for Disease Control and Prevention: Elevated blood lead levels in refugee children—New Hampshire, 2003-2004, *MMWR Morb Mortal Wkly Rep* 54:42-46, 2005.
12. NIEHS: Endocrine disruptors. *National Institute of Environmental Health Sciences* (website). www.niehs.nih.gov/health/topics/agents/endocrine/index.cfm. Accessed September 1, 2012.
13. Sutton P, Woodruff TJ, Perron J, et al: Toxic environmental chemicals: the role of reproductive health professionals in preventing harmful exposures, *Am J Obstet Gynecol* 207(3):164-173, 2012.
14. Duderstadt KG: Chemicals in daily life: emerging evidence on the impact on child health, *J Pediatr Health Care* 26:155-157, 2012.

CHAPTER **6**

SKIN

Renee P. McLeod

It is easy to underestimate the importance of a thorough examination of the skin. Careful inspection of the skin gives the examiner clear insight into the overall health of the child. Examination of the skin, hair, and nails provides clues to oxygenation, tissue perfusion, nutritional and hydration status of the child, and any underlying disease pathology or injury.[1] The skin of an infant, child, and adult share similarities in structure and function, but a child's skin reacts differently to environmental demands because of the unique skin properties of each age group. All skin, regardless of age, is affected by seasonal factors such as the heat and humidity of summer or the dryness and low humidity of winter; but the differences in an infant's skin and ability to sweat compared with an adult's skin can create many more problems associated with these seasonal changes. Therefore, the manifestations of a skin disorder observed in an infant or child may vary widely from what may be seen in an adult.[2]

The skin is the largest organ in the body and has five distinct functions. The skin controls fluids, regulates temperature, protects against invasion from microbial and foreign bodies, and protects against damage from the ultraviolet (UV) rays of the sun. Finally, the skin is an organ of communication. Touch and skin-to-skin contact is one of the ways we bond with our mothers and families at birth and later bond with our sexual partners. Research conducted over the past 50 years has proven that touch is more important to humans than food in regard to optimal development.[3-6] Having a disease of the skin, hair, or nails that prevents or decreases human touch can be devastating to a child's self-esteem.

ANATOMY AND PHYSIOLOGY

The skin consists of three layers: the *epidermis,* the *dermis,* and the *subcutaneous layer* (Figure 6-1). The *epidermis* is the outermost layer of the skin and consists of two main layers: the *stratum corneum,* and the *cellular stratum.* The *stratum corneum* is the very top layer of the skin and is composed of stacked, overlapping nonnucleated keratinized cells called *corneocytes.* The thickness of this layer depends on the region of the body, being thinnest on the face and thickest over the soles of the feet.[2] This layer forms the protective barrier of the skin and contains the waterproofing protein *keratin,* which restricts water loss and penetration of a variety of substances through the skin. The innermost layer of the epidermis consists of a single row of columnar cells called *basal cells,* which reside in the *stratum basale.* These cells divide to form the *keratinocytes* that move to the surface through the *stratum spinosum, stratum granulosum,* and

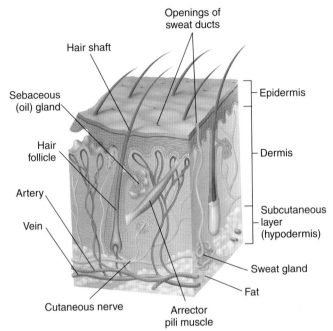

FIGURE 6-1 Anatomy of the skin. (From Thibodeau GA, Patton KT: *Anatomy and physiology*, ed 5, St. Louis, 2003, Mosby.)

stratum lucidum to replace the cells that are sloughed off every day in the stratum corneum.[2,7] The stratum basale also contains *melanocytes*, which synthesize melanin to provide color and protect the skin from damage by the UV rays of the sun. The dermal-epidermal junction lies beneath the stratum basale and is an important site of attachment in the skin. This junction allows nutrients to pass through the dermis to the avascular epidermis.

The *dermis* is a richly vascular layer consisting largely of fibroblasts and collagen. The collagen matrix of the dermis supports and separates the epidermis from the subcutaneous fat layer. Papillae project up into the epidermis to provide nourishment to the living epidermal cells. In addition, the dermis contains a large network of sensory nerve fibers. These fibers provide sensations of pain, itch, and temperature. *Meissner corpuscles* are encapsulated end organs of touch found in the dermal papillae close to the epidermis. They are most numerous in hairless portions of the skin such as the volar surfaces of the hands, fingers, feet, toes, lips, eyelids, nipples, and tip of the tongue. The dermis also contains autonomic nerve fibers that innervate blood vessels, the *arrectores pilorum* muscles, the sweat glands, sebaceous glands, hair, and nails.

The *sweat glands* in the dermis control thermoregulation by releasing water through the skin. The *eccrine sweat glands* are distributed throughout the body except for the lip margins, eardrums, nail beds, inner surface of the prepuce, and the glans penis.[8] The *apocrine sweat glands* are larger and deeper than the eccrine glands and secrete an odorless white fluid (sweat) in response to emotional or physical stimuli. They are located in the axillae, around the nipples, areolae, anogenital area, eyelids, and external ears. Body odor in adolescence comes from bacterial decomposition of the sweat produced by these glands; activation of these glands earlier than adolescence should be investigated. Neonates have the ability to respond to thermal stress by sweating, though it requires a greater thermal stimulus. This response is less developed in premature infants and increases with postnatal age.[9] Full-term infants are also able to respond to emotional stress by sweating, though this is not developed in the premature infant. This has clinical implications related to increased insensible water loss and thermoregulation in infants at risk.[9]

The *sebaceous glands* arise from the hair follicles deep within the dermis. The oil produced by these glands is called *sebum*, a lipid-rich substance that helps lubricate the skin and hair. The level of oil produced is related to hormonal levels in the bloodstream (primarily testosterone) and therefore varies throughout the life span. In the newborn, the production of sebum is accelerated while still under the influence of maternal hormones, and the glands themselves become hyperplastic until maternal hormones wane in the infant's body. This stimulated activity results in skin conditions in the newborn such as *neonatal acne*. Overactive sebaceous glands appear again in adolescence and contribute to the common skin conditions *acne vulgaris* and *tinea versicolor*.[2]

The nail bed starts to keratinize to form a hard, protective plate around 8 to 10 weeks of gestation. It sits on a highly vascular bed that gives each nail its color. The *cuticle*, or *eponychium*, the white crescent-shaped area at the end of the nail matrix, is the root and site of nail growth. It is covered by a layer of stratum corneum that pushes up and over the lower part of the nail body. The *parionychium* is the soft tissue that surrounds the nail border on each digit.

The *subcutaneous* layer of the skin is composed of adipose tissue. This layer connects the dermis to underlying organs, provides insulation and shock absorption, and generates heat for the body. It also provides a reserve of calories for use by the body.[9] Premature and small for gestational age infants often lack this critical layer of insulation, which causes difficulty with thermoregulation.

Hair, eyebrows, and nails are part of the anatomical structure of the skin. Hair is formed by epidermal cells that go deep into the dermal layer of the skin and consists of a *root*, a *shaft*, and a *follicle*. The loop of capillaries at the base of the follicle, known as the *papilla*, supplies nourishment to the hair to promote growth. *Melanocytes*, which lie in the hair shaft, supply color to the hair.

DEVELOPMENTAL VARIATIONS

In the newborn, all the hair on the body consists of fine *lanugo* hair—all of the hair is in the same phase of growth. As the lanugo is shed, it is replaced by hair that is increased in diameter and coarseness; the first to form are *vellus* hairs, which are short, fine, soft, and nonpigmented hairs on the body. Then adult-type *terminal* hairs, which are coarse, thick, longer, and pigmented, grow on the scalp and eyebrows. During adolescence, vellus hairs located in androgen-sensitive areas, pubic area, axillae, and the face in males, undergo a similar transition to terminal hairs.

PHYSIOLOGICAL VARIATIONS

The stratum corneum does not develop until between 23 and 25 weeks of gestation. Extremely premature infants are born without this critical top layer of skin and therefore have no protective barrier and are not able to control water loss. They need protection from the environment and can tolerate only the least amount of touching. The term newborn has a fully functional stratum corneum, but it is only about 60% of the thickness of adult skin depending on the location. A thin stratum corneum with the larger body surface area/weight ratio of the newborn may allow substances placed on the skin to pass more easily through to the bloodstream.[9,10]

The blood vessels continue to mature into a more adult pattern until 3 months after birth. The nerves in the skin are small and poorly myelinated at birth. The growth and myelination of the nerve fibers continue on into puberty (Table 6-1).

TABLE 6-1   STRUCTURAL AND FUNCTIONAL DIFFERENCES OF SKIN

Structure	Preterm Infant	Term Newborn Infant	Child	Adolescent	Significance/Implications
Epidermis	Thinner Cells more compressed Fewer layers of stratum corneum Increased transepidermal water loss	Stratum corneum appears as adherent cell layer Greater absorption because of higher skin surface/body weight ratio	Stratum is getting thicker, starts to appear as separate sheet of cells	Stratum corneum appears as separate sheet of cells Adult-like pattern	Thin skin of infant and child allows for easy absorption of products placed on skin Apply thin layer of topical medications
Dermis	Less cohesion between layers Fewer, immature elastin fibers Thinner than in older infants	Fewer immature elastin fibers Thinner than adult	Elastin fibers are maturing	Full complement of elastin fibers	Decreased elasticity Increased tendency to blister
Melanosomes	Melanin production low	Melanin production low Final overall skin tone is shown in genitalia where the scrotum, labia have darker pigment	Melanin production after 6 months of age like adult	Adult pattern of melanin production	Infants, young children need sunscreen/complete sun block because can sunburn easily
Eccrine sweat glands	May be more typical of fetus than adult Ducts are patent but do not produce sweat	Equivalent in structure to adult Dense distribution due to body surface area	Distribution starts becoming less dense as child grows, but has decreased neurological control until 2-3 years old	Distribution is less dense than in infant, child	Reduced sweating capability, especially first 13-24 days of life Decreased response to thermal stress
Apocrine sweat glands	Not present	Small, nonfunctional Devoid of secretory granules	Start to appear but generally nonfunctional in childhood	Apocrine sweating in response to mechanical, pharmacological stimuli	Secrete oily substance in adolescent

Continued

TABLE 6-1   STRUCTURAL AND FUNCTIONAL DIFFERENCES OF SKIN—CONT'D

Structure	Preterm Infant	Term Newborn Infant	Child	Adolescent	Significance/Implications
Sebaceous glands	Large and active	Large and active but diminish rapidly in size and activity several weeks after birth	Decreased activity throughout childhood	Large, active, produce sebum in large amounts	Infants get acne and tinea versicolor as do teens because of hormone activity and large active sebaceous glands
Nervous and vascular systems	Vascular system not fully organized Most nerves are small in diameter Sensory and autonomic nerves are unmyelinated, typically fetal in structure Meissner touch receptors* not fully formed	Vascular system fully organized after 3 months Most nerves are small in diameter Sensory autonomic nerves are unmyelinated Cutaneous nerve network not fully developed Meissner touch receptors not fully formed	Cutaneous network continuing to develop	Cutaneous network of nerves may continue to develop into adolescence Rest of nervous, vascular systems are in adult pattern	
Hair	Lanugo may be present Hair growth is synchronous	Lanugo covering body often shed within 10-14 days Vellus and terminal hairs appear quickly after birth Hair growth is synchronous	Vellus and terminal hairs present Hair growth is asynchronous	Vellus and terminal hairs present Hair growth is asynchronous	Dry, dull, and brittle hair may indicate protein-calorie malnutrition

*Meissner touch receptors are encapsulated end organs of touch found in dermal papillae close to epidermis.

FAMILY, CULTURAL, RACIAL, AND ETHNIC CONSIDERATIONS

Recent research has shown skin *pigmentation* or *melanin* should be considered as a factor for understanding some underlying skin properties and characteristics, particularly in children of multiracial ancestry. Understanding how underlying skin color and pigmentation may affect the examination and diagnosis of skin conditions allows the clinician to adjust assessment techniques and interventions using the child or adolescent's physiological characteristics rather than racial or ethnic categorization to guide care.[1]

Assessing skin pigmentation allows the health care provider to make clinical decisions based on tissue perfusion, jaundice, pallor, cyanosis, and blanch response. The *blanch test* differs widely based on underlying skin color. The blanch test differentiates healthy skin from erythematous skin that is nonblanchable when gentle pressure from fingertips is exerted on the skin, blood is temporarily forced out of the region, causing the skin to appear lighter than the normal skin color. In individuals with lighter skin pigmentation, the skin color returns swiftly as the blood refills the dermal capillaries. It may be difficult to determine this response in a darker pigmented or darker skinned individual. Individuals with darker skin often have a purplish tinge rather than a reddish tinge when erythema is present and often have a more follicular pattern.

Postinflammatory hypopigmentation, absence of normal melanin, and hyperpigmentation, increased melanin, occur more frequently in darker skinned individuals, and conditions such as acne or eczema can produce significant skin color changes from postinflammatory hyperpigmentation. African-Americans, Asians, and Hispanic children are also at higher risk of *keloid* scarring. A keloid is a type of scar at the site of a healed skin injury resulting from an overgrowth of granular tissue composed of collagen (see Table 6-4). Lighter skinned individuals may have more recognizable signs of skin breakdown, sun exposure, and tissue perfusion than darker skinned individuals. Looking at the sclerae, conjunctivae, buccal mucosa, lips, tongue, and nail beds will assist the health care provider in assessing children and adolescents with significant clinical variations in pigmentation and skin color. Variations of skin pigmentation with darker skinned individuals normally occur on the palms, soles of feet, nail beds, and the genital area. Freckling of the buccal cavity, gums, and tongue is also common. Areas that get regular exposure to the sun may have much darker pigmentation.

Other variations related to skin pigmentation or melanin may exist in the barrier properties of the skin and in the distribution of hair follicles. Variations in barrier properties and hair follicle distribution are significant because skin in darker pigmented individuals may provide more of a barrier against absorption of topically applied drugs and cosmetics. The barrier function may also prevent the penetration of some toxins.[10-12] The variation in barrier properties of the skin contributes to darker skinned individuals having an increased incidence of *xerosis,* abnormal dryness of the skin with a loss of natural skin shine, which presents as a whitish visual appearance in darkly pigmented skin.[11,12]

Hair follicle distribution and hair quality differ greatly with racial and ethnic background. African-Americans have hair that is often coated in natural oils, and the frequent use of oils, hair products, and braiding may make it more challenging to assess lesions on the scalp. African-Americans are more prone to scalp infections such as *tinea capitis* and require more prolonged medical management. Some of these hair qualities are present in multiracial children, and it may be confusing to a mother or parent who does not have similar hair qualities. Hair, skin, and nail care practices vary widely among cultures and within cultures. Timing of a child's first haircut is one such cultural variation. In many Asian and Latino cultures, it is common to shave the infant's head between 3 and 9 months of age in the belief the hair will grow in thick and long. In some cultures, shaving of the head is part of a religious ceremony. Some African-American communities believe an infant's hair should not be cut until he or she begins walking.

Health care providers should be sensitive and attentive to the differences in skin quality and skin integrity when caring for children, adolescents, and families from diverse racial and ethnic backgrounds and should encourage and support cultural practices that preserve the family culture except when a skin care practice or treatment is harmful and impacts the healthy development of the skin.

SYSTEM-SPECIFIC HISTORY

A careful age-appropriate history is critical to making an accurate assessment of the skin (see the Information Gathering table). The health care provider needs to gather information related to current skin conditions, any significant past medical history, and family history of chronic skin conditions. Skin care routines and any recent changes in skin, hair, or nail care habits should be assessed. Sun exposure habits and application of sunscreen are also important considerations in the assessment of the skin. Box 6-1 presents symptom-focused information gathering for skin conditions in children.

BOX 6-1   SYMPTOM-FOCUSED INFORMATION GATHERING OF SKIN CONDITIONS

- Any recent changes in skin, hair, or nails? Any dryness, pruritus, sores, rashes, lumps, color changes, or changes in texture or odor noted?
- What signs or symptoms are present (rash, single or multiple skin lesions, itching, pain, exudates, bleeding, color changes)? Other symptoms of fever, malaise, loss of appetite? Upper respiratory symptoms?
- Where is the skin problem located?
- When did it start, sequence of occurrence, rapidity of onset? Is this a recurrence? Any known allergies? Any history of recent illness?
- Any recent exposure to drugs, new skin products, detergent products, new foods, other environmental or occupational toxins, or family member or contact with similar condition? History of recent travel?
- What has been done to treat the problem, including medications (over-the-counter [OTC] or prescription) and/or lotions or other emollients applied? Did the problem get better or worse?

INFORMATION GATHERING AT KEY DEVELOPMENTAL STAGES

Age-Group	Questions to Ask
Newborn	*At birth:* History of skin trauma at birth or significant bruises to face/body? Presence of skin tags, dimples, cysts? Any extra digits? Moles or nevus? Hair or nail variations present at birth? Received any phototherapy?
Infant to 6 months of age	*Diaper history:* Type of disposable wipes used? Type of diapers used? *Skin care history:* Types of soap, moisturizing/cleansing lotion, other lotions, emollients, creams, oils? *Dressing habits:* Amounts/types of clothing in relation to environmental temperature, how clothing is washed, use of detergents, fabric softeners, dryer sheets? *Home environment:* Temperature, humidity, type of home heating? Air conditioning? *Feeding history:* Breast or bottle, type of formula, what foods introduced and when?
6 months to 2 years of age	History of eating large amounts of yellow fruits, vegetables? History of prolonged crawling on hands, knees without protective clothing? History of rubbing head against furniture/walls?

INFORMATION GATHERING AT KEY DEVELOPMENTAL STAGES—CONT'D

Age-Group	Questions to Ask
Early childhood	Eating habits/types of food? History of exposure to communicable diseases? Pets/animal exposure? History of dry skin, eczema, urticaria, pruritus, nasal allergy, asthma? History of nail biting, hair twisting?
Middle childhood	History of skin injuries: cuts, falls, fractures, need for sutures? Any unexplained scarring or bruises? Outdoor exposure to plants during hiking, camping, picnics? Bee stings, contact with plants resulting in allergic reactions, dog bite? Undiagnosed rashes?
Adolescence	History of skin/hair changes, acne? Acne treatments used? Sports-related injuries? Body tattooing, ritual scarring, piercing? Were they done professionally using sterile techniques/supplies? Problems/infections related to these practices?
Environmental risks	Exposure to tobacco smoke? Contact with chemical cleaning agents/other chemicals at home, school, work? Exposure to chemicals, toxins from parent's work?

PHYSICAL ASSESSMENT

The skin is one of the most accessible and easily examined organs of the body and is often the organ of most concern to children, adolescents, and parents. A complete examination of the skin using a consistent, systematic approach will increase the likelihood that important findings critical to making a diagnosis will not be missed. Always avoid making a quick diagnosis after only a brief inspection of an area of exposed skin or examining only the lesion of concern. A deliberate and methodical assessment of the skin will lead to a correct diagnosis and prevent missing important clues.

Dermatology has its own language. Using the correct terminology facilitates accurate description of skin lesions. A *skin lesion* refers to any variations or skin changes. If the inspection and palpation of the skin reveal a lesion, more examination is necessary. Skin lesions may be *primary* or *secondary* (Tables 6-2 and 6-3). A *primary lesion* is the initial lesion of a skin condition, and identifying the *primary lesion* is the most important step in assessing skin conditions in children and assists clinicians in diagnosis. A *secondary lesion* often develops as a skin condition progresses.

A rash cannot be diagnosed by listening to a description over the phone, and pediatric health care providers should avoid this type of assessment. It is important to conduct a complete skin examination before making a diagnosis. It is usually very easy to do a complete skin assessment on a newborn, but there may be a great deal of resistance from many adolescents to the idea of a complete skin exam. When the child or adolescent is uncomfortable being completely undressed because of developmental stage or cultural belief, then the assessment of the skin must be conducted using a systematic approach that divides the skin into areas that are sequentially uncovered, examined, and then re-covered before going on to the next area. In infants and young children, this may also prevent unnecessary cooling of the skin.

Inspection

Inspection of the skin is best conducted using natural light. If that is not available a well-lit room with fluorescent or incandescent lighting may be satisfactory. A magnifying glass and a measuring tool such as a flat, clear ruler will be helpful for examining small skin lesions and moles. It may be necessary to follow a lesion's progress for several weeks. A light for transillumination of lesions or for closer inspection also may be helpful. A photo inserted in the medical chart or electronic medical record may be useful when following a skin condition. In addition, a photo showing a ruler next to the skin lesion can assist evaluation of changes over time.

Nails should be examined for shape, color, and texture. Nail changes may be an early sign of systemic disease. Artificial nails or nail polish can interfere with the assessment. Inspect the curvature of the nail for *clubbing* or spooning and feel the surface for ridges. Changes in coloration or splinter hemorrhages in the nail should be noted. Finally, check the periungual tissue of the nail and note any redness, edema, induration, or tenderness. Absence or atrophy of the nails in the newborn period may indicate a congenital syndrome and should be evaluated further.

Hair should be examined carefully. Be sure to assess terminal and vellus hairs for changes. Note distribution, color, and quantity. If there are areas of hair loss, determine whether the hair is broken or burned off or whether the hair is absent. Check for any lesions, dryness, oiliness, scaling, or infestation on the scalp.

TABLE 6-2   PRIMARY LESIONS

Name	Photo	Description	Examples of Conditions
Macule/patch		Flat, circumscribed lesion of any size, <1 cm is macule; >1 cm is patch; lesions usually rounded but may be oval, can be vascular, hyperpigmented, or hypopigmented	Freckle, café au lait spots, vitiligo, flat mole (nevus), blue-gray macules of the neonate (Mongolian spots), port-wine stain
Papule		Circumscribed elevated lesions <1 cm	Molluscum contagiosum, papular urticaria, elevated moles, wart
Plaque		Circumscribed, elevated, disc-shaped lesion >1 cm; commonly formed by confluence of papules	Atopic dermatitis, lichen simplex chronicus (neurodermatitis), tinea corporis
Nodule		Circumscribed, elevated, usually solid lesion that measures 0.5-2 cm; may be in epidermis or extend deeper	Fibromas, neurofibromas, intradermal nevi, erythema nodosum, hemangioma, pyogenic granuloma

TABLE 6-2   PRIMARY LESIONS—CONT'D

Name	Photo	Description	Examples of Conditions
Cyst		Elevated, circumscribed, encapsulated lesion in dermis or subcutaneous layer filled with liquid/semisolid material	Sebaceous cyst, cystic acne
Vesicle		Sharply circumscribed, elevated, fluid-containing lesion that measures ≤0.5 cm	Herpes simplex, varicella, insect bite, herpes zoster
Bulla		Sharply circumscribed, elevated, fluid-containing lesion that measures ≥1 cm	Contact dermatitis, epidermolysis bullosa, pemphigus vulgaris, burn, bullous impetigo
Wheal		Distinctive type of solid elevation formed by local, superficial, transient edema; white to pink–pale red in color; blanches with pressure, varies in size, shape	Urticaria, insect bite, dermographia, erythema multiforme

Continued

TABLE 6-2 PRIMARY LESIONS—CONT'D

Name	Photo	Description	Examples of Conditions
Comedones		Plugged secretions of horny material retained within pilosebaceous follicle; may be flesh-colored, closed (white-heads); brown/black, open (blackheads)	Acne
Burrows		Linear lesion produced by tunneling of animal parasite in stratum corneum	Scabies, cutaneous larva migrans (creeping eruption)
Telangiectasia		Fine, irregular, red lines produced by capillary dilation	Rosacea

Papule, vesicle, and bulla images are from Weston W, Lane A, Morelli J: *Color textbook of pediatric dermatology*, ed 4, St. Louis, 2007, Mosby.
Cyst image is from Habif T: *Clinical dermatology*, ed 5, St. Louis, 2010, Mosby.
Wheal image is from Eichenfield L, Frieden I, Esterly NB: *Neonatal dermatology*, ed 2, Philadelphia, 2008, Saunders.
Comedone image is from Brinster NK, Liu V, Diwan AH, et al: *Dermatopathology: high-yield pathology*, Philadelphia, 2011, Saunders.
Burrow image is from White G, Cox N: *Diseases of the skin*, ed 2, St. Louis, 2006, Mosby.
Telangiectasia image is from Paller A, Manicini A: *Hurwitz clinical pediatric dermatology: a textbook of skin disorders of childhood and adolescence*, ed 4, Philadelphia, 2011, Saunders.

Palpation

Palpation of the skin should be done with warm hands. Use gloves if you think the child or adolescent may have an infectious lesion. Palpate skin temperature using the back of your hand, and compare the temperature of one area of skin to another area of skin using both hands. Temperature cannot be assessed accurately through gloves, and presence of a fever should always be checked using a thermometer. Check for *skin turgor,* resiliency or elasticity of the skin, by gently pinching a fold of the child's skin over the abdomen between your thumb and forefinger then releasing it. *Skin turgor* can give important clues to the hydration and nutritional status of a child. How long the skin remains tented after it is released will provide clues to the degree of dehydration (Table 6-4).

TABLE 6-3   SECONDARY LESIONS

Name	Photo	Description	Example of Diseases
Scale		Formed by accumulation of compact desquamation of stratum corneum layers; may be greasy, yellowish; silvery, fine, barely visible or large, adherent, and lamellar	Seborrheic dermatitis Psoriasis Pityriasis alba Tinea versicolor Ichthyosis
Fissure		Dry, moist, linear, often painful, cleavage from epidermis to dermis that results from marked drying; long-standing inflammation, thickening, loss of elasticity of integument	Chronic dermatoses Intertrigo Atopic dermatitis Ichthyosis
Licheni-fication		Rough, thickened epidermis secondary to persistent rubbing, itching, or skin irritation; often involves flexor surface of extremity	Atopic dermatitis Chronic dermatitis
Scar		Permanent fibrotic skin changes that develop following damage to dermis; initially pink/violet, fading to white, shiny, sclerotic area *Keloid:* pink, smooth, rubbery; often traversed by telangiectatic vessels; increases in size long after healing of lesion; differentiated from hypertrophic scars because surface of keloid scar tends to be beyond original wound area	Surgery Healed wound Stretch marks Keloid Herpes zoster Burn

Continued

TABLE 6-3   SECONDARY LESIONS—CONT'D

Name	Photo	Description	Example of Diseases
Crust		Dried exudate on epidermis composed of serum, blood, or pus overlying a ruptured bulla or vesicle; caused by staphylococcal or streptococcal bacteria	Impetigo Epidermolysis bullosa
Erosions		Moist, slightly depressed vesicular lesion in which all or part of epidermis has been lost; may have surrounding erythema or edema; heals without scarring	Impetigo Eczematous diseases Intertrigo Candidiasis Methicillin-resistant *Staphylococcus aureus* (MRSA)
Purpura		Flat lesion; petechiae if pinpoint; does not blanch to pressure; larger areas of bruising may be present	Henoch-Schönlein Purpura fulminans

Data from Eichenfield L, Frieden I, Esterly NB: *Neonatal dermatology*, ed 2, Philadelphia, 2008, Saunders; Seidel HM, Ball JW, Dains JE, Benedict GW: *Mosby's guide to physical examination*, ed 7, St. Louis, 2010, Mosby; Infoderm.com, Galderma Laboratories, LP, 2012. Scale and fissure images are from Paller A, Manicini A: *Hurwitz clinical pediatric dermatology: a textbook of skin disorders of childhood and adolescence*, ed 4, Philadelphia, 2011, Saunders.
Lichenification image is from Rudikoff D: Differential diagnosis of round or discoid lesions, *Clin Dermatol* 29(5):489-497, 2011.
Scar image is from Arndt K: *Procedures in cosmetic dermatology series: scar revision*, Philadelphia, 2006, Saunders.
Purpura image is from Marx J, Hockberger R, Walls R, et al: *Rosen's emergency medicine: concepts and clinical practice*, ed 7, Philadelphia, 2010, Mosby. Courtesy of Marianne Gausch-Hill, MD.

TABLE 6-4	ESTIMATING DEHYDRATION IN AN INFANT OR YOUNG CHILD	
Return to Normal After the Pinch	Degree of Dehydration
<2 seconds	<5% loss of body weight
2-3 seconds	5%-8% loss of body weight
3-4 seconds	9%-10% loss of body weight
>4 seconds	>10% loss of body weight

Data from Seidel HM, Ball JW, Dains JE, Benedict GW: *Mosby's guide to physical examination*, ed 7, St. Louis, 2010, Mosby.

SKIN CONDITIONS

Skin Lesions

The *morphology* or characteristic form and structure of skin lesions should be identified when any condition is noted during the assessment of the skin. Attention to the distribution and pattern of lesions will assist in making a diagnosis. The *distribution* refers to the location of skin findings, whereas *pattern* refers to the specific anatomical or physiological arrangement of the lesions. Note the shape of skin lesions and whether they are clustered together or scattered. The border or margin, any associated findings such as central clearing, and the pigmentation of the lesion also should be identified. Find and study the primary lesion and examine the distribution of any skin lesions or skin variations. Skin lesions should be classified as primary or secondary (see Tables 6-2 and 6-3). Box 6-2 illustrates the color, borders, configuration, and distribution of lesions. Common newborn and infant skin conditions are presented in Table 6-5.

BOX 6-2	BORDERS, CONFIGURATION, AND DISTRIBUTION OF LESIONS

Border

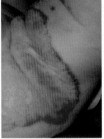

Acrodermatitis enteropathica

Borders of lesion may be raised or indurated, as in granuloma annulare and neonatal lupus, or indistinct, as in cellulitis or atopic dermatitis.

Configuration

Blaschko (Linear)

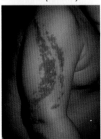

Linear epidermal nevus

Linear lesions do not follow any known vascular, nervous, or lymphatic pattern. V- and S-shaped lines may represent patterns of neuroectodermal migration, and distribution indicates a cutaneous mosaicism.

Continued

| BOX 6-2 | BORDERS, CONFIGURATION, AND DISTRIBUTION OF LESIONS—CONT'D |

Dermatomal/Zosteriform (Linear)

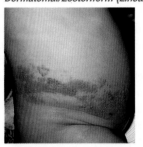

Herpes zoster

Lines demarcating a dermatome supplied by one dorsal root ganglia.

Segmental Patterns

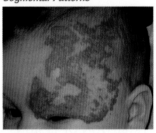

Infantile hemangioma

The configuration of segmental lesions is thought to be determined by the location of embryonic placodes or other embryonic territories, as can be seen in PHACE(S) syndrome.

Annular

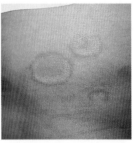

Annular lesions of neonatal lupus

A round, ring-shaped lesion, where the periphery is distinct from the center, as in tinea corporis or neonatal lupus.

Nummular

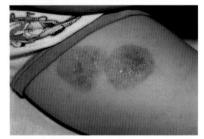

Nummular eczema

A coin-shaped lesion, with homogenous character throughout, as in nummular eczema.

BOX 6-2 BORDERS, CONFIGURATION, AND DISTRIBUTION OF LESIONS—CONT'D

Targetoid

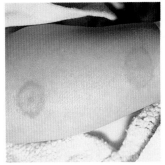

Early lesions of erythema multiforme

Concentric ringed lesions, often with a dusky or bullous center characteristic of erythema multiforme.

Herpetiform

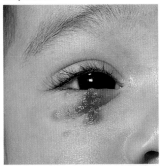

Herpes simplex infection

Clusters of erythematous occasionally scabbed lesions, as in herpes simplex.

Corymbiform

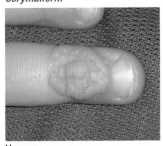

Verrucae

Defined as a central cluster of lesions surrounded by scattered individual lesions, as in verrucae.

Adapted from Eichenfield L, Frieden I, Esterly NB: *Neonatal dermatology*, ed 2, Philadelphia, 2008, Saunders.
Acrodermatitis enteropathica, linear epidermal nevus, herpes zoster, infantile hemangioma, neonatal lupus, erythema multiforme, herpes simplex, and verrucae images are from Eichenfield L, Frieden I, Esterly NB: *Neonatal dermatology*, ed 2, Philadelphia, 2008, Saunders.
Nummular eczema image is from Weston W, Lane A, Morelli J: *Color textbook of pediatric dermatology*, ed 4, St. Louis, 2007, Mosby.

TABLE 6-5   COMMON CONDITIONS IN NEWBORN AND INFANT SKIN

Condition	Photo	Description	Significance/Treatment
Acrocyanosis		Bluish coloration of hands and feet present at birth; may persist up to 24 hours; circumoral cyanosis also may be present	Benign color variation in newborn; no treatment needed if gone after 24 hours
Accessory tragi		Pedunculated, flesh-colored, soft, round papules usually arising on or near the tragus	May occur anywhere from corner of ear to mouth and require removal by careful surgical dissection; do not confuse with skin tags, do not tie off with suture
Cutis marmorata		Reddish-blue mottling or marbling of skin in response to changes in temperature; caused by dilation of capillaries and venules	Benign color variation; no treatment needed unless it does not disappear with skin warming
Erythema toxicum		Small white to yellow papules, vesicles with erythematous base; occurs in response to rubbing; starts as early as 24 hours of life, may continue until 2 weeks old	Common benign skin lesion in newborn; eosinophils in smear from papule confirms diagnosis
Miliaria rubra, m. crystallina, m. pustulosa		Clear, thin vesicles or discrete erythematous papules seen primarily over forehead, neck, in creases, or groin; occurs as a result of obstructed sweat glands in humid environment	Benign skin lesion in newborn; can be treated by eliminating precipitating factors such as heat, humidity, too many clothes
Transient neonatal pustular melanosis		Vesicles that rupture leaving collaret of scale and pigmented macule; macules may remain for up to 3 months after birth	Benign skin lesion requiring no treatment

CHARTING

Accurate charting using the correct terminology allows other health care providers to "visualize" the skin lesions and provide the necessary follow-up to evaluate whether there is change or improvement in lesions. Avoid the use of a specific diagnosis when describing a lesion in the objective physical findings, such as diaper rash or candidiasis, a common fungal infection in infants.

One advantage of moving to an electronic medical record (EMR) system of charting is the ability to use templates. Customizing a template for assessment of the skin using appropriate dermatological terms or adding a glossary of dermatological terms with definitions to the EMR provides accurate, consistent descriptions of lesions by different clinicians, and saves time when charting. This system allows evaluation of a lesion over time. Some EMRs allow photos to be inserted. These photos may be taken by the clinician at the time of the exam or by the patient and submitted by text message or e-mail to the provider for insertion into the medical record. The wide use of smartphones with high-resolution digital cameras by individuals and families from all economic and social backgrounds make the tracking of skin lesions and skin conditions at home a possibility for health care providers. The ability to accurately visualize a lesion digitally may prevent the child and family from returning to the clinical setting for frequent follow-up visits.

SUMMARY OF EXAMINATION

- Skin disorders may vary widely when observed in an infant or child as compared to the same skin disorder when seen in an adult.
- Extremely premature infants are born without the *stratum corneum,* have limited ability to control water loss, and can tolerate a limited amount of touch.
- Term newborns have a fully functional stratum corneum, which is about 60% the thickness of adult skin.
- Skin pigmentation or melanin should be considered as a factor for understanding some underlying skin properties and characteristics.
- A careful age-appropriate history is critical to making an accurate assessment of the skin (see the Information Gathering table and Box 6-1).
- On inspection of the skin, note distribution or location of skin findings and pattern of the skin lesions. A skin lesion refers to any variations or skin changes.
- Identify primary lesions, the initial lesion of a skin condition, and secondary lesions, which develop over time as a skin condition progresses.
- Palpation of the skin should be done with warm hands or with gloves when infection is suspected.
- Assessment of the skin must be conducted using a systematic approach that divides the skin into areas that are sequentially uncovered, examined, and then re-covered.
- Avoid making a quick diagnosis after only a brief observation of the skin.
- A rash in children cannot be diagnosed by listening to a description over the phone.
- Accurate charting using the correct terminology allows other health care providers to "visualize" the skin lesions and provide the necessary follow up.
- Avoid the use of a specific diagnosis when describing a lesion in the objective physical findings.

Charting
14-Month-Old with Candidiasis

Skin: Discrete, red papules and pustules over the perineum with satellite lesions over the legs and abdomen; otherwise skin lightly pigmented and clear.

Charting
15-Year-Old with Moderate Acne Vulgaris

Skin: Moderate amount of open and closed comedones over nose and cheeks, discreet pustular lesions on forehead, no nodules or cyst noted. Skin oily with moderate papular, erythematous lesions over upper back.

REFERENCES

1. Everett JS, Budescu M, Sommers MS: Making sense of skin color in clinical care, *Clin Nurs Res* 21(4):495-516, 2012.
2. Paller AS, Mancini AJ: *Hurwitz clinical pediatric dermatology: A textbook of skin disorders of childhood and adolescence*, ed 4, Philadelphia, 2011, Saunders.
3. Bowlby J: The nature of the child's tie to his mother, *Int J Psychoanal* 39(5):350-373, 1958.
4. Bowlby J: *Attachment and loss*, New York, 1969, Basic Books.
5. Klaus MH, Kennell JH: *Maternal-infant bonding: the impact of early separation or loss on family development*, St Louis, 1976, Mosby.
6. Spitz RA: *The first year of life: a psychoanalytic study of normal and deviant development of object relations*, New York, 1965, International Universities Press.
7. Habif TP: *Clinical dermatology*, ed 5, 2010, Mosby.
8. Seidel HM, Ball JW, Dains JE, et al: *Mosby's guide to physical examination*, ed 7, St. Louis, 2010, Mosby.
9. Eichenfield LF, Frieden IJ, Esterly NB: *Neonatal dermatology*, ed 2, 2008, Saunders.
10. Telofski LS, Morello III AP, Mack Correa MC, et al: The infant skin barrier: can we preserve, protect, and enhance the barrier? *Dermatol Res Pract* 2012:198789, 2012
11. Mangelsdorf S, Otberg N, Maibach HI, et al: Ethnic variation in vellus hair follicle size and distribution, *Skin Pharmacol Physiol* 19(3):159-167, 2006.
12. Muizzuddin N, Hellemans L, Van Overloop L, et al: Structural and functional differences in barrier properties of African American, Caucasian and East Asian skin, *J Dermatol Sci* 59(2):123-128, 2010.

CHAPTER 7

HEART AND VASCULAR SYSTEM

Elizabeth Tong; Patricia O'Brien

EMBRYOLOGICAL DEVELOPMENT

The heart begins to form in the fetus by the end of the third week after conception. A crescent-shaped structure is formed that fuses at the midline to create a single linear heart tube (Figure 7-1). As the primitive heart tube elongates, it differentiates into the *atria, ventricles, bulbus cordis,* and *truncus arteriosus.* The conduction system also begins to form during this time and by day 23 after conception the heart begins to beat. Valve formation begins around the fourth to fifth week after conception, and the formation of the heart is complete by the eighth week after conception. Any early changes in this process caused by genetic, maternal, or external environmental factors can lead to structural malformations of the heart.

During fetal life, the lung sacs are collapsed and blood is oxygenated through the placenta. Oxygenated blood travels from the placenta to the heart via the umbilical veins and *ductus venosus* to the *inferior vena cava* (IVC) and into the *right atrium* (RA). Blood then streams to the *left atrium* (LA) through a *patent foramen ovale* (PFO) and into the *left ventricle* (LV), which pumps it out the *aorta* (Figure 7-2). The less saturated venous blood traveling from the *superior vena cava* (SVC) and *coronary sinus* also flows to the right atrium, but is directed toward the *right ventricle* (RV) and *pulmonary artery* (PA). High pulmonary vascular

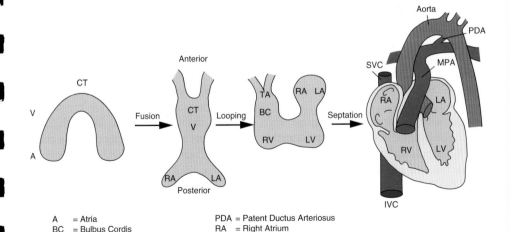

A = Atria
BC = Bulbus Cordis
CT = Conotruncus
IVC = Inferior Vena Cava
LA = Left Atrium
LV = Left Ventricle
MPA = Main Pulmonary Artery

PDA = Patent Ductus Arteriosus
RA = Right Atrium
RV = Right Ventricle
SVC = Superior Vena Cava
TA = Truncus Arteriosus
V = Ventricle

FIGURE 7-1 Fetal development of the heart.

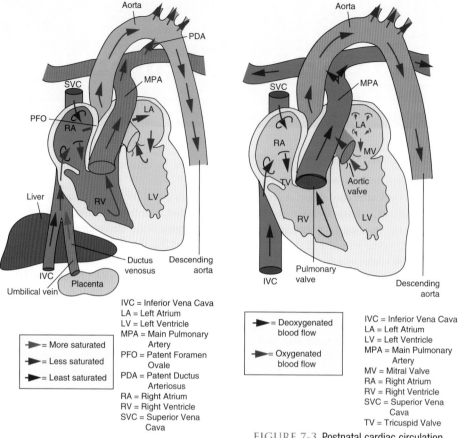

FIGURE 7-2 **Fetal cardiac circulation.**

IVC = Inferior Vena Cava
LA = Left Atrium
LV = Left Ventricle
MPA = Main Pulmonary
        Artery
PFO = Patent Foramen
        Ovale
PDA = Patent Ductus
        Arteriosus
RA = Right Atrium
RV = Right Ventricle
SVC = Superior Vena
        Cava

➤ = More saturated
➤ = Less saturated
➤ = Least saturated

FIGURE 7-3 **Postnatal cardiac circulation.**

➤ = Deoxygenated
    blood flow
➤ = Oxygenated
    blood flow

IVC = Inferior Vena Cava
LA = Left Atrium
LV = Left Ventricle
MPA = Main Pulmonary
        Artery
MV = Mitral Valve
RA = Right Atrium
RV = Right Ventricle
SVC = Superior Vena
        Cava
TV = Tricuspid Valve

resistance limits blood flow into the lungs, which are not yet involved in ventilation, and redirects it through the *patent ductus arteriosus* (PDA) to the descending aorta and lower body.

With a baby's first breaths, pulmonary vascular resistance falls, causing a dramatic increase in pulmonary blood flow. The ensuing increase in pulmonary venous return to the heart raises LA pressure, causing closure of the PFO. Arterial oxygen saturation increases as a result of improved oxygenation by the lungs. This higher saturation promotes functional closure of the PDA by 48 to 72 hours after birth, with complete anatomical closure occurring by 2 to 3 weeks of age.[1]

ANATOMY AND PHYSIOLOGY

Anatomy of the Postnatal Heart

The heart is composed of four chambers. The upper chambers (atria) are low-pressure receiving chambers, and the lower chambers (ventricles) are high-pressure pumping chambers. The heart is further divided into right and left sides. The *RA* receives deoxygenated blood from the body, and the *RV* pumps it out the pulmonary artery to the lungs to become oxygenated. The *LA* receives oxygenated blood from the lungs, and the *LV* pumps it out the aorta to the body (Figure 7-3). The LV operates at a higher pressure than the RV. This normal circulation occurs in series, and there is no mixing of deoxygenated and oxygenated blood.

There are four valves in the heart that regulate blood flow between the atria and ventricles. The atrioventricular (AV) valves regulate blood flow between the atria and ventricles, and the semilunar valves regulate blood flow between the ventricles and great vessels. The *tricuspid valve* on the right and the *mitral valve* on the left are the AV valves (see Figure 7-3). The *pulmonic valve,* located at the base of the pulmonary artery between the right ventricle and the pulmonary artery, and the *aortic valve,* located at the base of the aorta between the aorta and left ventricle, are the semilunar valves. Closure of these valves produces the heart sounds commonly referred to as "lub-dub" (S_1, S_2).

PHYSIOLOGICAL VARIATIONS

In preterm infants, the ductus arteriosus may remain open for several weeks after birth causing hemodynamic instability. Medical intervention with a prostaglandin inhibitor, such as the drug indomethacin, or surgical ligation of the ductus is required to stabilize the infant.[1]

SYSTEM-SPECIFIC HISTORY

A careful and systematic history needs to be performed at each developmental stage to monitor the overall health status of infants and children, to identify those with cardiac symptoms, and to recognize signs of cardiac disease. The Information Gathering table presents the relevant age-related questions to ask about the cardiovascular system and questions related to maternal infections and maternal medical conditions that place infants at high risk for *congenital heart disease* (CHD).

PEDIATRIC PEARLS

Infants with CHD may have tachypnea (rapid, shallow breathing) and tachycardia but typically do not present in respiratory distress (i.e., retractions, grunting, nasal flaring) unless there is a significant increase in pulmonary blood flow or poor systemic output with acidosis.

INFORMATION GATHERING FOR ASSESSING THE CARDIOVASCULAR SYSTEM AT KEY DEVELOPMENTAL STAGES

Age-Group	Questions to Ask	Rationale
Prenatal, infancy, early childhood	Any family history of CHD/chromosomal abnormalities, sudden/premature death; maternal illness/infections (both chronic and during pregnancy); maternal medications/drug use	CHD caused by interaction between genetic and environmental factors (systemic lupus, rubella, diabetes mellitus, anticonvulsants, alcohol, etc.)
	Apgar scores	Usually normal with CHD except for color if cyanotic
	Any problems with poor feeding, sweating (especially on the forehead) during feeding, weight loss/gain, FTT, decreased activity level	Symptoms of CHD often occur with feeding because of increased oxygen consumption and need for greater cardiac output
	Any pallor or blueness in color; any changes in color, especially when crying	Babies with cyanotic heart disease turn dark blue or ruddy in color when crying because of prolonged expiratory phase and resulting increase in right-to-left shunting. Hypercyanotic spells are often associated with extreme irritability and rapid, deep, and sometimes labored respirations.

Continued

INFORMATION GATHERING FOR ASSESSING THE CARDIOVASCULAR SYSTEM AT KEY DEVELOPMENTAL STAGES—CONT'D

Age-Group	Questions to Ask	Rationale
	Any pattern of rapid breathing; frequent respiratory infections	Left-to-right shunting lesions (VSD, AVSD, PDA) cause increased blood flow to the lungs, resulting in frequent respiratory infections, FTT, and decreased exercise tolerance.
Middle childhood and adolescence	Any inability to keep up with the activity level of peers, need for frequent periods of rest, anorexia, cough, wheezing, rales, chest pain, leg cramps, syncope, light-headedness, palpitations; any history of drug use; any family history of sudden death, syncope, or arrhythmias	CHD can decrease exercise intolerance. Left ventricular outflow obstructive lesions (AS, coarctation of the aorta) can cause CHF. Undetected coarctation of the aorta can cause leg cramps. Coronary artery abnormalities (including Kawasaki disease) and cocaine use can cause chest pain. Structural and dysrhythmic heart disease can first present as syncope. Some dysrhythmias are genetic in origin and run in families.
	Any history of recent infections, prolonged fever or malaise, recent dental work	Untreated streptococcal infections, Kawasaki disease, and subacute endocarditis can result in CHF or acquired heart disease.

AS, Aortic stenosis; *AVSD,* atrioventricular septal defect; *CHD,* congenital heart disease; *CHF,* congestive heart failure; *FTT,* failure to thrive; *PDA,* patent ductus arteriosus; *VSD,* ventricular septal defect.

PHYSICAL ASSESSMENT

The cardiac examination must be systematic and tailored to the child's developmental level (Figures 7-4 and 7-5). A complete assessment of the cardiac system must be done in order to make conclusions about the significance of any single abnormality. Cardiac findings should not be taken in isolation.

It is important to consistently plot height, weight, and head circumference in infants and children up to age 2 years of age to evaluate whether the growth rate is proportional and to monitor for failure to thrive (FTT). For infants, any drop-off in weight percentiles as compared to length and head circumference values should raise the suspicion of CHD.[1] Temperature, heart rate, and respiratory rate should be measured and assessed. Fever and respiratory distress both can elevate heart rate.

Blood pressure should be measured whenever possible during physical examinations, but

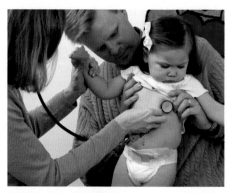

FIGURE 7-4 Cardiac examination of the toddler.

definitely once in infancy and then routinely after age 3.[2] *Coarctation of the aorta* and systemic *hypertension* can go undetected if blood pressure measurements are omitted during well-child visits. If measured, blood pressure in infants should be taken in all four extremities or at a minimum in the right arm and in one leg

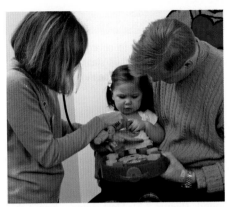

FIGURE 7-5 Decreasing fear of the cardiac examination through play.

to detect a coarctation of the aorta. In children, simultaneous palpation of the radial and femoral pulses is also important in assessing whether a coarctation may be present.

Inspection

Note general appearance and activity level and whether the child is alert, lethargic, or acutely ill. Note nutritional status and the proportion of weight to height and head circumference. Also, note whether any unusual facial or other external features are present that may indicate the presence of a syndrome or chromosomal anomaly, and any surgical scars on the sternum and chest area that would indicate a previous surgical procedure.

Color

Note whether the child is pale or cyanotic, and assess color under natural light if possible. Pallor can occur in infants who are anemic, who have vasoconstriction due to *congestive heart failure* (CHF), or who are in shock. Children with cyanotic heart disease will appear blue or ruddy, especially around the perioral area because of right-to-left shunting of blood at the arterial level.

Clubbing

Clubbing occurs when arterial desaturation has been present for at least 6 months or longer. The fingers and toes become red and shiny, and

progress to wide, thick digits with eventual loss of the normal angle between the nails and the nail beds[2] (Figure 7-6). It should be noted that infants born with cyanotic heart disease are being treated earlier than in the past, and this has resulted in a decreased incidence of clubbing in children and adolescents.

Palpation

Pulses need to be evaluated for their presence or absence, intensity, timing, symmetry, and whether the pulse is regular or irregular, weak or bounding. A comparison also should be made as to right and left symmetry and quality of pulses in the upper and lower extremities. A pulse that is absent or weaker in the lower extremities compared to the upper extremities is diagnostic of *coarctation of the aorta*. A strong pedal pulse is a good indication that there is no coarctation. Irregular pulses may be due to an *arrhythmia*. Weak and thready pulses may indicate poor perfusion or shock, whereas bounding pulses are usually noted with aortic run-off lesions such as a PDA, AV malformation, or aortic insufficiency.[2] *Peripheral perfusion* is also important to assess, especially in infants. Normally, extremities should be warm to the touch and have a brisk capillary refill time (CRT) of less than 3 seconds—a quick

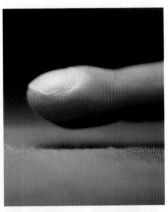

FIGURE 7-6 Clubbing of nails resulting from arterial desaturation. (Adapted from Hochberg MC, Silman AJ, Smolen JS, et al: *Rheumatology*, ed 3, St. Louis, 2003, Mosby.)

measure of cardiac output. Older children with cardiac conditions may have weak distal pulses on one side or the other because of previous cardiac catheterizations or cardiac surgeries.

Normal liver size is usually 1 to 2 cm below the right costal margin. In conditions of abnormal cardiac position, or situs (positional abnormalities), the liver edge is midline or on the left side of the abdomen. *Hepatomegaly,* or liver engorgement, is a consistent indicator of right heart failure when noted in conjunction with other cardiac findings.

The precordium should be palpated to determine the location of the *point of maximal impulse,* or PMI. The PMI is important in determining ventricular overload, cardiomegaly, and the presence or absence of thrills. Normally, the PMI is felt at the apex in the left midclavicular line, indicating LV dominance. However, it is normal for newborns and infants to have a greater RV impulse, with the PMI felt at the left lower sternal border (LLSB). A PMI that is diffuse and rises slowly is called a *heave,* and a PMI that is sharp and well localized is known as a *tap.*[2]

A *thrill* indicates turbulent blood flow and is never normal. It is felt as a vibratory sensation and should be examined not only on the precordium but also in the suprasternal notch and over the carotid arteries. Precordial thrills are best felt with the palm of the hand, whereas thrills in the suprasternal notch and over the carotid arteries are best felt with the fingertips.[2]

PEDIATRIC PEARLS

Palpation of the liver for enlargement is a critical indicator of overall fluid status in infants and children with congestive heart failure.

Auscultation

Auscultation of heart sounds in children should be done in a stepwise fashion and with both the diaphragm and the bell of a stethoscope to elicit both high (diaphragm) and low (bell) frequency sounds (Figure 7-7). Most children have a thin chest wall and heart sounds are louder than in adults. However, the faster heart rate can make it difficult to accurately distinguish the heart sounds from other adventitious sounds, particularly in early infancy. Thus it is recommended that the individual heart sounds be identified and analyzed before identifying murmurs.

Heart Sounds

The *first heart sound* is called S_1 and is created by the closure of the tricuspid and mitral valves. It is usually heard best at the LLSB or at the apex. A split S_1 can be a normal but uncommon finding in children.[2]

The *second heart* sound is called S_2 and is created by the closure of the aortic and pulmonic valves. It is usually heard best at the left upper sternal border (LUSB). Evaluation of S_2 is critical in children because it provides important clues as to the presence of structural

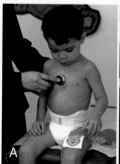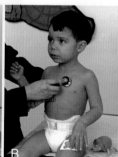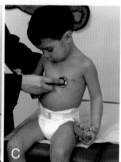

FIGURE 7-7 Auscultation of the heart sounds.

defects and to the pressures in the heart. S_2 normally varies with respiration—split with inspiration and single or narrowly split in expiration. A fixed split, single S_2, or loud S_2 warrants further evaluation by a cardiologist. Abnormal splitting of the S_2 may indicate increased pulmonary blood flow, pulmonary valve abnormality, or a cyanotic heart condition. A loud single S_2 may indicate pulmonary hypertension or malposition of the great arteries.[2]

A *third heart sound* (S_3) can be a common finding in children and young adults. S_3 can be heard at the apex and is caused by vibrations in the ventricle as it fills rapidly during diastole.

A *fourth heart sound* (S_4 or *gallop rhythm*) is rare in infants and children. An S_4 is an abnormal finding and suggests decreased ventricular compliance in conditions such as CHF.[2]

Ejection clicks are extra heart sounds that occur between S_1 and S_2. They are heard best at the upper sternal border and are usually associated with stenotic semilunar valves or dilated great arteries.[2]

Murmurs

Murmurs are produced when blood flows across an area that has a pressure difference and causes turbulence or disturbed flow. Murmurs should be assessed and evaluated according to their timing in the cardiac cycle, location, transmission, intensity, frequency, and quality.[2] It is always important to note whether a murmur radiates to the lung fields, axillae, clavicles, or neck. A normal grading scale is used to describe a murmur's intensity (Table 7-1).

Murmurs are described in relation to their timing during the cardiac cycle—systolic, diastolic, or continuous. Systolic murmurs occur between S_1 and S_2, and diastolic murmurs are heard after S_2. Systolic murmurs are further described as *ejection* crescendo-decrescendo, or *regurgitant* long systolic-decrescendo. Figure 7-8 illustrates the difference between ejection and regurgitant murmurs in relation to when they occur in the cardiac cycle.

Systolic ejection murmurs begin shortly after the first heart sound, are due to semilunar valve

TABLE 7-1	GRADING SCALE FOR CARDIAC MURMURS
Grade	Sound
1	Barely audible and softer than usual heart sounds
2	Still soft, but about as loud as usual heart sounds
3	Louder than usual heart sounds, but without a thrill
4	Louder than usual heart sounds, and with a thrill
5	Can be heard with stethoscope barely on chest (rare)
6	Can be heard with stethoscope off chest, or with naked ear (extremely rare)

Data from Park M: *Pediatric cardiology for practitioners,* ed 5, St. Louis, 2008, Mosby.

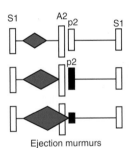

Ejection murmurs
Diamond-shaped crescendo–decrescendo

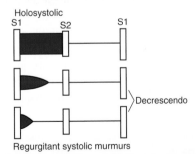

Regurgitant systolic murmurs

FIGURE 7-8 Systolic ejection and regurgitant murmurs. (Adapted from Park M: *Pediatric cardiology for practitioners,* ed 5, St. Louis, 2008, Mosby, p. 28.)

or great vessel stenosis, usually vary in intensity, and are diamond-shaped. They can be short or long in duration but usually end before S_2. Regurgitant murmurs typically begin with S_1, although they usually do not obscure it; are the result of mitral or tricuspid valve insufficiency; and can be long or short in duration. Holosystolic murmurs obscure S_1 at their maximal or loudest point and are usually caused by a *ventricular septal defect* (VSD).[2]

Diastolic murmurs occur between S_2 and S_1 and are described as early, mid, or late. Diastolic murmurs are usually caused by aortic or pulmonic regurgitation or mitral stenosis and are never normal.[2]

Continuous murmurs begin in systole and continue without interruption through S_2 and into diastole. They are usually caused by conditions in which vascular shunting occurs throughout the cardiac cycle, such as in PDA or a surgical aortopulmonary shunt. A continuous murmur from a PDA has a machinery-like quality, is best heard in the left clavicular area or back, and has a crescendo-decrescendo shape.[2]

The origin of a murmur is usually found at the point where the murmur is heard the loudest. This provides valuable information regarding the cardiac malformation. If a murmur is heard throughout the chest, the area of highest frequency will define its origin. For example, a systolic ejection murmur that radiates to the axillae and back is usually pulmonary in origin, and one that radiates to the neck and carotid arteries is typically aortic in origin. The frequency or pitch of a murmur is a good indicator of the pressure gradient across a valve or septal defect. The higher the pressure gradient, the higher the frequency of the murmur.

PEDIATRIC PEARLS

Innocent murmurs occur in up to 50% of normal children.[1] They are a common finding in infants and children and do not always signify heart disease.

Physiologic versus Pathologic Murmurs

It is important to distinguish physiologic, or innocent, murmurs from pathologic ones (Table 7-2). Innocent murmurs occur in up to 50% of normal children.[1] They are systolic ejection murmurs that are usually heard best at the LLSB and have a vibratory or musical quality (Figure 7-9). They tend to be short and well located. They are usually no louder than grade 2 to 3 in intensity and are often accentuated during high output states such as exercise, stress, anemia, or febrile illness. Innocent murmurs are never purely diastolic except in the case of a venous hum, which is a continuous physiologic murmur. Innocent murmurs are usually not associated with a diastolic murmur, a thrill, abnormal electrocardiogram (ECG) or chest x-ray, cyanosis, or other symptoms of heart disease. Although innocent murmurs usually begin around 3 to 4 years of age, they also may be heard in the newborn period.

COMMON DIAGNOSTIC TESTS

Pulse Oximetry

Pulse oximetry is used to verify and document the degree of central cyanosis and is an accurate way to assess arterial oxygen saturation, especially in infants. Using pulse oximetry to screen newborns in the well infant and intermediate care nurseries for critical CHD has now been recommended in the United States.[3,4] Pulse oximetry readings from the right hand and one foot (together or in sequence), taken on the second day of life before discharge, and using a motion tolerant pulse oximeter approved by the U.S. Food and Drug Administration are recommended. Box 7-1 presents the criteria for a positive result for pulse oximetry screening. A positive screening result is defined as any identified low oxygen level, and requires follow-up with a comprehensive history and physical examination to determine the cause of hypoxia. Critical CHD is excluded using a diagnostic echocardiogram, and it should be read and interpreted by a pediatric cardiologist.

Pulse oximetry is also commonly used to monitor oxygen saturations in children with known cardiac disease. Infants and children who

TABLE 7-2 PHYSIOLOGIC OR INNOCENT MURMURS

Murmur	Characteristics/Evaluation	Age of Occurrence
Still's murmur	Localized between LLSB and apex Grade 1-3/6 systolic ejection (outflow murmur), decreasing with inspiration, when upright, or disappearing with Valsalva maneuver Low frequency, vibratory, musical in quality Often confused with VSD murmur	Most commonly heard at 2-7 years old
Peripheral pulmonic stenosis (PPS)	Also known as *newborn pulmonary flow murmur* Heard at LUSB with radiation to back, axillae Grade 1-2/6 systolic ejection, crescendo-decrescendo	Often heard in premature infants, infants with low birth weight, and infants up to 4 months of age Need to document resolution by 4-5 months of age to rule out organic cause or valve involvement
Pulmonary ejection	Well localized to LUSB Grade 1-3/6 systolic ejection crescendo-decrescendo Heard loudest when supine and decreases or disappears with Valsalva maneuver Does not radiate Similar to ASD murmur, but S_2 is normal	Common in 8- to 14-year-olds with greatest frequency in adolescents
Venous hum	Heard best just below clavicles at either RUSB or LUSB Grade 1-3/6 low-frequency continuous murmur Loudest when sitting, diminishes or disappears when supine; can be increased by turning patient's head away from the side of the murmur, and can be obliterated by light jugular vein compression; can be mistaken for PDA	Common in 3- to 6-year-olds
Supraclavicular carotid bruit	Heard above the right or left clavicle with radiation to the neck Grade 1-3/6 holosystolic, crescendo-decrescendo Decreases or diminishes with shoulder hyperextension Can be confused with murmur of aortic stenosis	Common at any age

Data from Park M: *Pediatric cardiology for practitioners*, ed 5, St. Louis, 2008, Mosby.
ASD, Atrial septal defect; *LLSB*, left lower sternal border; *LUSB*, left upper sternal border; *PDA*, patent ductus arteriosus; *RUSB*, right upper sternal border; *VSD*, ventricular septal defect.

have complex cyanotic heart defects in which blood mixes in a common ventricle, or who are dependent on a surgically placed aorta-to-pulmonary artery shunt to supply pulmonary blood flow, normally have oxygen saturation levels between 75% and 85%. It is important to know an infant's baseline oxygen saturation to accurately assess their oxygen status. Pulse oximeters are increasingly being used at home to monitor changes in oxygen saturation in infants with hypoplastic left heart syndrome (HLHS) as part of home surveillance programs.[5,6]

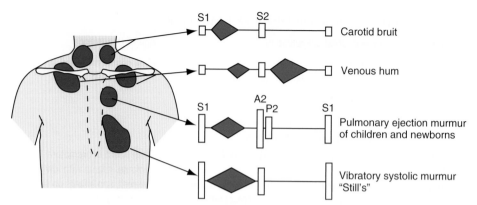

FIGURE 7-9 Anatomical locations of physiologic murmurs. (Adapted from Park M: *Pediatric cardiology for practitioners*, ed 5, St. Louis, 2008, Mosby, p. 37.)

BOX 7-1   CRITERIA FOR A POSITIVE PULSE OXIMETRY SCREENING RESULT

- Any oxygen saturation measure <90%
- Any oxygen saturation <95% in both extremities on three measures taken 1 hour apart
- Greater than 3% absolute difference between readings in the upper extremity (right hand) and lower extremity (foot) on three measures taken 1 hour apart (e.g., 96% right hand and 93% foot, or 88% right hand and 92% foot)

Data from Kemper AR et al: Strategies for implementing screening for critical congenital heart disease, *Pediatrics* 128(5):e1259-1267, 2011.

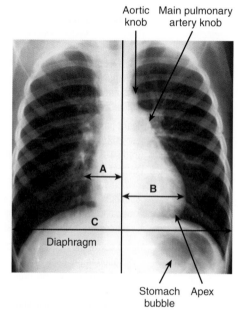

FIGURE 7-10 Anatomical landmarks for chest radiographs. (Adapted from Zitelli BJ, McIntire SC, Nowalk AJ: *Zitelli and Davis' atlas of pediatric physical diagnosis*, ed 6, Philadelphia, 2012, Elsevier; Park M: *Pediatric cardiology for practitioners*, ed 5, St. Louis, 2008, Mosby, p. 66.)

Chest X-Ray

A chest x-ray is helpful in determining overall heart size and shape, enlargement of specific heart chambers, size and position of the great vessels, degree of pulmonary blood flow, and abdominal situs. Heart size is determined by comparing the width of the cardiac silhouette at its widest diameter to the width of the chest at its maximal internal dimension (Figure 7-10). This is referred to as the cardiothoracic (CT) ratio. A CT ratio greater than 0.65 is considered cardiomegaly.[2] It is important to have a good inspiratory x-ray, because one taken on expiration may make the heart appear larger than it is. Thymic tissue in newborns also may distort the normal cardiac silhouette, giving the false impression of cardiomegaly.

The position of the cardiac apex provides information about ventricular enlargement. Normally, the apex points down and to the left.

An upward turned apex is indicative of right ventricular enlargement, whereas an apex that is pushed more downward and leftward than normal is caused by left ventricular enlargement. The *main pulmonary artery* (MPA) is normally seen as a small knob at the LUSB (see Figure 7-10). The prominence or absence of this shadow provides clues about the size, position, and presence of the MPA.[2]

Pulmonary vascular markings provide important information about the degree of pulmonary blood flow and should be noted as normal, increased, or decreased. It is also important to note the heart size and shape, position of the heart apex, and determination of abdominal situs. The location of the cardiac apex is normally on the left and should be on the same side as the stomach bubble and opposite the liver shadow. When these structures are misaligned (with the stomach bubble on the right and the apex on the left), or the liver is midline, then heterotaxy or situs abnormality is present, which is often associated with serious heart defects.

Electrocardiogram

An ECG provides information about the rhythm, conduction, and forces of contraction in the heart and is particularly useful in the diagnosis of arrhythmias and ventricular hypertrophy. However, ECG patterns vary within diagnostic groups, and it is entirely possible for an ECG to be normal in infants with serious heart disease such as in transposition of the great arteries (TGA). **Therefore, except for arrhythmias, ECGs are used most often to confirm a diagnosis of structural CHD as opposed to establishing one.**

Echocardiogram

Cardiac ultrasound, or *echocardiogram,* has become the primary diagnostic tool for patients suspected of having CHD. An echocardiogram can be done safely and noninvasively in the outpatient setting or at the bedside and provides accurate information for all age groups including premature infants. The addition of Doppler ultrasound and three-dimensional (3-D) techniques now make it possible to evaluate valve anatomy, function, and flow patterns throughout the heart and proximal vessels. This is particularly useful in quantifying degrees of shunting and obstruction. Advances in technical resolution have made fetal cardiac echocardiography an accepted prenatal evaluation tool for parents with a family history of CHD or other risk factors. Echocardiograms are expensive, however, and should only be ordered by a cardiologist after a thorough evaluation has been done to determine whether one is warranted. All referrals to a cardiologist should be as complete as possible and include data about the history, physical examination, chest x-ray, ECG, and oxygen saturation that have raised suspicion of CHD. Table 7-3 presents the common tests used to diagnose CHD.

CARDIAC SYMPTOMS

Arrhythmias and Palpitations

It is not unusual for children to complain of skipped heartbeats, a fast heart rate, or extra heartbeats. Most complaints are benign in origin, but a history of chest pain, light-headedness, or syncope can be indicative of a serious arrhythmia.[2] Family history should be directed toward any structural heart disease or history of sudden death, and the patient history should include any association of symptoms with exercise, food intake (especially caffeine), medications (especially cough preparations), or specific positioning. Physical findings, except the arrhythmia, are usually not present. Evaluation begins with an ECG. Documentation of the rhythm on an ECG is essential for determining diagnosis and treatment; however, obtaining this documentation can be challenging, especially if the symptoms are infrequent. For a complete evaluation, referral to a pediatric cardiologist or electrophysiologist is essential, and if the symptoms persist or worsen, additional testing with continuous Holter monitoring or event recording is recommended.

TABLE 7-3   OVERVIEW OF COMMON DIAGNOSTIC TESTS IN CHD

Test	Applications/Specific Modalities
Chest x-ray	Information on heart size and shape, enlargement of cardiac chambers, size and position of the great vessels, degree of pulmonary blood flow, position of abdominal organs
Electrocardiogram (ECG)	Graphic measure of electrical activity with information on rhythm, conduction, and force of contraction, chamber hypertrophy **Holter:** 24-hour continuous ECG recording used to assess arrhythmias
Echocardiogram	Noninvasive imaging using high frequency ultrasound to assess cardiac structures and ventricular function **Transthoracic echocardiogram (TTE):** Transducer is on the chest, most common. Infants and toddlers may need sedation for full study. • *M-mode:* one-dimensional graphic display to estimate chamber size and ventricular function, assess valve motion and pericardial fluid • *2-D:* real-time cross-sectional images to assess cardiac anatomy • *3-D:* imaging primarily to assess valve anatomy • *Doppler:* demonstrates blood flow patterns and pressure gradients **Transesophageal echocardiogram (TEE):** Transducer placed in esophagus to obtain images of posterior cardiac structures, used in patients with poor thoracic imaging. Widely used in the operating room after cardiac surgical repairs. Patient must be sedated or under general anesthesia. **Fetal:** Images fetal cardiac structures in utero
Cardiac MRI	Provides real time 3-D imaging and measurement of intracardiac structures and extracardiac vascular anatomy, assesses function • Often used in adolescents or young adults with limited imaging by echo. Takes an hour or more in a confined magnet • Children younger than 8 years of age or those with claustrophobia or anxiety may need anesthesia or sedation
Exercise (stress) test	Monitors heart rate, blood pressure, ECG, oxygen saturation, oxygen consumption and presence of symptoms (i.e., chest pain, dizziness) at rest and with progressive exercise on bicycle or treadmill • Done with physician supervision, emergency equipment available • 6-minute walk test: Assess maximum distance walked in 6 minutes while monitoring heart rate and oxygen saturation; used in patients with severe exercise limitations or those with pulmonary HTN
Cardiac catheterization	Invasive imaging modality using radiopaque catheters placed in peripheral vessels (femoral access most common) and advanced into the heart to visualize cardiac structures, measure chamber pressures and oxygen levels, and assess blood flow patterns **Hemodynamics:** Assessment of pressures and oxygen levels in cardiac chambers **Angiography:** Injection of contrast material to image heart structures and flow patterns under fluoroscopy **Biopsy:** Bioptome catheters used to obtain tiny samples of heart muscle for microscopic examination; used to assess for infection, inflammation or muscle dysfunction disorders, and post-transplant rejection **Electrophysiology:** Special catheters with electrodes used to record electrical activity from inside the heart and assess rhythm abnormalities

CHD, Congenital heart disease; *HTN*, hypertension; *MRI*, magnetic resonance imaging.

Syncope

Syncope is a common complaint in older children and adolescents (especially adolescent females).[2] It is usually characterized by a loss of consciousness, falling, and then a quick recovery once the child or adolescent is lying down. The episodes are usually preceded by dizziness, light-headedness, pallor, weakness, blurred vision, or cold sweats. The majority of syncopal events are benign, but a careful evaluation is always warranted, because it may be the first symptom of serious cardiac, neurologic, or metabolic disease. Syncope is unusual in children less than 6 years of age unless it is related to seizures, breath-holding, or cardiac arrhythmias.[2] The most common neurological cause is a seizure disorder, and possible metabolic causes include hypoglycemia, electrolyte imbalance, or profound anemia. In toddlers, the causes include breath-holding, and in adolescents, hyperventilation.

Cardiac etiologies include vasovagal syncope, which is also called *simple syncope* and is the most common. Arrhythmias, long QT syndrome, and *hypertrophic cardiomyopathy* (HCM) are additional cardiac causes of syncope. Information gathering should include careful details of the event and a family history of similar events or sudden cardiac death. Medication history and past medical history are important to elicit. Often the only evidence of HCM on physical examination may be the increased intensity of a cardiac murmur from supine to standing. If the neurological examination is negative, an ECG should be obtained, and referral to a cardiologist is warranted if there is a family history of sudden death, cardiomyopathy, murmur, and or abnormal ECG.[2]

Chest Pain

Chest pain in children is a common complaint causing anxiety in both patients and their parents. However, chest pain due to a cardiac cause is rare, occurring in less than 4% of cases.[2,7] The most common causes of chest pain are musculoskeletal (including muscle strain and trauma), pulmonary (especially asthma or illnesses associated with coughing), gastrointestinal (esophagitis or gastroesophageal reflux), or psychogenic (less often in children <12 years of age but more frequent in adolescent females).[2]

A careful history is instrumental in leading to a diagnosis. It is important to elicit the onset and duration of the pain, how long the child has been experiencing pain, and review sports activities or injuries that may have preceded the onset of chest pain. Document the severity, location, and radiation of the pains. Is the pain related to breathing or activity, does it occur with exercise or at rest? Ascertain factors that improve the pain and those that make it worse. Is the chest pain accompanied by palpitations or syncope? Has the child had a fever or recent illness? Chest pain with exertion, associated with dizziness or fainting, and chest pain that radiates to the back, jaw, or left arm could be indicative of cardiac disease and requires prompt evaluation by a cardiologist. A family history of sudden death, CHD, cardiomyopathy, or a hypercoagulable state is concerning for cardiac disease. Chest pain associated with fever may have an infectious cause. Illicit drug use, particularly cocaine, can cause myocardial ischemia with chest pain as a presenting symptom.

The physical exam should note the child or adolescent's color, perfusion, pulses, respiratory effort, and degree of acute pain. Auscultation includes the evaluation of breath sounds and their symmetry, as well as the identification of abnormal heart sounds, murmurs, rubs, gallops, or muffled heart sounds. If an acute chest pain of cardiac origin is suspected, an ECG should be obtained along with a referral to a pediatric cardiologist.

Cardiac origins of chest pain include ischemic causes (coronary artery abnormalities or cardiomyopathies), inflammatory conditions such as pericarditis or myocarditis, and arrhythmias. *Costochondritis* is an inflammation of the chest wall causing sharp, short, and well-localized pain that can be reproduced with pressure on palpation. *Pericarditis,* an inflammation of the pericardium, is characterized by chest pain that is worse lying down and improves with sitting and leaning forward.[2]

CARDIOVASCULAR DISEASE

Cardiovascular disease in children is normally divided into two categories: congenital or acquired. Congenital heart disease comprises the majority of cardiovascular disorders in the pediatric population. CHD is not a singular entity, but rather a myriad of structural anomalies in the heart that develop during fetal life and thus present at birth. Acquired heart disease (Kawasaki disease, hypertrophic cardiomyopathy, myocardial infections, rheumatic fever, hypertension) occurs after birth and develops during an individual's lifetime.

Congenital Heart Disease

CHD is prevalent in at least 10 per 1000 live births, with 40% of these malformations diagnosed during a child's first year of life.[8] Maternal infections such as rubella, coxsackie virus, and other viruses contracted during pregnancy can be associated with CHD or myocarditis. Medications, alcohol, and other drugs may act as teratogens on the developing fetus. Maternal medical conditions associated with an increased risk of the fetus developing CHD include diabetes mellitus (cardiomyopathy, transposition of the great vessels) and systemic lupus erythematosus (congenital heart block).[2] Common presentations of CHD are presented in Table 7-4.

CHD is caused by the interaction between genetic and environmental factors, with single gene mutations accounting for 3% of CHD, gross chromosomal anomalies accounting for 5%, environmental factors (rubella, fetal alcohol syndrome, other maternal illness/infections) accounting for 3%, and multifactorial genetic random event mediation for the remainder.[1] Genetic etiologies include genetic syndromes, deletion/duplication syndromes, and both syndromic and non-syndromic single gene disorders (i.e., *NKX2.5*). At least one or more additional congenital malformations can be found in 20% to 30% of infants with CHD.[1] Although knowledge and understanding of the role of genetics in CHD has advanced significantly, it is still an evolving science and current data can change or become outdated quickly. Table 7-5 presents

TABLE 7-4	COMMON PRESENTATIONS OF CONGENITAL HEART DISEASE		
Presentation	Physiology	Signs and Symptoms	Potential Diagnoses
Cyanosis (infants)	• Central, arterial (vs. peripheral) desaturation • Desaturated blood mixes with saturated blood in the heart due to right-to-left shunting	• Bluish or deeply ruddy color around mouth/lips • Usually not visible unless O_2 saturations are <85% • O_2 saturations for infants with cyanotic heart disease are normally 75%-85% • Supplemental O_2 will not raise saturations to normal levels of 95%-100% • Hct usually higher than normal • Cyanosis not evident if patient is anemic and will be greater with polycythemia • Can be tachypneic without respiratory distress	• TOF • PA

TABLE 7-4	COMMON PRESENTATIONS OF CONGENITAL HEART DISEASE—CONT'D		
Presentation	**Physiology**	**Signs and Symptoms**	**Potential Diagnoses**
Congestive heart failure (CHF)	• Heart is unable to meet metabolic demands (output) of the body • Etiologies can be both cardiac and noncardiac related	• Tachycardia • Tachypnea with or without respiratory distress (grunting, wheezing, rales) • Cough, wheezing, rales (older children) • Gallop rhythm • Hepatomegaly (liver palpable >2 cm below right costal heart margin) • Peripheral edema plus hepato-megaly (older children) • Pallor due to vasoconstriction • Poor feeding, failure to thrive (infants) • Sweating, especially on fore-head, during feeding (infants) • Anorexia, somnolence (older children) • Frequent respiratory infections • Fatigue, exercise intolerance, inability to keep up with peers	• VSD • HCM • Decreased ventricular function post-CHD surgical repair or intervention • Arrhythmia • Myocardial infection • Anemia
Shock	• Severe obstruction of blood flow out of the heart • Can occur suddenly in newborn infants with undetected coarctation of the aorta or interrupted aortic arch when the PDA closes at 2-3 weeks of age	• Hypotension • Extreme pallor • Poor ventricular function, circulation • Hypovolemia • Weak pulses • Poor urine output	• Coarctation of the aorta • Interrupted aortic arch

CHD, Congenital heart disease; *HCM,* hypertrophic cardiomyopathy; *PA,* pulmonary atresia; *PDA,* patent ductus arteriosus; *TOF,* tetralogy of Fallot; *VSD,* ventricular septal defect.

some examples of the more common syndromes associated with CHD diagnoses.

Common Presentations of Congenital Heart Disease

Cyanosis in Infants
Cyanosis indicative of CHD is due to arterial desaturation and may not be visible unless the oxygen saturation is 85% or less.[1,2] Arterial desaturation or *central cyanosis* is best detected in the perioral area, the mucous membranes of the mouth, the lips, and the gums. Central cyanosis should be distinguished from *peripheral cyanosis,* which can occur in a cold environment, and *acrocyanosis,* which in newborns is due to sluggish circulation in the fingers and toes.[1]

TABLE 7-5   COMMON PEDIATRIC SYNDROMES ASSOCIATED WITH CONGENITAL HEART DISEASE

Type	Clinical Entity	% CHD	Associated CHD Diagnosis
Chromosomal	Trisomy 21 (Down syndrome)	40-50	AVSD, VSD, ASD, PDA, TOF
	Deletion 22q11 (DiGeorge syndrome; velocardiofacial syndrome)	75	IAA-B, TA, aortic arch abnormalities, TOF, VSD
	Deletion 7q11.23 (Williams-Beuren syndrome)	50-85	Supravalvar AS and PS, PPS
	Deletion 20p12 (Alagille syndrome)	85-94	PPS, pulmonary artery hypoplasia, PS, TOF
	Turner syndrome (45 XO)	25-35	CoA, BAV, valvar AS, aortic dissection, mitral atresia, HLHS
Single gene disorders	CHARGE (Hall-Hittner syndrome)	60-90	Conotruncal malformations, ASD, VSD, PDA
	Holt-Oram syndrome	75	Secundum ASD, VSD, progressive AV conduction delay
	LEOPARD syndrome	85	PS, HCM, rhythm abnormalities
	Marfan syndrome	80	Ascending aorta dilation/ dissection, MVP, MPA dilation

Data from Ruppel K: Disorders of the cardiovascular system. In Rudolph C et al: *Rudolph's pediatrics*, ed 22, New York, 2011, McGraw-Hill.

AS, Aortic stenosis; *ASD*, atrial septal defect; *AV*, atrioventricular; *AVSD*, atrioventricular septal defect; *BAV*, bicuspid aortic valve; *CoA*, coarctation of the aorta; *HCM*, hypertrophic cardiomyopathy; *HLHS*, hypoplastic left heart syndrome; *IAA-B*, interrupted aortic arch type B; *MPA*, main pulmonary artery; *MVP*, mitral valve prolapse; *PDA*, patent ductus arteriosus; *PPS*, peripheral pulmonic stenosis; *PS*, pulmonic stenosis; *TOF*, tetralogy of Fallot; *VSD*, ventricular septal defect.

PEDIATRIC PEARLS

The intensity of cyanosis is dependent on the concentration of desaturated hemoglobin and not on the actual arterial oxygen saturation.

An infant who has *polycythemia,* an abnormal increase in circulating erythrocytes, will appear more cyanotic than an infant who is anemic in the presence of the same degree of arterial desaturation. Therefore, it is important to follow a cyanotic infant's hemoglobin (Hgb) and hematocrit (Hct) levels, particularly at 2 to 3 months of age, the time of normal physiological anemia.

Congestive Heart Failure
CHF is the inability of the heart to adequately meet the metabolic demands of the body. It occurs in 15% to 25% of children with CHD, and about 40% of patients with cardiomyopathy can have CHF so severe that it results in death or the need for heart transplantation.[9] Causation can be related to both cardiac disease (VSD, AV septal defect, aortic stenosis, coarctation of the aorta, cardiomyopathy, myocarditis, arrhythmia, Kawasaki disease) and noncardiac disease (anemia, sepsis, hypoglycemia, and renal failure). This multiple causation of CHF manifests in a variety of clinical presentations that are usually age related. Infants most commonly present with pallor, tachycardia, tachypnea, poor feeding, FTT, and hepatomegaly. Older children are often unable to keep up with their peers, and may exhibit peripheral edema, hepatomegaly, anorexia, and respiratory symptoms such as cough, wheezing, and rales.[9]

Acquired Heart Disease

Hypertension (HTN)

HTN is increasing in children and adolescents in the United States, and is in part related to the increase in childhood obesity. HTN is more prevalent in non-Hispanic blacks and Mexican-American youth and occurs more often in males than females.[10] There is now evidence that blood pressure in childhood tracks into adulthood, so children who are hypertensive in their younger years are frequently hypertensive as adults.[11] Screening for HTN in childhood and effective management is aimed at decreasing the risk of cardiac disease in adulthood.

EVIDENCE-BASED PRACTICE TIP

HTN is more prevalent in non-Hispanic blacks and Mexican-American youth, and it occurs more often in males than females.[10]

EVIDENCE-BASED PRACTICE TIP

Both blood pressure and lipid levels track from childhood to adulthood. Elevated blood pressure and elevated lipid levels in childhood frequently remain elevated in adulthood.[10,11]

The definition of HTN is derived from blood pressure percentile tables that are based on gender, age, and height[12] (Table 7-6). Chapter 2 reviews the proper method for obtaining blood pressure measurements, and both the systolic and diastolic values are of equal importance.

HTN can be classified as primary (without a clear cause) or secondary to an underlying disorder (often related to renal or vascular disease). In secondary HTN, treatment of the underlying cause can cure the HTN. Secondary HTN has a higher incidence in prepubertal children and likely underlies the more severe or stage 2 HTN. Primary HTN is more often seen in older school-age children and adolescents and is often associated with excess weight, obesity, and a positive family history of HTN.[10]

The goal of HTN screening is to identify children and adolescents with HTN and distinguish between primary and secondary causes. Evaluation of HTN includes a comprehensive history and physical examination, as well as baseline laboratory studies including complete blood count, serum electrolytes, blood urea nitrogen, creatinine, lipids, glucose, and urinalysis. Renal and cardiac ultrasounds are performed to assess for secondary causes or to document end-organ involvement such as increased left ventricular mass.

TABLE 7-6   CLASSIFICATIONS OF HYPERTENSION

Classification	Criteria
Normal	Both systolic and diastolic BP are <90th percentile
Pre-hypertension	Systolic and/or diastolic BP ≥90th percentile but <95th percentile OR BP exceeds 120/80 mm Hg
Hypertension	Systolic and/or diastolic BP measures ≥95th percentile measured on three separate occasions
	Stage 1 hypertension: Systolic and/or diastolic BP falls between 95th percentile and 5 mm Hg above 99th percentile
	Stage 2 hypertension: Systolic and/or diastolic BP ≥99th percentile + 5 mm Hg

Data from National High Blood Pressure Education Program Working Group on High Blood Pressure in Children and Adolescents: The fourth report on the diagnosis, evaluation, and treatment of high blood pressure in children and adolescents, *Pediatrics* 114(2 Suppl 4th report):555-576, 2004.
BP, Blood pressure.

It is also important to identify those with other risk factors for premature atherosclerosis such as HTN, smoking, overweight/obesity, dyslipidemia, family history of premature cardiovascular disease, diabetes, and chronic renal disease. The target blood pressure for children with other cardiovascular risk factors is a systolic and diastolic blood pressure <90%[12] (Table 7-6).

Dyslipidemia

Recent evidence supports the correlation between lipid disorders in childhood and the onset and severity of atherosclerosis in children and young adults.[10] Like HTN, elevated lipid levels track from childhood to adulthood. In the past, children with a strong family history of lipid disorders or premature cardiovascular disease were screened for lipid disorders, but the increase in childhood obesity has contributed to a larger population of children at risk for dyslipidemia. Dyslipidemia, genetic factors, and childhood obesity are contributing factors to coronary artery atherosclerosis along with diabetes, nephrotic syndrome, chronic renal disease, post-cardiac transplant, history of Kawasaki disease with aneurysms, and chronic inflammatory disease.

Lipid screening is now recommended for all children at 9 to 11 years of age, and selective screening is advised for children over the age of 2 years who have a family history of high cholesterol or early heart disease in a first- or second-degree relative, or who have individual health risk factors.[10] The initial screen can be either a fasting lipid profile or a nonfasting blood test measuring total cholesterol and high-density lipoprotein (HDL) cholesterol. Non-HDL cholesterol level is then calculated from these two values (non-HDL cholesterol = total cholesterol − HDL cholesterol).[10] Normal values are a non-HDL cholesterol value less than 145 mg/dL with an HDL cholesterol above 40 mg/dL. If the non-HDL cholesterol is abnormal, children should have a fasting lipid profile and further evaluation and follow-up.

SUMMARY OF EXAMINATION

- Obtain a thorough history, including gestational history, birth history, family history, and any presenting symptoms.
- Routine cardiac assessment begins with evaluation of growth with weight, height, head circumference (infants), and body mass index.
- Assess temperature, heart rate, respiratory rate, color, activity level, and oxygen saturation *when indicated.*
- Accurately assess blood pressure in all children whenever possible and definitely once in infancy and routinely from 3 years of age and up using the National High Blood Pressure Education Program percentile tables (see Table 7-6).
- Approach the examination systematically, starting from the periphery and moving inward and upward towards the chest.
- Assess color, perfusion, and pulses in upper and lower extremities.
- Palpate liver edge for enlargement and position. NOTE: 1 to 2 cm below the right costal margin is normal in infants.
- Inspect for head and neck for signs of any syndromes; inspect the chest for scars, signs of respiratory distress, and pectus excavatum.
- Palpate cardiac area for any heaves and presence of a thrill.
- Auscultate lungs for quality of breath sounds, any wheezing, grunting, or rales.
- Auscultate systematically through the four precordial areas (see Figure 7-7) moving from LLSB to apex listening for *first heard sound* to the LUSB listening for *second heart sound*, noting variation with respiration and any *third* or *fourth heart sounds* or *ejection clicks.*

- Findings of tachypnea, respiratory distress, tachycardia, bradycardia, low oxygen saturation with pallor or hypoperfusion, hepatomegaly, and syncope require immediate further evaluation and consultation.
- Diagnostic chest x-ray and ECG are performed *as indicated.*

- Refer to cardiology for further evaluation *as indicated* by examination findings, diagnostic results, or parental anxiety/concern and before echocardiogram.

Charting

1-Month-Old Infant with Murmur

Cardiac: Increased RV (right ventricular) impulse, normal S_1, split S_2, 2-3/6 low frequency SEM (systolic ejection murmur) heard best at lower left sternal border. No diastolic murmur, extra heart sounds, thrill, or clicks.

REFERENCES

1. Clyman R, Hoffman J, Gutgesell HP, et al: Newborn (section 5) and disorders of the cardiovascular system (section 26). In Rudolph C, Rudolph AM, Lister G, First L, Gershon A (editors), *Rudolph's pediatrics*, ed 22, New York, 2011, McGraw-Hill.
2. Park M: *Pediatric cardiology for practitioners*, ed 5, St. Louis, 2008, Mosby/Elsevier.
3. Kemper AR, Mahle WT, Martin GR, et al: Strategies for implementing screening for critical congenital heart disease, *Pediatrics* 128 (5):e1259-1267, 2011.
4. Mahle WT, Sable CA, Matherne PG, et al: On behalf of the American Heart Association Congenital Heart Defects Committee of the Council on Cardiovascular Disease in the Young. Key concepts in the evaluation of screening approaches for heart disease in children and adolescents: a science advisory from the American Heart Association, *Circulation* 125:2796-2801, 2012.
5. Ghanayem NS, Hoffman GM, Mussatto, KA, et al: Home surveillance program prevents interstage mortality after the Norwood procedure, *J Thorac Cardiovasc Surg* 126(5): 1367-77, 2003.
6. Petit CJ, Fraser CD, Mattamal R, et al: The impact of a dedicated single-ventricle home monitoring program on interstage somatic growth, interstage attrition and 1-year survival, *J Thorac Cardiovasc Surg* 142:1358-66, 2011.
7. Saleeb SF, Li WYV, Warren SZ, et al: Effectiveness of screening for life-threatening chest pain in children, *Pediatrics* 128:e1062-e1068, 2011.
8. Pierpoint ME, Basson CT, Benson DW, et al: Genetic basis for congenital heart defects: current knowledge (AHA Scientific Statement), *Circulation* 115: 3015-3038, 2007.
9. Madriago E, Silverbach M: Heart failure in infants and children, *Pediatr Rev* 31(1): 4-11, 2010.
10. Danielson SR et al: National Heart Lung and Blood Institute, Expert panel on integrated guidelines for cardiovascular health and risk reduction in children and adolescents: summary report, *Pediatrics* 128(Suppl 5):S212-S256, 2011.
11. Chen X, Wang Y: Tracking of blood pressure from childhood to adulthood: a systematic review and meta-regression analysis, *Circulation* 117(25): 3171-3180, 2008.
12. National High Blood Pressure Education Program Working Group on High Blood Pressure in Children and Adolescents: The fourth report on the diagnosis, evaluation, and treatment of high blood pressure in children and adolescents, *Pediatrics* 114(2 Suppl 4th Report):555-576, 2004

CHAPTER 8

CHEST AND RESPIRATORY SYSTEM

Concettina (Tina) Tolomeo

EMBRYOLOGICAL DEVELOPMENT

Knowledge of lung development is critical when performing a respiratory assessment in early childhood, especially in a newborn infant who is born preterm. This information along with an understanding of respiratory anatomy and physiology will provide you with a foundation for interpreting pulmonary symptoms.

Lung development begins in utero at approximately 4 weeks' gestation. It occurs in five stages: embryonic, pseudoglandular, canalicular, saccular, and alveolar. During the embryonic phase, the lungs form from a sac on the ventral wall of the alimentary canal. Right and left branches form through budding and dividing. During the pseudoglandular stage, branching of the lung bud occurs, as the trachea, bronchi, and bronchioles are formed by 16 to 17 weeks' gestation. During the canalicular stage, branching of the bronchioles continues and alveoli begin to form. By approximately 25 weeks, the number of bronchial generations with cartilage is the same as the adult lung. Growth of the pulmonary parenchyma and *surfactant* system occurs during the saccular phase. Maturation and expansion of the alveoli occur during the alveolar period and persist through early childhood.[1,2]

Breathing movements occur in utero. The movements are irregular, range from 30 to 70 breaths per minute, and become more frequent as gestation progresses. These movements are thought to train the respiratory muscles and promote lung development.[2] Fetal gas exchange occurs via the placenta. At birth, the lungs fill with air for the first time and take on the role of ventilation and oxygenation.

The fluid in the lungs moves into the tissues surrounding the alveoli and is absorbed into the lymphatic system. At this point, gas exchange occurs via diffusion across the alveolar-pulmonary capillary membranes.[1,2]

ANATOMY AND PHYSIOLOGY

Thorax

The thorax is the bony cage that surrounds the heart, great vessels, lungs, major airways, and esophagus.[3] It is composed of the sternum and ribs (Figure 8-1). The *sternum* is a flat, narrow bone made up of three parts, the *manubrium,* the body, and the *xiphoid process.*[4] The *manubrium* is roughly triangular and attaches to the body of the sternum; the angle at which the manubrium and body meet is termed the *manubriosternal angle* or the *angle of Louis.* This angle is in line with the second rib and therefore serves as an important landmark. The *xiphoid process* is the small, thin, cartilaginous end of the sternum, which varies greatly in shape and prominence in infants and children because of the influence of heredity, intrauterine environment, and nutrition. It sits at the level of T9.[4,5] *Pectus carinatum,* pigeon breast, is the abnormal protrusion of the xiphoid process and sternum, and *pectus excavatum,* funnel chest, is the abnormal depression of the sternum[6,7] (Figure 8-2). The chest cavity is divided, with the middle portion known as the *mediastinum.*

There are 12 pairs of ribs; the first 7 pairs attach anteriorly via their corresponding costal cartilages to the sternum. Ribs 8, 9, and 10 are attached to the costal cartilage on the rib above

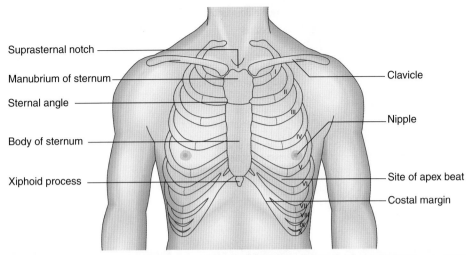

Suprasternal notch

Manubrium of sternum

Sternal angle

Body of sternum

Xiphoid process

Clavicle

Nipple

Site of apex beat

Costal margin

FIGURE 8-1 Anatomy of the rib cage and thorax. (From Revest P: *Medical sciences*, Edinburgh, 2009, Saunders Ltd.)

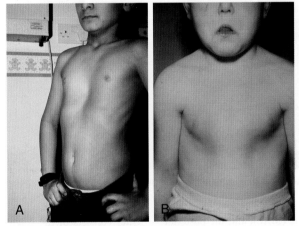

FIGURE 8-2 **A,** Pectus excavatum. **B,** Pectus carinatum. (**A,** From Chaudry B, Harvey D: *Mosby's color atlas and text of pediatrics and child health,* St. Louis, 2001, Mosby. **B,** From Lissauer T, Clayden G: *Illustrated textbook of paediatrics,* ed 2, St. Louis, 2001, Mosby.)

them; ribs 11 and 12 do not attach anteriorly and are known as floating ribs. All 12 pairs of ribs attach posteriorly to the thoracic vertebrae. The diaphragm sits at the bottom of the rib cage and is the major muscle of respiration. There are 11 intercostal muscles anteriorly and posteriorly and 8 thoracic muscles, all of which help to increase the volume of the rib cage with inspiration and decrease the thoracic volume with expiration[3-5] (Figure 8-3).

The following landmarks are often used in describing the location of physical findings of the chest: the midsternal line (MSL), which runs down the middle of the sternum; the midclavicular line (MCL), located on the right and left sides of the chest, runs parallel to the MSL and through the middle of the clavicles (midway between the jugular notch and acromion) bilaterally. Laterally, there are three lines on each side, the anterior axillary line (AAL),

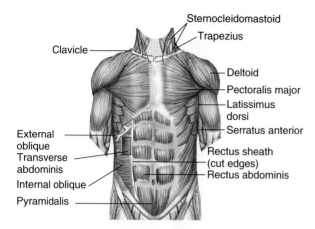

Sternocleidomastoid

Trapezius

Clavicle

Deltoid

Pectoralis major

Latissimus dorsi

Serratus anterior

External oblique

Transverse abdominis

Internal oblique

Pyramidalis

Rectus sheath (cut edges)

Rectus abdominis

FIGURE 8-3 Anterior thoracic muscles.

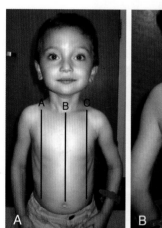
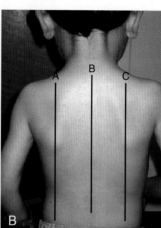
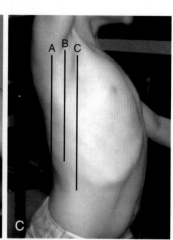

FIGURE 8-4 Anatomical landmarks of the chest. **A,** Anterior chest. **B,** Posterior chest. **C,** Lateral chest.

the midaxillary line (MAL), and the posterior axillary line (PAL). The AAL begins at the anterior axillary folds, the MAL begins at the middle of the axilla, and the PAL begins at the posterior axillary folds. Posteriorly is the vertebral line that runs down the middle of the spine and the scapular line, which runs down the inferior angle of each scapula[4,5] (Figure 8-4).

Lower Respiratory Tract

The respiratory system is divided into two parts, the *upper respiratory tract* and the *lower respiratory tract*. The upper respiratory tract consists of the nasal cavity, pharynx, and larynx and is reviewed in Chapter 13. The *lower respiratory*

tract consists of the trachea, bronchi, bronchioles, alveolar ducts and sacs, and alveoli (Figure 8-5). The *trachea* is a tube that lies anterior to the esophagus. The distal end of the trachea splits into the right and left mainstem/primary *bronchi*. This bifurcation occurs at the level of T3 during infancy and childhood. By the time the child is an adult, this bifurcation occurs at T4 or T5. The right mainstem bronchus is shorter and more vertical than the left and, therefore, more susceptible to aspiration of foreign bodies in the young child. Beyond the bifurcation, the bronchi continue to branch into lobar/secondary bronchi. There are three branches on the right and two on the left; each branch supplies one of the lung lobes. These branches

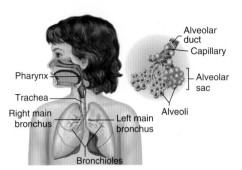

FIGURE 8-5 Lower respiratory tract.

further divide into segmental/tertiary smaller bronchi to supply each segment of the lungs and finally the terminal *bronchioles*. Ultimately, the respiratory tract terminates with the alveolar ducts, alveolar sacs, and alveoli where gas exchange takes place. The bronchial arteries branch from the aorta and supply blood to the lung parenchyma. The blood supply is returned primarily by the pulmonary veins.[1,3,5]

Lungs

The lungs are positioned in the lateral aspects of the thorax, separated by the heart and the mediastinal structures. The right lung has three lobes (upper, middle, and lower), and the left lung has two lobes (upper and lower). The *apex* is the top portion of the upper lobes, which extends above the clavicles. On the right side, the minor or horizontal fissure, located at the fourth rib, divides the right upper lobe (RUL) from the right middle lobe (RML). On the left side, there is a tongue-shaped projection that extends from the left upper lobe (LUL), called the *lingula*. Laterally, the right lower lobe (RLL) and the left lower lobe (LLL) occupy most of the lower lateral chest area. Only a small portion of the RML extends to the midaxillary line, and it does not go beyond that point. Posteriorly, the vertebral column helps in identifying the underlying lung lobes. T4 marks the inferior portion of the upper lobes and the superior portion of the lower lobes. The *base* is the bottom portion of the lower lobes and is marked by T10 or T12 depending on the phase of respiration.[4] The principle function of the

lungs is gas exchange between the atmosphere and the blood. Oxygen is carried into the lungs and carbon dioxide is eliminated. The lungs play a significant role in acid-base balance.

PHYSIOLOGICAL VARIATIONS

Table 8-1 presents variations in growth and development that impact the function of the respiratory system in the infant and young child.

SYSTEM-SPECIFIC HISTORY

Complete and accurate information gathering is essential when assessing an infant, child, or adolescent with respiratory symptoms (see the Information Gathering table). Questions should be open-ended and age-specific to allow the parent or caregiver the opportunity to give a full explanation of past and present concerns. In addition, always obtain information directly from the older child or adolescent when possible. Table 8-2 presents a symptom-focused assessment of respiratory conditions for children and adolescents.

EVIDENCE-BASED PRACTICE TIP

The Childhood Asthma Control Test (C-ACT) for children 4 to 11 years of age is a seven-item questionnaire that assesses asthma control over the previous 4 weeks. The first four questions are completed by the child and the last three by the parent/guardian. Each question has four response levels. The Asthma Control Test (ACT) for children 12 years of age and older is a five-item questionnaire that assesses asthma control over the previous 4 weeks. Each question has five response levels. Questions for both pertain to daytime and nighttime symptoms, activity limitations, use of short-acting beta agonists, and perception of asthma control. Both questionnaires have been validated to measure asthma control (well controlled, not well controlled, and very poorly controlled) in accordance with the National Heart, Lung, and Blood Institute's *Expert Panel Report 3: Guidelines for the Diagnosis and Management of Asthma.*[8] The questionnaires are available in print and Web format (www.asthmacontroltest.com) in a number of languages.

TABLE 8-1   PHYSIOLOGICAL VARIATIONS OF THE CHEST AND LUNGS

Age-Group	Physiological Variation
Preterm infant	Respiratory muscles are weak, poorly adapted for extrauterine life; periodic breathing occurs that is similar to fetal breathing; preterm infants become easily hypoxic and apnea occurs
Newborn	Diaphragm is flatter, more compliant; paradoxical breathing occurs in the neonate with inward movement of chest during inspiration; predominantly nose breathers until 4 weeks of age; chest circumference very close in size to head circumference at birth
Infancy	Smaller airways with increased resistance to airflow; rapid respiratory rate; minimal nasal mucus causes mild to moderate upper airway obstruction
Early childhood (1 year to 4 years of age)	Rapid growth and maturation of alveoli improve ventilation; respiratory rate decreases dramatically from newborn period
Middle childhood (5 years to 10 years of age)	Alveoli continue to increase in number; lung development is complete by 5-6 years of age
Adolescence	Alveolar size matures to adult capacity

TABLE 8-2   SYMPTOM-FOCUSED ASSESSMENT OF RESPIRATORY CONDITIONS

Symptom	Questions to Ask
Cough	History: Onset of cough symptoms? Was onset sudden or gradual? Coughing for how long? Is cough worsening or changing character? Is cough wet, dry, hacking, barking, whooping? Worse during day or at night? Worse with feeding, sleeping, running? Any other symptoms: Shortness of breath, chest pain/tightness, or wheeze? Choking episodes? History of aspiration (small toy, food, etc.)? Rhinorrhea or nasal congestion? In older child/adolescent: Is cough productive with sputum or nonproductive? Pattern: Occasional, persistent, or coughing spasms?
Wheeze	History: Onset of wheezing? Was onset sudden or gradually worsening? Any other symptoms: Cough? Shortness of breath? Chest pain/tightness? History of aspiration (small toy, food, etc.)? Pattern: Occasional, increase with exercise?
Shortness of breath	History: Onset of shortness of breath? Was onset sudden or gradual? Does it occur with activity or rest? Is it difficult to get air in, out, both? History of aspiration (small toy, food, etc.)? Accompanying symptoms of cough, wheezing? History of breath-holding spells, seizures?
Chest pain	History: Onset of chest pain? Was onset sudden or gradual? Is it difficult to get air in, out, or both? Chest pain occurs with movement or rest? Type of pain (sharp, dull)? Ask verbal child to point to area of pain. History of trauma or recent sports injury or weight lifting? Any other symptoms: Cough, wheezing, shortness of breath? Pattern: Occasional with respirations or persistent?

INFORMATION GATHERING FOR CHEST AND LUNG ASSESSMENT AT KEY DEVELOPMENTAL STAGES

Age-Group	Questions to Ask
Preterm infant	How many weeks' gestation? Admitted to newborn intensive care unit? Length of stay? Any episodes of apnea or tachypnea? Need for oxygen? Need for ventilation? For how long? Infant discharged to home on a ventilator/on oxygen? Infant discharged home on any medications? Any maternal substance abuse?
Newborn	How many weeks' gestation? Birth weight? Any birth complications? Meconium aspiration? Breathing problems at birth? Any episodes of apnea or tachypnea?
Infancy	History of respiratory infections as infant (respiratory syncytial virus [RSV], rhinovirus, etc.)? Frequent upper respiratory infections (URIs)? History of wheezing? Hospitalizations? History of intubations? History of eczema/skin allergy? In daycare? Immunization status? Frequent vomiting after feeds/"choking" episodes? Arches back after feeding?
Early childhood	History of apnea/breath-holding spells? Does child's speech have a nasal or congested sound? History of nasal congestion, chronic URIs, allergy symptoms, tonsillitis, frequent ear infections? In daycare or preschool? Does child frequently put objects in mouth/nose? Exposure to group A streptococcal infection? Does child snore at night? Exposure to ill contacts? Foreign travel/recent immigrant?
Middle childhood	History of nasal congestion, chronic rhinorrhea, sinusitis, tonsillitis, chronic URIs, recurrent pneumonia? Does child snore at night? Exposure to group A streptococcal infection? History of asthma? Exposure to ill contacts? Foreign travel or recent immigrant?
Adolescence	History of chronic URIs, allergic rhinitis/asthma, recurrent tonsillitis? History of oral sex? Tobacco use? How many cigarettes per day? Marijuana use? Any oral piercings?
Environmental risks	Year home was built? Location (inner city, suburb, rural, near highway/high traffic areas)? Is there a basement? Number of people in home? Anyone smoke in home? Pets in home? Type of heating system? Wood burning stove? Humidifier? Mold? Carpets? Drapes? Mice or roaches? Presence of chemicals/fumes in home or near home?

PHYSICAL ASSESSMENT

Equipment

When auscultating breath sounds, use the diaphragm of the stethoscope. The size of the stethoscope being used is extremely important when evaluating respiratory sounds. Stethoscopes with a smaller diaphragm should be used on infants and toddlers. Isolating cardiac and respiratory sounds is difficult in small children with too large a diaphragm, and using a diaphragm that is too small on adolescents or on children who are overweight or obese causes practitioners to miss findings of cardiac and respiratory sounds on auscultation.

Positioning

If possible, the child should sit upright for the respiratory assessment. Young children, especially toddlers, may be more relaxed on their parent's lap during the examination of the chest. Children should be allowed to help as much as possible during the exam. Have them hold the stethoscope in place once you position it in the appropriate location. Other techniques include letting children role-play by allowing them to listen to their parent, a doll, or stuffed animal.

School-age children are very curious. Therefore, explain what you will be doing during the exam and why, using developmentally appropriate vocabulary. Taking a few extra minutes to incorporate the child's developmental level into your exam will result in more thorough and reliable findings. In addition, pictures of lungs in the exam room can be helpful with older children when you are explaining what you are looking for and listening to during the examination.

PHYSICAL EXAMINATION

Pediatric health care providers should begin the physical examination by assessing the chest. The "quieter" parts of the exam, the cardiac and respiratory exam, require astute listening skills and less active participation of the child. Therefore, they are best performed first—an effective approach to assessing children among pediatric experts. The pediatric provider must take a systematic approach to examining the chest and use all the components of physical assessment. This includes inspection, palpation, percussion, and auscultation. Examination of the chest should always include both the anterior and the posterior chest.

A thorough assessment of the chest and lungs is not complete without examination of the upper airway and the extremities. Nasal passages should be examined for the appearance of the nasal turbinates as well as the presence of rhinitis, nasal secretions, nasal polyps, or a foreign body. When looking at the oropharynx, note the presence of postnasal drip and tonsillar size. Tonsillar size is often graded on a scale of 0 to 4+, where 0 indicates tonsils that fit in the tonsillar fossa and 4+ indicates tonsils that occupy >75% of the oropharyngeal width. An abnormal finding in any of these areas can be a cause of respiratory symptoms. Finally, you need to examine the extremities for signs of digital clubbing. *Clubbing* is the bulbous-shaped enlargement of the soft tissue of the distal phalanges (Figure 8-6). To assess for *clubbing,* ask the child to place the first phalange of each thumb together (nails facing each other). Normally, this position results in a diamond shape between

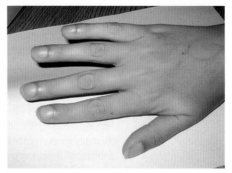

FIGURE 8-6 Digital clubbing.

the two thumbs. With clubbing, the diamond shape disappears and the space between the two thumbs is decreased or absent, depending on the degree of clubbing. Clubbing can be hereditary or can be the result of cardiac disease, respiratory disease, or severe malnutrition.

EVIDENCE-BASED PRACTICE TIP

Atopic dermatitis/eczema, rhinitis, and nasal mucosal swelling along with symptoms of airway reactivity increase the probability of a diagnosis of asthma.[9]

Inspection

Ideally, start the exam by visually inspecting the infant or child undressed from the waist up. This allows you to make general observations about the child's respiratory rate, breathing pattern, respiratory effort, accessory muscle use, inspiratory to expiratory ratio (I:E ratio), skin color, presence of noisy breathing, chest symmetry, and chest shape. In an irritable, ill, or fearful child, observation of respiratory pattern and rate may be the most helpful part of the examination if the child exhibits resistance to auscultation.

Assess the shape of the chest and note any abnormalities. The normal anterior-posterior (AP) to transverse ratio is 1:2. In the infant, the chest is round with a diameter roughly equal to the head circumference until 2 years of age and has a 1:1 AP/transverse ratio, giving a barrel chest appearance. As the child grows, the chest takes on the shape of the adult chest.[4,6] A barrel

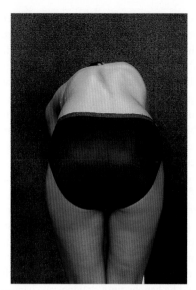

FIGURE 8-7 Scoliosis. (From Zitelli B, Davis H: *Atlas of pediatric physical diagnosis,* ed 5, St. Louis, 2007, Mosby.)

TABLE 8-3	EXPECTED RANGE OF RESPIRATORY RATES FOR AGE
Age	Rate
Preterm neonate	40-70
0 to 12 months	24-55
1 to 5 years	20-30
5 to 9 years	18-25
9 to 12 years	16-22
12 years and older	12-20

Data from Hughes DM: Evaluating the respiratory system. In Goldbloom RB: *Pediatric clinical skills,* ed 4, Philadelphia, 2011, Elsevier/Saunders; Hartman ME, Cheifetz IM: Pediatric emergencies and resuscitation. In Kleigman RM, Stanton BD, St. Geme JW, Schor NF, Behrman: *Nelson textbook of pediatrics,* ed 19, Philadelphia, 2011, Elsevier/Saunders; Tschudy MM, Arcara KM: *The Harriett Lane handbook: a manual for pediatric house officers,* Philadelphia, 2012, Elsevier/Mosby.

chest shape also can be seen when chronic air trapping is present, such as in advanced stages of *cystic fibrosis.* Other deformities of the chest that can have an impact on the child's respiratory status and decrease expansion of the lungs include *pectus carinatum, pectus excavatum,* or *scoliosis* (Figure 8-7).

Assessment of Respirations

Resting respiratory rates vary with the age of the child: the younger the child, the higher the respiratory rate (Table 8-3). The child's rhythm of breathing should be regular. Many factors can increase or decrease the respiratory rate, such as fever, pain, exercise, and medications.

PEDIATRIC PEARLS

Assess respiratory rate before the physical exam portion of the visit when the child is calm; this is best accomplished when the child is in the parent's/guardian's arms.

Periodic breathing is characterized by rapid breathing followed by periods of *apnea,* cessation of breathing. This is normal in the first few hours of life in healthy full-term newborns. Periodic breathing is more likely to persist in preterm infants, but the episodes of apnea should improve as infants approach term age.[10] *Apnea* is considered clinically significant if it lasts >20 seconds or >10 seconds if it is associated with bradycardia (heart rate <80 beats per minute) or oxygen desaturation (oxygen saturation <80% to 85%). There is no consensus on the duration of apnea that is considered pathologic.[11] If the apnea is prolonged (>20 seconds) or it is accompanied by central cyanosis, it is abnormal and requires immediate further evaluation.[11] *Paradoxical breathing,* or seesaw breathing, is often seen in newborns and infants because they use abdominal muscles more than intercostal muscles.[3,10,12] *Cheyne-Stokes breathing* is characterized by cycles of increasing and decreasing tidal volume separated by apnea. It occurs in children with congestive heart failure and increased intracranial pressure.[7,10,12]

Noisy breathing includes stridor, grunting, and snoring. *Stridor* is a high-pitched, loud, inspiratory sound produced by upper airway obstruction. Causes of upper airway obstruction include edema status postintubation, subglottic stenosis, laryngotracheobronchitis, and foreign body aspiration. *Grunting* is a low-pitched expiratory sound present with respiratory distress and is the result of a partial closure of the glottis. Snoring is a rough, snorting sound that can be present on inspiration or expiration. It may be present during sleep in healthy children who have an upper respiratory infection. Snoring is often heard in the presence of adenoidal and tonsillar hypertrophy or congenital anomalies that involve the upper airway or facies.[6,13]

Inspect for nasal flaring and use of accessory muscles in the infant and toddler. Mild nasal flaring can be seen in newborns because they are obligate nose breathers in the first month of life. However, increased nasal flaring should be investigated because it is a sign of labored breathing. Other signs of increased effort and respiratory distress include retractions, bulging of the intercostal muscles, and head bobbing.[14] Although mild retractions may be seen in some healthy young children, increased retractions can be a sign of airway obstruction. The chest wall of newborns and infants is more compliant than that of older children, making them more prone to retractions. Bulging of the intercostal spaces also may be seen with airway obstruction as a consequence of increased expiratory effort.[6,12] *Head bobbing,* the forward movement of the infant's head, is a sign of respiratory distress due to the contraction of the scalene and *sternocleidomastoid* muscles.

An abnormal inspiratory to expiratory (I:E) ratio is an additional sign of respiratory distress. A normal I:E ratio in the infant is 1:2 seconds except in the newborn, when it is variable. Obstructive diseases such as cystic fibrosis or an acute asthma exacerbation can increase the expiratory time. Restrictive diseases can give a ratio of 1:1, and acute upper airway obstruction can produce a ratio of 2:2 to 4:2.

Assess for *cyanosis,* a bluish color to the skin or mucous membranes. *Acrocyanosis,* cyanosis of the hands and feet, is normal in the newborn and can persist for days if the infant is in a cool environment. *Central cyanosis,* which occurs in the conjunctiva, lips, mucous membranes, and nail beds, is an abnormal finding at any age and warrants immediate further evaluation. In the anemic child, it may be difficult to detect cyanosis early on because the arterial oxygen saturation at which cyanosis becomes apparent varies with the total hemoglobin level.[6,12] In addition, in a dark-skinned child, cyanosis is best assessed by looking at the mucous membranes and/or nail beds.

Auscultation

Auscultation is best performed at the beginning of the examination when the infant/child is more cooperative and attentive. Auscultation is performed with the diaphragm of the stethoscope placed firmly on the chest. The child's chest should be bare because clothing can change the quality of the breath sounds. You want to auscultate moving from side to side across the chest so that you can compare one side to the other. Be sure to listen at each location for one full breath (Figure 8-8). Breath sounds are identified by their intensity, pitch, and duration. In children breath sounds tend to be louder because of the thinness of the chest wall.[6] There has been much confusion about the terminology used to describe breath sounds. Table 8-4 presents the most accurate description of normal breath sounds in the respiratory cycle.

Transmitted voice sounds or an infant's cry (vocal fremitus) also can be assessed with a stethoscope. Voice sounds are typically muffled on auscultation. If you hear the voice sound or cry loud and clear, it is termed *bronchophony.*

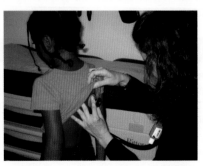

FIGURE 8-8 Auscultation of middle lobe.

TABLE 8-4   NORMAL BREATH SOUNDS

Sound	Description	Duration of Inspiration and Expiration	Sound Diagram
Vesicular	Soft, low-pitched sound heard over entire surface of lungs; inspiration louder	Inspiration > expiration	
Bronchovesicular	Moderately loud and pitched sounds heard over intrascapular area; heard on inspiration and expiration	Inspiration = expiration	
Bronchial (tubular)	Loud and high-pitched sounds heard over trachea near suprasternal notch; louder on expiration	Inspiration < expiration	
Tracheal	Loudest and highest pitched sounds heard over the trachea; heard on inspiration and expiration	Inspiration = expiration	

Data from Hughes DM: Evaluating the respiratory system. In Goldbloom RB: *Pediatric clinical skills,* ed 4, Phildelphia, 2011, Elsevier/Saunders; *Lippincott manual of nursing practice series: assessment,* Philadelphia, 2007, Lippincott, Williams & Wilkins; Aylott M: Observing the sick child: part 2c respiratory auscultation, *Paediatr Nurs* 19(3):38-45, 2007.

This technique can be used to examine an infant or uncooperative child even while he or she is crying. If the verbal child speaks the sound "ee" and it sounds like "ay," it is called *egophony.* If the child whispers a word and it is heard loud and clear, it is called *whispered pectoriloquy.* If any of these signs are positive, it is evidence of a consolidation indicated by fluid or exudate in the alveolar spaces.[7]

Abnormal Lung Sounds

In addition to normal lung sounds, you may hear adventitious or abnormal breath sounds (Table 8-5). Adventitious lung sounds are sounds that are superimposed on normal breath sounds.

Palpation

Palpation is performed to identify anatomical landmarks, respiratory symmetry, and areas of tenderness or abnormalities. Begin by counting the ribs, locate the *angle of Louis,* and move your fingers laterally to feel the second rib and corresponding costal cartilage. Directly below this rib is the second intercostal space.

From there, count downward to the other ribs and their respective intercostal spaces.[4,5]

To assess chest excursion, place your hands along the lateral rib cage and squeeze the thumbs toward each other so that you gather a small amount of skin in between your thumbs. As the child inhales, note the symmetry of the chest excursion. Again, this should be done both anteriorly and posteriorly. Asymmetry is an abnormal finding. In the newborn period, asymmetrical chest excursion may be a sign of a diaphragmatic hernia. Other possible abnormalities associated with asymmetrical chest excursion during the newborn period or later include diaphragmatic dysfunction, pneumothorax, mass, foreign body, or abnormal chest wall shape. An important part of the exam that should not be ignored is palpation of the trachea to assess for a mediastinal shift. To perform this exam, place fingers in the suprasternal notch on both sides of the trachea. The distance between the trachea and the sternocleidomastoid tendons should be equal on both sides. A shift in the trachea occurs when there is a difference in volume or pressure between the

TABLE 8-5 ABNORMAL BREATH SOUNDS

Sound	Description
Crackles	Discontinuous sounds, heard primarily on inspiration, do not clear with cough; associated with pneumonia, pulmonary edema, cystic fibrosis • Fine crackles—soft and higher in pitch, generally indicative of fluid in smaller airways in infants, children • Coarse crackles—loud and lower in pitch, usually signify fluid in larger airways
Wheezes	Continuous, high-pitched musical sounds heard primarily on expiration; associated with foreign body aspiration, bronchiolitis, asthma
Rhonchi	Continuous low-pitched sounds; clears with coughing; caused by secretions/mucus in larger airways as in bronchitis and lower respiratory tract infections
Stridor	High-pitched, harsh sounds; heard primarily with inspiration; associated with laryngotra-cheobronchitis, laryngomalacia, subglottic stenosis, and vocal cord dysfunction

Data from Hughes DM: Evaluating the respiratory system. In Goldbloom RB: *Pediatric clinical skills*, ed 4, Phildelphia, 2011, Elsevier/Saunders; *Lippincott manual of nursing practice series: assessment*, Philadelphia, 2007, Lippincott, Williams & Wilkins; Tschudy MM, Arcara KM: *The Harriett Lane handbook: a manual for pediatric house officers*, Philadelphia, 2012, Elsevier/Mosby; Aylott M: Observing the sick child: part 2c respiratory auscultation, *Paediatr Nurs* 19(3):38-45, 2007; Murphy RLH: In defense of the stethoscope, *Respir Care* 53(3):355-369, 2008.

two sides of the chest, as is seen in a pneumothorax or pleural effusion.[4,5,7]

To complete the palpation portion of the exam, assess for tactile fremitus. To do this, place your palms, the ulnar surface of your hands, or your fingers depending on the size of the chest wall on the child's back (right and left side), and ask the verbal child to say "1-2-3." In an infant or uncooperative child this technique can be performed while the child is crying. Perform this exam both anteriorly and posteriorly. Vibrations/fremitus should be of equal intensity bilaterally. A pneumothorax or hyperinflation can decrease fremitus; a mass or pneumonia can increase fremitus.[7]

Percussion

Percussion is used to determine the sounds of the underlying organs and tissues. It helps to distinguish whether the tissue is air filled, fluid filled, or solid. There are five sounds that are produced with percussion: *resonance, hyperresonance, dull, flat,* and *tympany.* The sounds are distinguished by their intensity, pitch, and duration. In infants and toddlers, the sound produced is more resonant because the chest wall is thinner than in older children and adolescents (Table 8-6). To perform percussion, hyperextend the middle finger of your nondominant hand and press the distal interphalangeal joint firmly on the chest. With the middle finger of your dominant hand, strike down on the hyperextended interphalangeal joint. The movement must be sharp and quick and the only portion of the nondominant finger that should be touching the chest should be the hyperextended joint. Strike each area two or three times and then move to the opposite side for comparison (Figure 8-9). Lastly, it may be necessary to repeat auscultation to confirm findings that were revealed during palpation and percussion. Percussion is often deferred in infants and young children.

DIAGNOSTICS

Pulse Oximetry

For a discussion on pulse oximetry, see Chapter 7.

Chest Radiograph

Chest radiography is often used to identify pulmonary pathology in the presence of pulmonary symptoms such as coughing,

TABLE 8-6	PERCUSSION SOUNDS			
Tone	Intensity	Pitch	Quality	Clinical Implication
Tympanic	Loud	High	Drumlike	Air collection (i.e., large pneumothorax)
Resonant	Loud	Low	Hollow	Normal lung
Dull	Moderate	Moderate	Dull thud	Solid area (i.e., mass)
Flat	Soft	High	Very dull	Consolidation (i.e., pneumonia)

Data from *Lippincott manual of nursing practice series: assessment,* Philadelphia, 2007, Lippincott, Williams & Wilkins.

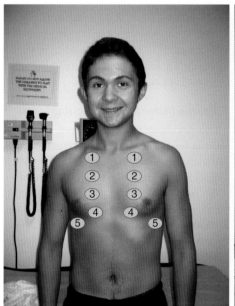
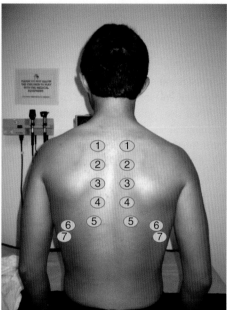

FIGURE 8-9 Sequence for percussion of the thorax.

wheezing, shortness of breath, and chest pain. A finding of hyperinflation is indicative of air trapping and is often seen in children with bronchiolitis or an acute asthma exacerbation. Atelectasis or collapse may indicate mucus retention and can be present in children with bronchiolitis, asthma, or bronchomalacia. Consolidation can be caused by pneumonia, and an area of hyperlucency without normal lung markings is indicative of a pneumothorax or other air-containing pathology such as a cyst.

Pulmonary Function Testing

Pulmonary function testing is performed to evaluate pulmonary symptoms and assess for obstructive and/or restrictive lung disease. It is also used to monitor disease progression and response to therapy. Although infant pulmonary function testing is available at specialized pediatric respiratory medicine centers, pulmonary function tests are generally reserved for children ≥ 5 years of age. Predicted values are based on a reference population and are dependent upon age, height, sex, and ethnicity.

There are specific guidelines for the performance of lung function testing; an experienced technician is of paramount importance in the testing process. An assessment of patient technique and effort is necessary when interpreting results; in addition, acceptability criteria must be met before a test can be considered interpretable.[15] Severity of lung dysfunction is categorized as normal, mild, moderate, moderately-severe, severe, and very severe.[16] While there are many types of pulmonary function tests available, this chapter will focus on the most common tests performed in the pediatric population.

Spirometry

The most common pulmonary function test is spirometry. Portable spirometers are available for office use. Spirometry is defined as "a physiological test that measures how an individual inhales or exhales volumes of air as a function of time."[17,p.320] Measures include 1) forced vital capacity (FVC), which is the maximum volume of air forcefully exhaled after a maximal inhalation; 2) forced exhaled volume in the first second (FEV_1), which is the maximum volume of air exhaled in the first second of FVC; 3) FEV_1/FVC which is the ratio of air exhaled in the first second to the total volume of air exhaled; and 4) forced expiratory flow 25-75 (FEF 25-75), which is the forced expiratory flow between 25% to 75% of FVC.[17] The FEV_1 is a measure of large airways and is effort dependent, while the FEF 25-75 is a measure of small airways and is effort independent. A reduced FEV_1 and FEV_1/FVC is indicative of an obstructive pattern as seen in asthma. A reduced FVC and FEV_1 and a normal FEV_1/FVC is indicative of a restrictive pattern as seen in chest wall abnormalities. A mixed pattern may be seen in someone with advanced cystic fibrosis. The *Expert Panel Report 3: Guidelines on the Diagnosis and Management of Asthma* recommends performing spirometry at the initial assessment, after treatments have been initiated and symptoms have stabilized, during

periods of loss of asthma control, and at least every 1 to 2 years.[9]

Lung Volumes

A restrictive pattern on spirometry must be confirmed with lung volume testing. Common lung volume measures include 1) total lung capacity (TLC), which is the volume of air in the lungs after a maximal inspiration; 2) functional residual capacity (FRC), which is the volume of air in the lungs at the end of expiration during tidal breathing; and 3) residual volume (RV), which is the volume of air in the lungs at the end of a maximal expiration. A decreased TLC is indicative of a restrictive pattern. An increased RV is indicative of an obstructive pattern.[18]

Bronchodilator Response Testing

Bronchodilator response testing is used to assess for the presence of reversible airflow limitation. To perform the test, the patient should first undergo baseline spirometry. This is followed by the administration of a short-acting beta agonist and repeat spirometry 15 minutes after medication administration. The American Thoracic Society considers a change in the FEV_1 and/or FVC of >12% and 200 mL from baseline as a significant response.[20,22] The *Expert Panel Report 3: Guidelines on the Diagnosis and Management of Asthma* considers an increase in FEV_1 of ≥12% from baseline or an increase of ≥10% of predicted after bronchodilator as significant reversibility.[9]

Quantitative Pilocarpine Iontophoresis Sweat Chloride Testing

The sweat test is the gold standard for diagnosing cystic fibrosis. The test measures the concentration of chloride in sweat after stimulation with pilocarpine. Specific guidelines for collection and analysis have been established by the Cystic Fibrosis Foundation and must be adhered to in order to ensure accuracy of results. A test is considered negative if the concentration of chloride is <40 mmol/L, borderline if it is 40 to 60 mmol/L, and consistent with cystic fibrosis if it is >60 mmol/L. In infants, values >30 mmol/L require further evaluation. In addition, values <40 mmol/L have been reported in some patients with genetic evidence of cystic fibrosis.[19]

CHEST AND RESPIRATORY CONDITIONS

Table 8-7 presents respiratory conditions seen in infants, children, and adolescents by the pediatric health care practitioner.

TABLE 8-7 CHEST AND RESPIRATORY CONDITIONS

Condition	Description
Bronchiolitis	Inflammatory obstruction of small airways caused by edema, mucus production; occurs during first 2 years of life with peak incidence at 6 months of age
	Etiology: Viral etiology common with a large percentage caused by respiratory syncytial virus (RSV)
	Symptoms: Wheezing, crackles, and cough; when severe, nasal flaring, retractions and tachypnea can be present
Epiglottitis	Obstructive inflammatory process of airway that is supraglottic; abrupt onset of high fever, sore throat, drooling, dysphagia, dyspnea, increasing airway obstruction; occurs between 2 and 6 years of age
	Etiology: Bacterial with marked decrease in incidence because of widespread use of *Haemophilus influenzae* vaccine; most cases post–*H. influenzae* due to streptococci and staphylococci
	Symptoms: Fever, difficulty swallowing, drooling, sore throat
Asthma	Inflammatory process characterized by airway obstruction and hyperresponsiveness; inflammation plays key role in factors leading to symptoms
	Symptoms: Cough, wheezing, tachypnea, chest tightness, and dyspnea with prolonged expiration
Croup/ laryngotracheobronchitis	Acute upper airway obstruction; inflammation and edema of the airway leads to symptoms
	Etiology: 50%-70% due to parainfluenza virus
	Symptoms: Hoarse, barky cough that is worse at night, stridor; respiratory distress can occur
Cystic fibrosis	A multisystem disease related to thick secretions that lead to airway obstruction
	Etiology: Inherited, autosomal recessive
	Symptoms: Chronic or recurrent cough, wheeze, recurrent pneumonia or bronchitis
Foreign body aspiration	Lodging of object in larynx, trachea, bronchi (most common site) with degree of obstruction dependent on size/location of object in respiratory tract
	Etiology: Food and small objects are the most common causes; possibility of foreign body must be considered in infants and young children with acute respiratory distress regardless of history; common in children <3 years of age
	Symptoms: Choking, prolonged cough, dyspnea, nonresolving pneumonia

Continued

TABLE 8-7   CHEST AND RESPIRATORY CONDITIONS—CONT'D

Condition	Description
Laryngomalacia	Immature cartilage of the supraglottic larynx leads to symptoms; it slowly resolves by 12 to 18 months of age
	Symptoms: Inspiratory stridor with activity/feeding that improves when the child is calm
Tracheomalacia	Weakened/"floppy" trachea that leads to symptoms
	Symptoms: Harsh noise/stridor on expiration caused by airway collapse; onset in early neonatal period; diagnosed by bronchoscopy.
Pneumonia	Infection of lung parenchyma or interstitium; may be primary condition or manifestation of another illness
	Etiology: Bacterial (streptococcus, staphylococcus, etc.) or viral (RSV, parainfluenza, adenovirus, etc.); most commonly caused by viral microorganisms—bacterial pneumonia is less common, but *Mycoplasma pneumoniae* accounts for ~70% of all pneumonias in 9- to 15-year-olds; noninfectious causes such as aspiration should be considered
	Symptoms: Crackles, decreased breath sounds; more severe cases may also see tachypnea, nasal flaring, and retractions
Neonatal respiratory distress syndrome	A condition related to decreased number of branching airways and alveoli, surfactant deficiency, atelectasis, impaired gas exchange, and hypoxemia
	Symptoms: Tachypnea, retractions, cyanosis, apnea

Data from Tolomeo C: *Nursing care in pediatric respiratory disease*, Ames, IA, 2012, Wiley-Blackwell.

SUMMARY OF EXAMINATION

- Obtain a detailed history (including onset, aggravating factors, associated symptoms, etc.) of the symptom(s) from the parent/guardian and, when possible, the child; a thorough family and past medical history should also be obtained.
- Start the physical examination with inspection of the chest wall for shape and symmetry as well as respiratory rate and effort. Also assess skin for cyanosis and atopy. Relate findings to child's age and symptoms.
- Systematically auscultate breath sounds bilaterally. Note any adventitious sounds and correlate findings with clinical history.
- Systematically palpate chest bilaterally. Note excursion and vocal fremitus; correlate findings with clinical history.
- Systematically percuss chest bilaterally. Note sounds; correlate findings with history.
- All respiratory findings should be related to the child's age and clinical symptoms.

Charting

3-Week-Old Infant

Chest: Respiratory rate 40, rate regular, respirations quiet. No nasal flaring, retractions or intercostal bulging. I:E 1:2, AP diameter 1:1. Chest excursion symmetrical. Trachea midline. Vesicular lung sounds across lung fields.

Charting

6-Year-Old with Acute Asthma Exacerbation

Chest: Respiratory rate 32. Audible wheeze present. Mild nasal flaring. Intermittent cough present. I:E 1:3. Mild intercostal retractions. Symmetrical chest excursion. Inspiratory and expiratory wheezes scattered throughout lung fields. No crackles noted.

REFERENCES

1. Nakra N: Pediatric pulmonary anatomy and physiology. In Tolomeo C: *Nursing care in pediatric respiratory disease*, Ames, IA., 2012, Wiley-Blackwell.
2. Porth CM: Respiratory tract infections, neoplasms, and childhood disorders. In Porth CM: *Pathophysiology concepts of altered health states*, ed 7, Philadelphia, 2008, Lippincott, Williams & Wilkins.
3. Porth CM: Control of respiratory function. In Porth CM: *Pathophysiology concepts of altered health states*, ed 7, Philadelphia, 2008, Lippincott, Williams & Wilkins.
4. Aylott M: Observing the sick child: part 2b respiratory palpation, *Paediatr Nurs* 19(1):38-45, 2007.
5. Morton DA, Foreman KB, Albertin KH: Anterior thoracic wall. In Morton DA, Forman KB, Albertin KH: *The big picture: gross anatomy*, New York, 2011, McGraw Hill.
6. Hughes DM: Evaluating the respiratory system. In Goldbloom RB: *Pediatric clinical skills*, ed 4, Philadelphia, 2011, Elsevier/Saunders.
7. *Lippincott manual of nursing practice series: assessment*, Philadelphia, 2007, Lippincott, Williams & Wilkins.
8. Liu AH, Zeiger RS, Sorkness CA, et al: The childhood asthma control test—retrospective determination and clinical validation of a cut point to identify children with very poorly controlled asthma, *J Allergy Clin Immunol* 126:267-273, 2010.
9. National Heart, Lung, and Blood Institute: *Expert Panel Report 3: guidelines for the diagnosis and management of asthma*. Available at http://www.nhlbi.nih.gov/guidelines/asthma/. Accessed July 29, 2012.
10. Tolomeo C: Pediatric respiratory health history and physical assessment. In Tolomeo C: *Nursing care in pediatric respiratory disease*, Ames, IA., 2012, Wiley-Blackwell.
11. Finer NN, Higgins R, Kattwinkel J, et al: Summary proceedings from the Apnea of Prematurity Group, *Pediatrics* 117(3):S47-S51, 2006.
12. Aylott M: Observing the sick child: part 2a respiratory assessment, *Paediatr Nurs* 18(9):38-44, 2006.
13. Mellis C: Respiratory noises: how useful are they clinically?, *Pediatr Clin North Am* 56:1-17, 2008.
14. Nitu ME, Eigen H: Respiratory failure, *Pediatr Rev* 30(12):470-478, 2010.
15. Miller MR, Crapo R, Hankinson J, et al: General considerations for lung function testing, *Eur Respir J* 26(1):153-161, 2005.
16. Pellegrino R, Viegi G, Brusasco V, et al: Interpretative strategies for lung function tests, *Eur Respir J* 26(5):948-968, 2005.
17. Miller MR, Hankinson J, Brusasco V, et al: Standardisation of spirometry, *Eur Respir J* 26(2):319-338, 2005.
18. Wanger J, Clausen JL, Coates A, et al: Standardisation of the measurement of lung volumes, *Eur Respir J* 26(3):511-522, 2005.
19. LeGrys VA, Yankaskas JR, Quittell LM, et al: Diagnostic sweat testing: the Cystic Fibrosis Foundation guidelines, *J Pediatr* 151(1):85-89, 2007.

CHAPTER 9

HEAD AND NECK

Karen G. Duderstadt

EMBRYOLOGICAL DEVELOPMENT

The rapid growth of the head begins during the fifth week of embryonic life, as the brain simultaneously undergoes a similar period of rapid growth. By the eighth week, the embryo is humanlike in form, but the head size is disproportionate to the body. During this early fetal development, the head is the fastest growing part of the body and constitutes 50% of the body length at 8 weeks' gestation. The head growth then slows during the period from the ninth to the twelfth week in the developing fetus while spine growth accelerates. During the thirteenth week, ossification of the cranium begins in the skull, which is one of the primary ossification centers of the skeletal system; the other is located in the long bones. The hair patterns on the scalp also develop during the thirteenth week of fetal development, and the scalp hair present in the term infant is established by the twentieth week.[1] During the second and third trimesters of pregnancy, the head size becomes proportional to the body. The fetus continues to grow and gains 85% of its birth weight during the final period of growth.

DEVELOPMENTAL VARIATIONS

The normal growth of the skull depends on placental function, familial and hereditary factors, growth potential within the uterus, and optimum nutrition during pregnancy and early childhood. The contour of the cranium of the newborn reflects fetal positioning and the effects of the delivery presentation. The cranial bones are pliable and are loosely connected by the sutures and the fontanels, which allow the head to be molded during delivery.[1] Skull fractures are rare because the cranium is adaptable, but they can occur with vacuum-assisted vaginal births, forceps delivery, or a prolonged, difficult labor. The head is slightly flattened during the normal birth process then becomes ovoid by 1 to 2 days of age. If growth retardation does occur in the fetus as a result of either intrinsic or extrinsic factors, skull growth and brain development are impacted. Depending on the timing of the insult during fetal development, the infant can suffer long-term consequences of delayed growth and development.

ANATOMY AND PHYSIOLOGY

The cranium or *skull* provides a protective housing for the brain and parts of the central nervous system. There are eight skull plates, or bones, in the cranium joined together by sutures (Figure 9-1). These skull plates are movable and separate at birth. The *fontanels* are the membranous spaces between the frontal and parietal bones and the parietal and occipital bones. The *anterior fontanel* lies along the *coronal* and *frontal* sutures (Figure 9-2). The *posterior fontanel* lies at the juncture of the *sagittal* and *lambdoidal* sutures. There are smaller fontanels located bilaterally in the lower skull. The *sphenoid fontanel* is located at the lower juncture of the frontal and parietal bones superior to the ear, and the *mastoid fontanel* is posterior to the ear at the juncture of the

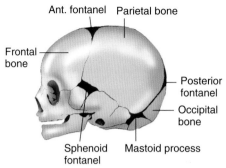

Ant. fontanel   Parietal bone

Frontal bone

Posterior fontanel

Occipital bone

Sphenoid fontanel   Mastoid process

FIGURE 9-1 **Anatomy of the skull in the newborn.**

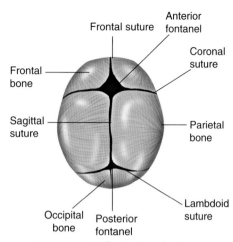

Frontal suture   Anterior fontanel

Coronal suture

Frontal bone

Sagittal suture

Parietal bone

Occipital bone   Posterior fontanel

Lambdoid suture

FIGURE 9-2 **Fontanels and sutures.**

occipital and posterior parietal bones. The cranial sutures accommodate brain growth. The cranium is supported by the first cervical vertebra, the *atlas*. The *atlas* is a solid vertebra and rests on the second vertebra, the *axis*. These bones form the rotational bones of the skull. Ossification of the skull continues throughout infancy and childhood and into adulthood.

The facial bones are also pliable at birth, except for the maxilla and the mandible, which are then very small and underdeveloped. The facial skeleton consists of the larger bones of the frontal area, zygomatic processes, *maxilla,* and *mandible* (Figure 9-3). The two *nasal plates* and the *lacrimal, ethmoid,* and *sphenoid* bones comprise the smaller bones in the head. The maxillary and ethmoid sinuses are present at birth but are small, and the sphenoid and frontal sinuses develop during infancy and childhood.

The muscular structure of the head and neck is an intricate part of the underlying fascia of the cranium and neck structures. The connections between the muscular fascia and the facial orifices control facial expressions such as smiling, raising the eyebrows, and wrinkling the forehead. The superficial and deep muscles of the neck support the pivotal rotation of the head. The *sternocleidomastoid* or *sternomastoid* muscle is the largest muscle in the neck, running from the mastoid area at the base of the ear to the clavicle and sternum, and is primarily responsible for turning the head from side to side. It can be particularly susceptible to the effects of viral infections and gastrointestinal conditions in the pediatric patient. The

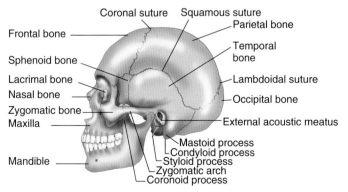

Coronal suture   Squamous suture
Parietal bone

Frontal bone

Temporal bone

Sphenoid bone

Lacrimal bone

Lambdoidal suture

Nasal bone

Occipital bone

Zygomatic bone

Maxilla

External acoustic meatus

Mandible

Mastoid process
Condyloid process
Styloid process
Zygomatic arch
Coronoid process

FIGURE 9-3 **Facial skeleton.**

trapezius muscle lies at the back of the neck and is triangular. The origin of the *trapezius* muscle is in the back at the twelfth thoracic vertebra extending to the lateral border of the clavicle and attaches at the posterior edge of the occipital bone. It supports the head movement from side to side and the shoulder movement.

The structures in the neck are protected by the deep vertebral muscles, which support the side movements of the head. The *trachea* is the cartilaginous tube that extends from the larynx to the bronchi in the upper chest beneath the sternum. In infants and children, it is more mobile and more deeply recessed in the vertebral muscles than in adults.

The *thyroid gland* lies in the anterior middle region of the neck just below the larynx surrounding the fifth or sixth tracheal ring. There are two lobes joined by an anterior *isthmus* connecting the lobes. The gland is composed of tiny follicles filled with *thyroglobulin,* which binds with iodine in thyroid synthesis. A dietary intake of 150 to 200 mcg of iodide is enough to produce sufficient quantities of thyroid hormone, and large reserves of iodide are concentrated in the thyroid gland. Thyroid hormone is necessary for normal growth and development in children and normal sexual maturation. The thyroid gland is extremely vascular and secretes *thyroxine* directly into the bloodstream, which promotes normal growth.

The four *parathyroid glands* are small endocrine glands generally located on the posterior side or dorsal surface of the thyroid gland. Like the thyroid gland, they do not contain ducts, and they secrete *parathyroid* hormone, which regulates calcium metabolism. Infants born with abnormal development of the parathyroid gland have an embryological defect known as DiGeorge syndrome caused by a chromosomal microdeletion (22q11). It is often associated with congenital heart defects, facial abnormalities, and other systemic defects.

The head and neck region are perfused by the *carotid arteries.* The *external carotid* supplies the head, face, and neck, and the *internal carotid* supplies the cranium. Blood from the cranium is drained through the *subclavian* and *jugular* veins. The thyroid and parathyroid are perfused by the superior and inferior *thyroid arteries.*

PHYSIOLOGICAL VARIATIONS

Rapid growth in the infant brings rapid changes in the head and neck. At birth, the *anterior fontanel* ranges in size from an average of 2 cm to 4 to 5 cm in the term infant. The anterior fontanel may be small at birth, about the size of a fingertip, because the skull is compressed during vaginal delivery, and then the fontanel enlarges in the neonatal period. The *posterior fontanel* may or may not be palpable at birth. It enlarges by a range of 0.5 to 1 cm and closes by 6 weeks to 2 months of age. Suture lines can be overlapping or protuberant after birth and often are palpable until 6 months of age from molding at birth. Slow progression of closure of the anterior fontanel occurs during the first year of life, and closure in some infants may begin by 9 months of age with only a fingertip concavity present at the crown of the scalp. However, closure of the *anterior fontanel* normally occurs by 18 months of age. Head growth in the first year is determined not by the size of the fontanel, but by the normal increase of the occipital-frontal circumference (OFC) of the head. *Microcephaly,* a small head for gestational age, is considered 1 to 2 standard deviations (SD) *below* the norm for age and size, and *macrocephaly,* a large head for gestational age, is 1 to 2 SD *above* the norm for age and size.

Cephalhematoma is a soft, fluctuating effusion of blood trapped beneath the pericranium caused by rupture of the blood vessels. It does not cross the sagittal suture at the crown. It is usually unilateral and occurs over the parietal area. The bleeding into the periosteum of the cranium may occur slowly and therefore may not be apparent until the infant is 24 to 48 hours old. A cephalhematoma may be associated with hyperbilirubinemia. Resolution of a cephalhematoma may be slow and it may persist until 6 weeks to 2 months of age. See Table 9-1 for developmental variations in the head and neck.

TABLE 9-1	PHYSIOLOGICAL VARIATIONS OF THE HEAD AND NECK DURING DEVELOPMENT
Age	**Physiological Variations**
Preterm infant	Symmetrical or asymmetrical head shape with a flattened temporal/parietal region giving head an elongated shape
	Craniotabes, abnormal softness of cranium, related to incomplete bone and ossification of widened sutures, is often present
Newborn	Symmetrical or asymmetrical head shape with head circumference > chest circumference; ridges over suture lines are common in neonate because of pressure on skull during vaginal birth
	Craniotabes may be present until 6 months of age
Infancy	Symmetrical brain growth is reflected in *occipital-frontal circumference* (OFC) of skull; abnormal growth patterns of skull are indicated by a misshapen cranium and/or a rapidly increasing OFC or slow growth of skull; closure of *anterior fontanel* is expected by 18 months of age in healthy term infant
Early childhood	After 18 months, chest circumference exceeds head circumference by 5-7 cm; brain reaches 80% of adult size by 2 years of age; cranium continues to ossify; sutures are proximate and immobile; neck lengthens at 3-4 years of age and neck-to-body proportion is closer to adult size
Middle childhood	Nasal sinus cavities widen and deepen with skull growth, and size approximates those of an adult; thyroid gland is more readily palpable and approximates adult size

FAMILY, CULTURAL, RACIAL, AND ETHNIC CONSIDERATIONS

African-American infants have a slightly larger anterior fontanel than do Caucasian infants secondary to familial and genetic factors. Native American infants have an additional horizontal suture line over the occipital bone.

SYSTEM-SPECIFIC HISTORY

Obtaining a thorough history of growth and development of the head and neck area, including any injury or insult to the skull during the growth process, is an important part of accurate diagnosis. Refer to the Information Gathering table for pertinent questions to ask about the growth and development of the head and neck.

INFORMATION GATHERING FOR HEAD AND NECK ASSESSMENT AT KEY DEVELOPMENTAL STAGES

Age-Group	Questions to Ask
Preterm infant	History of intraventricular insult? History of maternal substance abuse? Perinatal infections?
Newborn	Vaginal or cesarean birth? Prolonged labor with prolonged third stage? Precipitous delivery? Vacuum-assisted delivery? Shoulder presentation? Respiratory distress at birth? Head tilt? Newborn screening results? History of maternal hyperthyroidism, thyroid disease, gestational diabetes?

Continued

INFORMATION GATHERING FOR HEAD AND NECK ASSESSMENT AT KEY DEVELOPMENTAL STAGES—CONT'D

Age-Group	Questions to Ask
Infancy	Newborn screening results? History of maternal infection? Neonatal infections? Meningitis? Quality of muscle tone and strength, head control? Achieving developmental milestones?
Early childhood	History of falls, clumsiness? Stable gait? Head tilt, neck pain/stiffness? Persistent lymph gland swelling? History of head trauma or falls, neck pain/stiffness? Use of bike or scooter helmet?
Middle childhood	History of headache? Onset and duration? History of head injury? Neck pain/stiffness? Use of bike or skateboarding helmet? Other protective sports equipment?
Adolescence	History of head injury? Recurrent headaches? Blurred vision? Neck pain/stiffness? Weight loss or gain? Swelling of lymph glands? Use of bike or skateboarding helmet, other protective sports equipment?
Environmental risks	Maternal exposure to hazardous chemicals or hazardous waste materials? Childhood exposure to pesticides, chemical cleaning agents, hazardous chemicals, tobacco smoke, or radiation? Limiting exposure to bisphenol A (BPA) and other plasticizers in the environment?

PHYSICAL ASSESSMENT OF THE HEAD AND NECK

The examination of the head and neck area involves inspection and palpation. In infants and young children, examination of the head and neck region may follow the quieter parts of the examination, the cardiac and respiratory exam, because palpation around the head and neck region often makes young children very fearful and uncomfortable, or ticklish with a response of moving their shoulders upward. In the older child, the physical examination may proceed head to toe.

No specialized equipment is necessary for the examination of the head and neck area except good lighting to view the areas of the neck region during examination. Gloves can be worn if skin lesions are noted.

Inspection of the Head

Inspection of the head includes observation by the health care provider for head movement and head control. Head lag when pulling the infant to the sitting position is normal until 3 to 4 months of age in the term infant. Head lag should be evaluated in all infants in the first 6 months of life as an indicator of muscle tone. Persistent head lag between 4 and 6 months of age in the term infant is concerning, and the infant should be monitored closely for the attainment of developmental milestones and referred if indicated.

Head alignment should be evaluated in the infant and young child with the head at midline on the examining table or while being supported in a sitting position by the parent or caregiver. Persistent head tilt from the normal position may indicate *hypotonia, congenital torticollis,* muscular abnormalities, gastrointestinal reflux, or visual and hearing deficits. Range of motion and movement of the head should be examined to determine tone and flexibility. In examining the infant younger than 3 months, the provider should move the head passively on the examining table to the left and right to determine mobility and range of motion. At 3 to 4 months of age, the infant can begin to follow a light or small toy to determine the full range of motion of the head and neck and the function of the musculature.

Any limited range of motion, head bobbing or jerking, tremors, persistent downward gaze, or involuntary muscle contractions or spasms should be further evaluated and referred when indicated.

Observe the shape and size of the head in the infant and young child. Head shape varies widely in young infants and generally follows a normal growth pattern influenced by familial and genetic patterns and cultural influences. A flattened occipital region or a unilateral flattening of the parietal region can occur in young infants because of prolonged positional placement. Positional skull deformities are often benign and reversible and will normalize by 3 months of age.[2,3] However, there has been a large increase in reported cases of *plagiocephaly* in infants since the adoption of supine sleeping recommendations to prevent sudden infant death syndrome.[4] Plagiocephaly refers to an asymmetrical flattening or deformity of the skull.[5] Plagiocephaly occurs when external forces are applied to the developing skull of an infant and it becomes misshapen, often resulting in asymmetry of the ears and face.[3] *Deformational plagiocephaly* is most commonly seen on the lateral and central side of the occiput.[5] Plagiocephaly may be prevented by varying the head position frequently when putting the very young infant down to sleep on the back and by giving supervised tummy time when awake.

EVIDENCE-BASED PRACTICE TIP

Most positional skull deformities can be prevented by alternating the infant's head position when supine from the left to right occipital area during sleep and providing short periods of supervised tummy time while the infant is awake.[2]

Craniosynostosis is the premature closure or fusion of sutures in the skull of the young infant.[6] In contrast to deformational plagiocephaly, craniosynostosis causes a trapezoidal head shape with flattening of both the occiput and frontal regions on the affected side.[2]

Health care providers need to be able to properly differentiate infants with benign skull deformities from those with craniosynostosis, and educate parents on methods of proactively decreasing the likelihood of the development of occipital flattening.[2] *Lambdoidal craniosynostosis,* which occurs in 3 in 100,000 births, causes a parallelogram-shaped skull with the ear displaced posteriorly and inferiorly.[1] It is important for the health care provider to inspect the shape of the head from above the infant as well as with the infant supported in a sitting position with the head midline and verify the accuracy of the OFC of the head. If any significant abnormal shape of the head is noted, evaluation and referral are indicated.

On inspection, observe the level of the fontanel in the cranium. Normally there is a slight pulsation in the *anterior fontanel,* and it tenses or bulges slightly when the infant is crying but flattens when the infant calms. In the ill infant, a tense, bulging anterior fontanel can be a sign of increasing intracranial pressure due to *meningitis* or head trauma and is a medical emergency. Tumors in the brain and meninges also can cause increased intracranial pressure indicated by a bulging fontanel. Infants can have a mildly depressed fontanel, unaccompanied by other symptoms, which may indicate mild dehydration due to the metabolic demands of growth or fluid lost through heat and perspiration. A sunken fontanel, if accompanied by gastrointestinal symptoms, infection, or loss of normal turgor of skin and mucous membranes, may indicate severe dehydration and an urgent need for further evaluation and treatment.

Inspection of the Face

Examination of the facial area begins with initial observation of the infant, child, or adolescent for symmetry of facial features, ears, and facial movements. Observing the smile, laugh, facial creases, and facial wrinkles reveals normal function as well as innervation of the facial structures. Observing the symmetry of the facial features in the newborn and infant during crying will assist the health care provider in assessing any facial or neurological injury that occurred during birth. During vaginal deliveries, excessive lateral traction of the head and neck away from the shoulder may injure the brachial plexus, the ventral root of the fifth cervical nerve,[1] and cause paralysis of the arm and shoulder. Injury to the facial nerve before or during the birth process may cause asymmetrical nasolabial folds and/or asymmetrical facial expression. Any unusual facies with disproportional features, frontal bossing of the forehead, and small or low-set ears may be indicative of a genetic abnormality and require further evaluation and referral.

Inspection of the Neck

The neck should be inspected for symmetry, shape, and mobility. The neck is shortened in the newborn and very young infant and the musculature is underdeveloped; therefore, it is best to inspect the neck with the infant on a firm surface for examination. While supporting the neck and shoulders cradled with the thumb and forefingers, use the opposite hand to extend the head back slightly to expose the shortened neck region and conduct a full inspection. This position allows the examiner to determine the symmetry and strength of the musculature of the neck, the alignment of the trachea, and the condition of the skin in the infant and young child, who are vulnerable to fungal and bacterial infection in the anterior neck region. *Torticollis,* or wryneck, causes the head to tilt to one side and limits range of motion of the neck muscles. Congenital torticollis is the most common associated finding in infants with deformational plagiocephaly, and early referral is indicated to support repositional therapy for the head.[5] Acquired torticollis in the infant may be related to gastroesophageal reflux disease (GERD) associated with overfeeding, or it may be associated with hypotonia or neurological features including rotation of the head and extension of the neck.

Infants and young children with unexplained fever, irritability, or a bulging fontanel associated with increased intracranial pressure may indicate pain or neck stiffness during examination of the neck region. *Meningismus* or *meningitis,* inflammation of the brain and spinal cord, can manifest in the neck. Flexion of the head forward or ventrally with the infant or young child lying on a flat surface or examining table causes pain, irritability, resistance to movement and range of motion, a sign of *nuchal rigidity.* Often, flexion of the lower extremities will occur spontaneously with flexion of the head forward in an effort to guard or protect the body. The infant or young child with meningitis will resist extension of the knees and lower extremities when lying in the supine position. *Kernig sign,* pain or resistance to straightening legs or knees from flexed position, or *Brudzinski sign,* involuntary flexion of knees or legs when lying supine and neck is flexed, indicate a positive sign for meningeal irritation. *Opisthotonos,* hyperextension of the neck and spine, indicates severe meningeal irritation.

In the school-aged child, inspect the *thyroid gland* for size and symmetry, and note any swelling or masses. In children who are obese, adipose tissue in the neck region is common and should not be mistaken for an enlarged thyroid gland. Tilting the head back during inspection of the neck will assist the health care provider in evaluating the structures of the neck. In the older child, offering a sip of water to swallow may assist the provider in distinguishing the movement of the thyroid gland. The thyroid gland should rise as the child swallows.

Palpation of the Head and Sinuses

Begin palpation at the crown of the head and evaluate the scalp and the bony structures of the skull. In the infant, the fontanels should be palpated for size, level of tenseness, and pulsations (Figure 9-4). The length and width of the fontanel can be noted in the medical record to monitor head growth. Infants and young children who present with a bulging fontanel and signs of increased intracranial pressure may

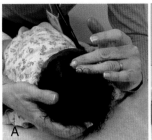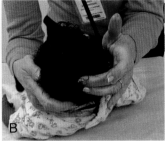

FIGURE 9-4 Palpation of the anterior **(A)** and posterior fontanels **(B)**.

have a resonant or cracked-pot sound, *Macewen sign*, when the scalp is tapped or percussed with the forefinger.

Overlapping sutures may occur in the first 6 months of life as a result of the birth process during a normal vaginal birth and are not considered abnormal in the presence of a normal OFC of the head (see Chapter 2). In the first few months of life, an infant may have a visible or palpable ridge at the crown of the head known as a *metopic ridge.* This is a normal variant when the head shape appears normal and the OFC is normal. Infants with a wide margin along the sagittal suture may have a communicating *anterior* and *posterior* fontanel, often referred to as a *metopic suture.* Suture lines are not normally palpable after 6 months of age in the term infant. Premature closure of the sutures may indicate *craniosynostosis,* or asymmetrical growth of the skull, which requires immediate evaluation and referral. Separation of the sagittal suture is one of the most common findings in infants with Down syndrome, along with a flattened occiput and a small rounded head.

When palpating the skull of an infant less than 6 months of age, an abnormal softness of the cranium known as *craniotabes* may be noted, and it is a normal variant resulting from incomplete ossification of bone in the cranium or widened sutures. If craniotabes is accompanied by abnormal facies or persists after 6 months of age, it may be associated with hydrocephalus or rickets, and further evaluation and referral is necessary.

Infants should be monitored closely for increasing head size or other indications of abnormal growth and development in the first year. If other tenderness, masses, skin lesions, or edema are detected on examination, note the size, location, and character of the mass or nodule. Evaluate for mobility and pain on examination. Any abnormal skull findings require diagnostic evaluation and referral as indicated. Any depression on the scalp indicating a skull fracture requires urgent evaluation.

Only the maxillary and frontal sinuses can be assessed by physical examination through inspection and palpation. The facial area over the maxillary and frontal sinuses should be evaluated for swelling and tenderness in school-age children and adolescents. Percuss or apply mild pressure with the thumb or forefinger over the maxillary and frontal sinus area (see Chapter 13).

Palpation and Auscultation of the Neck

If masses or nodules are noted during the inspection of the neck in the infant, then the provider should palpate the neck to evaluate the size, shape, and character of the mass or nodules. *Brachial cleft cysts* are smooth, nontender masses on the lateral neck area along the border of the sternocleidomastoid muscle. They may be fluctuant and require surgical removal. *Thyroglossal duct cysts* present higher in the neck region and require diagnostic evaluation and referral. Surgical removal may be indicated. Palpation of the lymph glands is reviewed in Chapter 10.

In the infant and young child, palpate the *sternocleidomastoid muscle* for masses, strength, and tone including the clavicular area at the base of the sternocleidomastoid muscle. Any sign of pain or irritability, or resistance to range of motion of the neck or arm in the infant, child, or adolescent indicates an abnormal finding and requires further evaluation. Resistance to lateral motion of the neck may indicate lymph gland swelling, infection, or trauma to the sternocleidomastoid muscle. If webbing of the neck is noted, it may indicate *Turner syndrome* (Table 9-2).

The jugular vein is not normally distended in children who are sitting or standing upright. Pulsations in the jugular vein in the neck can be seen when the child is lying supine on the examining table. The jugular vein should appear full but not bulging, and it is normal to observe jugular venous pulsations (JVPs). The JVP is normally a gentle undulation visible in good lighting. The pulsations should be of normal rate and amplitude, without bruits, or blowing sounds, heard on auscultation over the vessel. Abnormal pulsations can indicate right-sided heart failure or pericarditis.

In older children, *carotid pulsations* can be palpated with the finger pads of the second and third fingers in the area between the trachea and the sternocleidomastoid muscle. Evaluate for rate, rhythm, and intensity. Avoid significant pressure to the carotid artery, which may cause a vagal response or hypotension. Auscultation may be performed to detect bruits, although this is not routinely performed on children.

Palpation of the Thyroid Gland

Palpation of the thyroid gland is not usually performed in infants and young children unless masses or nodular lesions are noted on inspection of the neck. The neck is short with strong musculature and difficult to palpate. Thyroid disease in infants and young children often presents with systemic symptoms including hypotonia, lethargy, distended abdomen, and enlarged tongue as in *congenital hypothyroidism* (see Table 9-2). Newborn screening for thyroid disease is required in all states, and results should be confirmed by the pediatric health care provider on the initial postpartum or well-child visit.

Palpation of the *thyroid gland* in children is often performed beginning with school entry. The palpation of the thyroid gland is most easily approached from the front of the neck in the young child to minimize any fear that may occur during the examination. Tilt the head forward slightly while the child maintains a sitting position with the back straight. To guide the examination, the provider may gently support the child's head. Begin by using the forefinger to locate the prominent ring of the tracheal cartilage, the *cricoid cartilage,* which provides a landmark to determine the position of the thyroid gland (Figure 9-5, *A*). Just lateral to the carotid cartilage, palpate the thyroid gland by placing one hand on one side of the trachea and gently displacing the thyroid tissue to the contralateral side of the neck (Figure 9-5, *B*). Repeat this movement to examine both sides of the thyroid gland. Once positioned, extend the forefingers of both hands and apply slight pressure for deep palpation along both sides of the trachea and ask the child to swallow. Fingernails must be groomed short for effective examination of the thyroid. Tilting the head to one side, or rotating the neck very gently may help to evaluate the size, quality, and firmness of thyroid gland.

In the older school-age child, adolescent, and young adult, the thyroid gland can be examined from behind with the head tilted slightly forward. Using the *cricoid cartilage* as a landmark, the provider uses the forefingers of both hands to palpate deeply, laterally to the trachea and medial to the sternocleidomastoid muscle (Figure 9-5, *C*). A soft, mushy gland, or any masses or nodules noted on examination of the thyroid gland are abnormal and require prompt evaluation. A *goiter* is a firm, nontender, mobile, symmetrical mass in the neck. Enlargement of

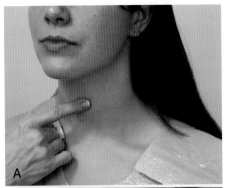

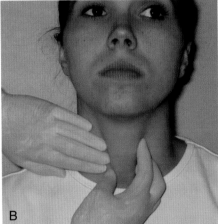

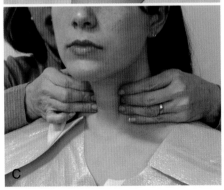

FIGURE 9-5 Examination of the thyroid gland. (**B** from Fehrenbach M, Herring S: *Illustrated anatomy of the head and neck*, ed 4, St. Louis, 2012, Elsevier.)

the thyroid gland may occur with *hyperthyroidism, Graves disease,* or *Hashimoto thyroiditis.*

DIAGNOSTIC PROCEDURES

For children presenting with a history of head injury, computed tomography (CT) scan may be indicated to aid in diagnosis. Children must remain immobilized during CT imaging. For diagnosis of possible tumors or malformations in the skull, magnetic resonance imaging (MRI) may be indicated. MRIs require sedation in children and may require injection of contrast for digital subtraction angiography. Skeletal radiography is used to evaluate cranial abnormalities such as craniosynostosis.

An ultrasound may be the most appropriate initial noninvasive test to perform in an infant, child, or adolescent with an abnormal mass in the neck region. CT imaging for differentiation of cysts or solid neck lesions may be indicated. Thyroid function test, thyroxine (T_4) and thyroid-stimulating hormone (TSH), should be performed in any child with an enlarged thyroid or signs and symptoms of thyroid disease such as weight loss, fatigue, or growth failure. Chapter 10 reviews the diagnostics for the lymph glands in the neck region and lymphatic system.

HEAD AND NECK CONDITIONS

Table 9-2 presents the most common acute and chronic conditions of the head and neck in infants, children, and adolescents.

TABLE 9-2   HEAD AND NECK CONDITIONS

Condition	Description
Bell palsy	Acute unilateral paralysis of cranial facial nerve VII related to postinfectious viral neuritis
Congenital hypothyroidism	Thyroid dysgenesis characterized by prolonged gestation, large for gestational age (LGA), delayed first stool and constipation, poor feeding; infant may have dysmorphic facial features, enlarged tongue, sparse hair/eyebrows with low-set hairline
Congenital syphilis	Bacterial infection transmitted placentally characterized by frontal bossing, depressed nasal bridge, chronic rhinitis, facial lesions circumorally
Congenital torticollis	Contracture of sternocleidomastoid muscle causing tilting of head to one side; occurs secondary to birth trauma, cervical spine or spinal cord congenital deformities
Craniosynostosis	Premature closure of the cranial sutures resulting in *craniostenosis*, narrowness of skull due to premature closure of sutures
Down syndrome	Microcephaly or small rounded head, thick epicanthal folds, almond-shaped eyes or oblique palpebral fissures; flattened nasal bridge, large protuberant tongue; ears are low-set, small, and protuberant
Facies of fetal alcohol syndrome	Fetal alcohol exposure characterized by dysmorphic features: microcephaly, short palpebral fissures, wide and flattened philtrum/thin lips; associated with developmental delay
Hydrocephalus	Ventricle enlargement in dura caused by increased production and blockage of or impaired absorption of cerebrospinal fluid; increased head circumference, bulging fontanel, widening fontanel
Hypothyroidism	Acquired thyroid condition usually caused by lymphocytic thyroiditis
Micrognathia	Underdeveloped mandible
Plagiocephaly	Asymmetrical head shape or flattening from persistent positioning of infant on one side during first 6 months of life
Potter syndrome	Renal agenesis characterized by low-set ears, broad nose, underdeveloped chin line, blank appearance
Sandifer syndrome	Acquired torticollis in the infant related to gastroesophageal reflux disease (GERD) associated with overfeeding, or associated with neurological features including rotation of the head and extension of the neck
Torticollis	Contraction of sternocleidomastoid muscle causing tilting of head toward involved side; can be sequela of upper respiratory infection
Turner syndrome	Genetic disorder, a female phenotype; characterized by short stature, webbed neck, pectus excavatum, primary amenorrhea, no development of secondary sexual characteristics

SUMMARY OF EXAMINATION

- Observe the infant for head control. Head lag when pulling the infant to the sitting position is normal until 3 to 4 months of age.
- Observe shape and size of the head in the infant and young child. Monitor head circumference. Note any misshapen skull or masses, nodules, or lesions on scalp.
- Fontanels should be palpated for size, pulsations, level of tenseness, or depression of fontanel.
- Inspect neck for symmetry, shape, and mobility.
- Palpate neck for any swelling, masses, or nodules.

- Palpation of the thyroid gland is often omitted in infants and young children unless masses or nodular lesions are noted on inspection.
- To examine the thyroid, begin by locating the cricoid cartilage as a landmark for examination of the thyroid gland. Palpate with pads of forefingers of both hands and exert pressure lateral to the trachea. Ask the child or adolescent to swallow to aid in examination of thyroid.
- Any masses or nodules on the scalp or masses in the neck area require diagnostic evaluation and referral when indicated.

Charting
Term Newborn

Head: Normocephalic, anterior and posterior fontanel patent and soft, overriding sagittal suture

Neck: Supple, no masses palpable.

Charting
9-Year-Old Male

Head: Normocephalic, no masses or nodules noted, nontender

Neck: Full range of motion (ROM), no lymphadenopathy, palpable adipose tissue over anterior neck region, thyroid gland: firm, without nodules or masses.

REFERENCES

1. Porth CM, Matfin G: *Pathophysiology: concepts of altered health status,* ed 8, Philadelphia, 2010, Lippincott, Williams & Wilkins.
2. Laughlin J, Luerssen TG, Dias MS: Prevention and management of positional skull deformities in infants, *Pediatrics* 128(6):1236-1241, 2011.
3. Miller LC, Johnson A, Duggan L, et al: Consequences of the "back to sleep" program in infants, *J Pediatr Nurs* 26(4):364-368, 2011.
4. Hutchison BL, Thompson JMD, Mitchell EA: Determinants of nonsynostotic plagiocephaly: a case-control study, *Pediatrics* 112(4):316-327, 2003.
5. Looman WS, Kack Flannery AB: Evidenced-based care of the child with deformational plagiocephaly, Part I: Assessment and diagnosis, *J Pediatr Health Care* 26(4):242-250, 2012.
6. Merritt L: Recognizing craniosynostosis, *Neonatal Netw* 28(6):369-376, 2009.

CHAPTER 10

LYMPHATIC SYSTEM

Karen G. Duderstadt

EMBRYOLOGICAL DEVELOPMENT

The lymphatic system is established in the mesoderm layer during the third week of embryonic development, and the development of the primary lymphoid organs, the thymus and bone marrow, begin during the fifth to sixth week of fetal development.[1] The secondary lymphoid organs—the spleen, lymph nodes, and lymphoid tissue—develop soon after the primary organs and are well developed at birth. The ectoderm gives rise to the epithelial linings of the glandular cells of the large organs that make up the lymphatic system.[1]

DEVELOPMENT VARIATIONS

The spleen, lymph nodes, and lymphoid tissue are small at birth and mature rapidly after exposure to antigens or microbes during the postnatal period. The thymus is the largest lymphoid tissue in the body at birth and continues to develop during the first year of life as the immune system develops. At puberty, the thymus begins slowly regressing as the immune system is well established in the lymphoid tissue.[1]

ANATOMY AND PHYSIOLOGY

Lymphatic System

The *lymphatic system* forms an extensive network throughout the body and is composed of capillaries, collecting vessels, lymph nodes, and lymphoid organs. The bone marrow and thymus, which are the central lymphoid organs, provide the center for the production and maturation of the immune cells.[1] The peripheral lymphoid organs—the spleen, tonsils, appendix, and lymphatic tissue in the respiratory, gastrointestinal,

and reproductive systems—concentrate *antigens* or *immunogens* and promote the cellular interactions of the immune response throughout the body to seek out and destroy microbes.[1]

Lymph is a clear, colorless fluid filtered and collected from the organs and tissues through the *lymphatic capillaries*. The fluid consists of white bloods cells and occasionally red blood cells. The *collecting vessels* carry the lymph from the lymphatic capillaries to the bloodstream. The *lymph* is deposited into the bloodstream through the jugular and subclavian veins in the neck. The lymphatic system also absorbs fat and fat-soluble substances from the intestinal wall. The lymph and fat are transported from the lymph glands to the larger ducts and through the venous return to the heart. The lymphatic system plays a major role in the maintenance of fluid balance, and filters fluid at the lymph nodes and removes bacteria. Obstruction of lymph flow or removal of lymph nodes causes lymphedema.

Lymph nodes are small aggregates of lymphoid tissue lying along lymphatic vessels throughout the body and consist of outer cortical layers and an inner medullary layer. The terms *lymph gland* and *lymph node* are often used interchangeably, and both terms can be applied to the lymphatic system. A *gland* is an organ that produces a substance or secretion, and a *node* is a swelling or protuberance. The lymph nodes throughout the body are filters for the collection vessels. Each lymph node processes lymph from the surrounding anatomical area. Lymph nodes remove antigens and microbes from the lymph before it enters the bloodstream, serve as the site of the body's immune response, and aid in the maturation of lymphocytes and monocytes.

The T lymphocytes are responsible for cell-mediated immunity and aid in antibody production. They are activated in the cortex of the lymph nodes and proliferate to fight antigens. The B lymphocytes are essential for humoral immunity. They interact with the T lymphocytes and migrate to the medulla to mature before releasing antibodies. Many interactions in the immune system depend upon the secretion of chemical mediators such as *cytokines* and *chemokines*. *Cytokines* are soluble proteins secreted by cells of the immune system and mediate many functions within the cell. *Chemokines* are cytokines that stimulate the immune system and activate inflammatory cells.[1] They are implicated in acute and chronic conditions such as inflammatory bowel disease, asthma, and rheumatoid arthritis. Figure 10-1 illustrates the lymph glands in the head and neck area and gives a view of the lymphatic chain in the body.

PEDIATRIC PEARLS

Occipital nodes are located high above the hairline in the infant and are often missed by the examiner palpating too low at the nape of the neck. Occipital adenopathy may be an indicator in the newborn of maternal infection during pregnancy or in the infant of an acute viral infection. They may be visible on inspection and are often noted by the parent of a young infant.

PEDIATRIC PEARLS

Visible swelling in the lymph glands on inspection is generally an ominous sign in the child or adolescent and indicates the need for further diagnostics and immediate intervention.

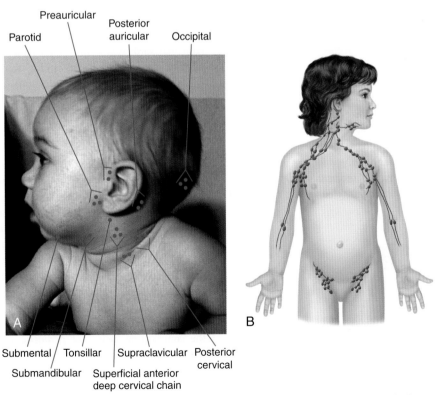

FIGURE 10-1 **A,** Lymph glands in the head and neck area. **B,** Lymph glands in the body.

The *tonsils* and *adenoids* are organs of the lymphatic system. The buds of *tonsillar tissue* are present in the oropharynx at birth, but are underdeveloped. As the immune system develops and reacts to respiratory triggers, such as viral, bacterial, and fungal infections and environmental toxins, the *tonsils* are the first line of defense. The tonsils harbor the immune cells needed to respond to the constant exposure of microorganisms. The adenoidal tissue is a mass of lymphoid tissue situated posterior to the nasal cavity. The *adenoids* are also known as a *pharyngeal tonsil* or *nasopharyngeal tonsil*. Significant hypertrophy of the adenoidal tissue can partially or completely block airflow through the nasal passages and impact the voice.

The *thymus gland* is embedded beneath the upper sternum above the heart and is a fully developed organ in the term infant. The thymus gland is prominent in the mediastinum of the newborn and infant in the first year of life, often shadowing the cardiac silhouette on radiographs (Figure 10-2). In the infant, the thymus begins to produce mature T lymphocytes and plays an important role in cell-mediated immunity. In puberty, when the immune system is well established, the thymus decreases in size and is gradually and almost entirely replaced by adipose tissue. Some thymus tissue persists, but is usually undetectable in the adult.

The *spleen* lies in the upper left quadrant of the abdomen protected by the rib cage. It is composed of lymphoid tissue and reticuloendothelial cells and is a densely vascular organ. The spleen acts to filter antigens in the bloodstream and responds to systemic infections. The spleen acts as a part of the immune system and hosts a sequence of activation events similar to the lymph nodes to fight blood-borne infection. In the infant and young child, the spleen stores erythrocytes and filters the blood through the large presence of phagocytes. The spleen plays an important role in the immune system and the storage of erythrocytes, but it is a nonvital organ in the body.

PHYSIOLOGICAL VARIATIONS

The lymphatic system is one of the most sensitive indicators of infection and toxins in children. The lymphatic tissue plays a role in the immune system as a first responder to fight infection through phagocytosis, the destruction of harmful cells, and the production of lymphocytes and antibodies.

In the newborn, the amount of lymphatic tissue is small, but *lymphadenopathy,* enlargement or disease of the lymph glands, can often be detected particularly in the occipital region as a result of perinatal infections. Lymphoid tissue increases throughout the first year of life, and cervical lymph nodes become more pronounced with respiratory infections by 12 months of age. In the young child, splenomegaly may also occur with episodic viral illness. By school age, tonsillar and adenoidal tissues are approximately the same size as in an adult, and then they increase in volume during pubertal development when tonsillar tissue becomes twice the adult size. During adolescence, the volume of lymphatic tissue begins to decrease and resumes an adult level, which is 2% to 3% of total body weight.

The variable size of the lymphoid tissue in early and middle childhood may be one of the contributing factors of *pediatric disordered breathing,* but other common causes include congenital craniofacial abnormalities, chronic nasal allergy, recurrent respiratory infections, and childhood obesity. All children

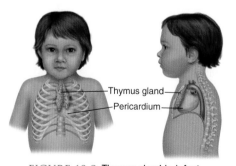

FIGURE 10-2 Thymus gland in infant.

INFORMATION GATHERING FOR LYMPHATIC SYSTEM ASSESSMENT AT KEY DEVELOPMENTAL STAGES

Age-Group	Questions to Ask
Preterm infant and newborn	History of maternal substance/alcohol abuse? Maternal infections or autoimmune disease? HIV+ mother? Neonatal sepsis? Meningitis? Immunization history in NICU?
Infancy	Neonatal screen results? History of maternal/neonatal infection? History of fever/respiratory infection? Poor growth or failure to thrive?
Early childhood	Lymphadenopathy? History of fever/respiratory infection, exposures? International travel? Persistent lymph gland swelling? Head tilt? Neck pain/stiffness? Anemia? Tonsilitis? Adenoiditis? Oral candidiasis or chronic diarrhea?
Middle childhood	Lymphadenopathy? History of fever/respiratory infection? Exposures? Fatigue? Loss of appetite? History of anemia? International travel? Family history of infections, tuberculosis? Snoring? Disrupted sleep from snoring?
Adolescence	Lymphadenopathy? Swelling to extremity? History of fever/respiratory infection? Neck pain/stiffness? Fatigue? Weight loss or gain? Neck swelling?
Environmental risks	Contact with chemical cleaning agents, hazardous chemicals, smoke, radiation, hazardous waste? Recent professional carpet cleaning?

NICU, Neonatal intensive care unit; *TORCH,* Toxoplasmosis, Other (congenital syphilis and viruses), Rubella, Cytomegalovirus, and Herpes simplex virus.

and adolescents should now be screened for snoring.[2] It is important to differentiate primary snoring from snoring associated with disordered breathing. Pediatric sleep-disordered breathing is characterized by prolonged partial upper airway obstruction and intermittent obstructive apnea that disrupts normal sleep patterns.[2] The prevalence of obstructive sleep apnea is currently 1% to 3% in the pediatric population, and the prevalence of primary snoring is estimated to be 3% to 12%.[3]

SYSTEM-SPECIFIC HISTORY

When a child presents with *lymphadenopathy* or enlarged lymph glands, obtaining a complete history is key to an accurate assessment of infection in the pediatric population. The Information Gathering table reviews the areas of assessment that are pertinent for each age-group and developmental stage and focuses on exposure to infection.

PHYSICAL ASSESSMENT

Lymph glands are distributed throughout the body and normally range in size from 3 mm in the head to 1 cm in the neck and inguinal area. In children, lymph glands are often palpable and the pediatric health care provider will often palpate small, firm, mobile lymph nodes along the *cervical* chain on physical examination. These are occasionally referred to as "shotty" nodes because of their pellet-like distribution. The provider must be an astute observer when examining the lymphatic system, because each region of the body has clusters or chains of lymph glands that can signal infection in adjacent areas (Table 10-1).

Inspection and Palpation

It is important to include the *inspection* and *palpation* of the lymph glands regionally during the physical examination. The examination includes palpating lymph glands

TABLE 10-1 SIZING OF LYMPH GLANDS ON EXAMINATION

Size	Description
1+	Shotty, firm, nontender, <1 cm to >1-1.5 cm, requires deep palpation
2+	Mobile, detectable on superficial-to-deep palpation, >2-2.5 cm
3+	Palpable superficially, visible on inspection, >3-3.5 cm
4+	Lymph glands are walnut size or larger, nonmobile, tender; skin can be reddened and warm; >4-4.5 cm; visible on inspection

accessible in four areas: the head and neck, arms, axillae, and inguinal areas of the body. Inspect enlarged lymph nodes for erythema or edema. Most effective for palpation are the pads of the examiner's second, third, and fourth fingers. It is important to distinguish between massage and palpation. Massaging an area superficially may not detect nodes, but superficial then deep palpation with the forefingers moving over the neck regions can better determine the size and mobility of a lymph gland. Lymph nodes are generally mobile, nontender, and do not feel warm to the touch. Lymph nodes that are immobile, tender, and warm to the touch indicate infection or an abscess and require further diagnostic evaluation and treatment.

Head and Neck

Assessment of the lymph glands begins with the inspection of the clusters of lymph glands in the head and neck area followed by palpation. The *cervical nodes* constitute the largest collection of lymph glands in the body. In children, the cervical glands are often palpable because of the frequency of respiratory infections. The *posterior auricular* and *preauricular nodes* are often not palpable in the presence of common respiratory infections but are enlarged and palpable with infection related to the external and internal ear, the *pinna,* and surrounding skin. The *occipital nodes* in the infant and young child lie on either side of the occiput just above the base of the skull. In the young infant, the occipital nodes are located well above the hairline adjacent to the occipital bony prominence and are commonly palpable with viral respiratory infections.

The *parotid* glands are located anterior to the ear and surround the oral cavity. The *mandibular, submandibular,* and *submental* glands are located along the anterior and posterior jaw line and under the anterior jaw. They are palpable when infection occurs in the tongue, mucous membranes of the mouth, sublingual area extending to the base of the tongue, or gums or when decay or abscess occurs in the teeth (Figures 10-3 and 10-4).

The *superficial cervical nodes* are palpable at the juncture of the *mandible* and *sternocleidomastoid muscle* at the neck. This examination requires both superficial

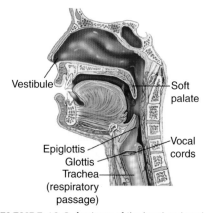

FIGURE 10-3 Anatomy of the head and neck.

Vestibule

Soft palate

Epiglottis
Glottis
Trachea
(respiratory passage)

Vocal cords

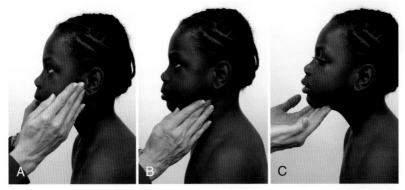

FIGURE 10-4 **A-C,** Palpation of the cervical chain in a school-age child.

and deep palpation depending on the age and developmental stage of the child or adolescent. These glands are almost always palpable during throat and respiratory infections, but may be missed due to incorrect positioning of the fingertips during the assessment of the neck (Figure 10-5). The *deep cervical nodes* are rarely palpable and are only identifiable with deep palpation in the older child. Visible swelling in the lymph glands on inspection is generally an ominous sign in the child or adolescent and indicates the need for further diagnostics and immediate intervention.

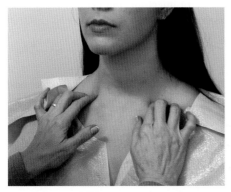

FIGURE 10-5 Palpation of the supraclavicular nodes.

Abdomen

Palpation of the *spleen* is an important part of the examination for the lymphatic system, and tenderness and enlargement of the spleen on deep palpation indicates the need for further diagnostic evaluation. The examination of the spleen is reviewed in Chapter 14.

The *inguinal nodes* can be palpated along the juncture of the thigh and abdomen and along the inguinal ligament and the saphenous vein. The horizontal chain of inguinal nodes runs along the inferior groin and the vertical chain can be palpated on deep palpation along the upper inner thigh. If lymph glands are enlarged in the inguinal area, they are often visible when the young child lies supine on the examining table. Figure 10-6 shows a young child in the supine position for examination of the inguinal nodes. Inguinal lymphadenopathy often occurs with systemic viral infection in the pediatric patient. Table 10-1 reviews commonly used sizing of the lymph nodes on physical exam.

Extremities

The *axillary, brachial,* and *subscapular* nodes lie anteriorly along the brachial artery and in the axillae along the lateral edge of the pectoralis major muscle. They are generally

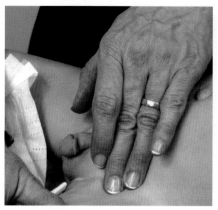

FIGURE 10-6 Palpation of inguinal nodes in a young child.

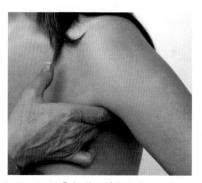

FIGURE 10-7 Palpation of the subscapular nodes of the axillary chain.

noted in children only on deep palpation unless enlarged. Examination of the subscapular nodes of the axillary chain is illustrated in Figure 10-7. The *epitrochlear* nodes lie along the medial aspect of the arm above the elbow and are palpable over the *humerus*. The *epitrochlear* and *popliteal* nodes are the only peripheral lymph nodes in the lymphatic system and act as collection ducts for the limbs.

DIAGNOSTIC PROCEDURES

Complete blood count (CBC), erythrocyte sedimentation rate, and blood and throat culture studies are commonly used for diagnostic evaluation of lymphadenopathy. However, biopsy of the lymph nodes may be indicated when an isolated, enlarged lymph node or nonmobile mass persists in children or adolescents and does not respond to antibiotic therapy. Children with primary snoring and symptoms of obstructive sleep apnea require a full-night polysomnography (PSG) for confirmatory diagnosis or pediatric sleep-disordered breathing.[4]

LYMPHATIC CONDITIONS

The extensive lymphatic system throughout the body provides the health care provider with a map in times of illness. The patterns of drainage leading to the regional lymph glands are indicative of infections that occur in different areas throughout the body. Accurate assessment and diagnosis may depend on the health care provider's knowledge of the lymphatic drainage system. The head and neck region is the area of the body with the highest concentration of lymph glands, and even mild infections in children cause swelling in the regional lymph glands. But generalized swelling of the lymph glands indicates a systemic source of infection, and general lymphadenopathy is more likely to occur in children than in adults.

Lymphadenopathy in children is generally episodic, benign, and self-limiting and is most often associated with viral infections. Table 10-2 reviews some of the causes of regional and systemic lymph node swelling in infants, children, and adolescents. Table 10-3 reviews common pediatric infectious conditions presenting with lymphadenopathy.

TABLE 10-2   REGIONAL AND SYSTEMIC CAUSES OF LYMPHADENOPATHY

Region	Related Causes
Occipital	Scalp infections such as seborrheic dermatitis, tinea capitis, pediculosis/head lice; viral syndromes such as varicella, measles, rubella, roseola; viral respiratory infections (i.e., rhinovirus, RSV, postimmunization)
Preauricular, parotid, postauricular, and superficial cervical	Infection of pinna (ear), otitis externa, middle ear infection; parotitis
Cervical glands—tonsillar, sublingual, submandibular, deep cervical	Tonsillitis, pharyngitis, stomatitis; tooth decay, dental abscess; ear infection; oral mucosa/mucous membrane infections, tongue; cervical adenitis from systemic infections; neoplasm or cancer; postimmunization response
Axillary	Breast infections, thoracic wall inflammation, infections of shoulder and arm, systemic infection, or neoplasm in lymphatic system
Supraclavicular and subclavian	Neoplasm or cancer—metastatic cancers from respiratory, gastrointestinal, or lymphatic system
Epitrochlear and popliteal	Forearm and finger infections, infection secondary to fractures, skin infections, neoplasm, or cyst in lower extremity, venous insufficiency, cardiac or renal disorder
Inguinal	Diaper rash, gluteal and perineal infections; skin infections in lower abdominal area; foot and leg infections, systemic viral infections
Generalized lymphadenopathy	Systemic disease occurring in lymphatic, circulatory, respiratory, gastrointestinal, or genitourinary system; infections such as tuberculosis, HIV

RSV, Respiratory syncytial virus.

TABLE 10-3   LYMPHATIC CONDITIONS

Condition	Description
Cat-scratch disease	Bacterial infection *(Bartenolla henselae)* caused by scratch or bite from contact with kitten or cat; initial lesion on face/arm area; fever may or may not be present; regional lymphadenopathy present after incubation period of 10-14 days or longer
Cervical lymphadenitis	Marked swelling most commonly in anterior cervical node, although other lymph glands can be involved; characterized by tenderness, >4+ swelling *Etiology:* Primarily streptococcal, 20% staphylococcal, 10% of viral origin
Hodgkin lymphoma	Malignant neoplasm of lymph system characterized by painless, enlarged lymph nodes, generally asymmetrical, nontender, firm along cervical/supraclavicular chain; onset common in adolescent or young adult; swelling in left clavicular node in adolescent males is ominous sign of disease
HIV seropositive, AIDS	HIV+ adolescent onset of severe fatigue, weight loss, fever, persistent lymphadenopathy with history of recurrent persistent infections including pneumonias

Continued

TABLE 10-3 Lymphatic Conditions—cont'd

Condition	Description
Infectious mononucelosis	Systemic viral etiology characterized by splenomegaly with accompanying tenderness, cervical adenopathy 3+ to 4+; may be tender/firm; tonsillar hypertrophy *Etiology:* Epstein-Barr virus 30% to 50% of time.
Leukemia	Most common malignancy of childhood characterized by fever, fatigue, lymphadenopathy, splenomegaly, pallor, loss of appetite; may present with purpura or petechiae
Lymphangitis	Acute onset of inflammation of lymphatic vessels or channels usually extending from finger, forearm, or upper arm infection; characterized by erythematous line extending from infection area along collecting vessels *Etiology:* Streptococcal or staphylococcal bacteria
Obstructive sleep apnea	Disordered breathing during sleep characterized by frequent snoring (≥3 nights/wk), labored breathing during sleep, gasps, snorting noises or observed episodes of apnea, and daytime sleepiness
Roseola infantum	Viral exanthem of infancy characterized by high fever for 3-4 days and swelling of occipital and postauricular nodes; with defervescence, mildly erythematous morbilliform rash appears over trunk
Streptococcal pharyngitis	Acute onset of bacterial pharyngitis with swollen anterior cervical nodes, fever, malaise, scarlatiniform rash may appear over trunk, abdominal pain

AIDS, Acquired immunodeficiency syndrome; *HIV,* human immunodeficiency virus.

SUMMARY OF EXAMINATION

- Examination of the lymphatic system includes *inspection* and *palpation* of lymph glands regionally (head and neck, arms, axillae, and inguinal areas of the body) during the physical examination.
- In the young infant, the *occipital nodes* are located well above the hairline adjacent to the occipital bony prominence and are commonly palpable with viral respiratory infections.
- The *inguinal nodes* can be palpated along the juncture of the thigh and abdomen over the inguinal area, along the inguinal ligament and saphenous vein.
- Lymph nodes are generally mobile, nontender, and do not feel warm.
- Lymph nodes that are immobile, tender, and warm indicate infection or an abscess and require further diagnostic evaluation and treatment.
- Visible swelling in the lymph glands on inspection is generally an ominous sign in the child or adolescent and indicates the need for further diagnostics and immediate intervention.

Charting

Adolescent with Lymphadenopathy

Neck: 3+ tonsillar lymph nodes, mobile, warm, tender to touch, neck supple with full ROM (range of motion), no meningismus noted.

REFERENCES

1. Porth CM, Matfin G: *Pathophysiology: concepts of altered health status*, Philadelphia, 2009, Lippincott, Williams & Wilkins.
2. Marcus CL, Brooks LJ, Draper KA, et al: Diagnosis and management of childhood obstructive sleep apnea syndrome, *Pediatrics* 130(3):576-584, 2012.
3. Church GD: The role of polysomnography in diagnosing and treating obstructive sleep apnea in pediatric patients, *Curr Probl Pediatr Adolesc Health Care* 42(1):2-25, 2012.
4. Baldassari CM, Kepchar J, Bryant L, et al: Changes in central apnea index following pediatric adenotonsillectomy, *Otolaryngol Head Neck Surg* 146(3): 487-490, 2012.

CHAPTER 11

EYES

Karen G. Duderstadt

When an infant is born, the eyes are anatomically complete, but the sense of vision develops over the first weeks and months of life. The development of normal vision depends on the reception of light rays that stimulate the internal structures of the eye during the early critical period after birth. Visual acuity is determined by an individual's heredity, as well as physical health and environmental factors. Any condition that limits or occludes the process of visual development in the first year of life affects the long-term visual health of the infant and child. A complete and thorough eye examination by the pediatric health care provider is critical to assure optimum visual development for infants and children.

EMBRYOLOGICAL DEVELOPMENT

The development of the eye fields begins in the third week of embryonic development with the optic groves forming in the neural tube, and by the end of the fourth week the optic vesicle is formed and lies close to the ectoderm surface. The surface ectoderm thickens and forms the lens placode. By the fifth week of gestation, the optic cup and the lens cavity are formed, and by the sixth week, invagination of the optic vesicle occurs forming the choroid layer and vasculature of the eye. The formation of the cornea, lens, and anterior chamber proceeds during the seventh and eighth week, and the eyelid folds develop and begin to cover the palpebral fissure. It is during this period of gestation that insults to the fetus, such as maternal rubella, cause the development of congenital cataracts. Development of the

retinal tissue continues with the differentiation of the nerve fiber layer, proliferative layer of the macula, and the pigmented layer of the retina that precedes the development of the iris and the ciliary body, which occurs between the ninth and twelfth weeks of embryonic development. The ciliary body gives rise to the ciliary muscles, which control the accommodative reflex and pupillary aperture (Figure 11-1). Development of the structures of the eye is complete by 15 weeks' gestation. At the fourth month of gestation, the development of the retinal blood vessels is initiated and full vascularization of the retina occurs just before birth in a term infant.[1] The pupillary light reflex, which requires intact optic and oculomotor nerves, can be elicited by 30 weeks' gestation.

DEVELOPMENTAL AND PHYSIOLOGICAL VARIATIONS

Visual development begins after birth at the very center of the *retina* in the *macula*. The macula is a circular area surrounding the *fovea*. At birth, the macula is not fully developed but holds the genetic potential for 20/20 vision. The retina predominantly consists of rods at birth, and the cones are located near the outermost layer of the retina. As the retina is exposed to light, the cones migrate toward the center to become the anatomical macula on the *fundus* at the posterior surface of the retina. The lens has a key role in focusing light on the neural layer of the retina, and the ciliary muscles assist in accommodation of the lens.

The *optic nerve* is also developing at the same time as the retina. There are as many as 8 million cells in the optic nerve and 5 million

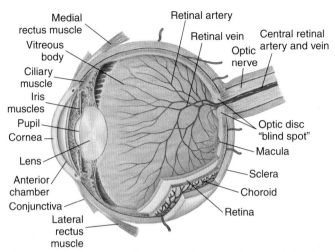

FIGURE 11-1 Anatomy of the human eye. (From Seidel H, Ball J, Dains J, et al: *Mosby's guide to physical examination*, ed 7, St. Louis, 2011, Mosby.)

retinal cells in the optic neuron at birth that compete for synaptic sites on the nerve. Cells that are not oxygenated do not develop. *Hypoxia* or *hyperoxia* in the preterm infant often impact the normal development of the retina, and cause a *retinopathy,* a disorder of the retinal vessels. Infants born prematurely have an avascular zone in the periphery of the retina that disrupts the normal proliferation of the retinal vessels and interrupts blood flow to the visual receptors. The disruption of blood flow may lead to retinal detachment from the choroid, causing visual impairment or blindness if left untreated. The gestational age of the infant at birth determines the area of the avascular zone.[1] Very low birth weight infants ($\leq$1500 g) are at high risk for *retinopathy of prematurity,* and infants born at 28 weeks' gestation or weighing $\leq$1000 g are at highest risk for developing macular folds and retinal detachment.[2] Refractive anomalies also occur approximately eight times more frequently in preterm infants than in term infants.[3]

Term infants from 36 to 40 weeks of gestation can perceive shape, color, motion, and patterns at birth. Visual development in the newborn is dependent upon development of

the visual pathways that link the eyes to the lateral geniculate nucleus in the thalamus to the visual cortex located in the occipital lobe of the brain. Exposure to light begins the synaptic development of the neurons at birth.[3] Central fixation is present shortly after birth in the term infant, and the human face at a distance of 8 to 12 inches holds the most visual interest for a newborn. The term infant is *hyperopic,* or farsighted, at birth. Visual images are focused behind and not on the retina, so the visual image is blurred. For the infant to see near objects, the *ciliary muscles* of the eye must work hard to accommodate, or shape, the lens; in time these efforts of the *ciliary muscles* result in thickening of the lens, which makes accommodation of the image onto the retina possible.

The term infant's eyes often wander or deviate in the first 6 weeks when trying to achieve visual fixation in the *central field* of vision. After 6 weeks of early visual stimulus, an infant is able to focus and visually follow an object or the parent's movements. Any inability to visually focus after 6 weeks of age in a term infant is considered suspect and at 3 months of age is considered abnormal. As the eyeball or *globe* grows, the hyperopia decreases and the lens hardens, but detailed visual acuity is not present until 3 to 4 months of age in the healthy eye and not until 3 to 4 months corrected age for preterm infants (Table 11-1). Differentiation and maturation of the retinal layers of the macula, which is responsible for colors and contrasts, precise visual acuity, and stereoscopic vision; and the fovea, which is responsible for central vision, continues until 8 months of age.[3] The critical window for normal development of full visual acuity is from birth to 5 to 6 years of age, and the synaptic development of the neuronal paths in the visual cortex continues until approximately 10 years of age. After this age, conditions that affect early visual development cannot be completely corrected (Table 11-2).

TABLE 11-1   Visual Development

Age	Developmental Stage of Vision
Birth	Awareness of light and dark
Neonatal	Rudiments of fixation on near object
2 weeks	Intermittent fixation
4 weeks	Follows moving objects
6 weeks	Fixates and follows moving objects
8 weeks	Convergence beginning to stabilize
4 months	Inspects hands and small held objects; vision 20/300
6 months	Retrieves small objects; hand-eye coordination appears
9 months	Binocular vision clearly established; beginning of depth perception
12 months	Vision 20/180; looks at pictures with interest; fusion is established
18 months	Convergence established; visual localization peripherally poor
2 years	Accommodation well developed; vision 20/40 in normal eyes

Anatomy and Physiology

External Eye

The *bony orbit* is the structure surrounding the eye in the cranium. Only one third of the eyeball, or optic *globe,* in the infant and child is exposed to the examiner, and the cranium protects the remainder of the globe in the orbital cavity. The *optic foramen* is the opening in the cranium that allows the passage of the optic nerve, ophthalmic artery, and ophthalmic vein to pass from the globe to the brain and visual cortex. The upper eyelid is shaped by connective tissue containing *tarsal plates.* The *meibomian glands* are located in the tarsal plates near the hair follicles of the eyelashes in the upper and lower lids. In infants and children with atopic or allergic reactions, the meibomian glands, one of the oil producing sebaceous glands in the body, exude a yellowish sebaceous material onto the base of the eyelids. The eyelashes add further protection to the surface of the eye.

The *lacrimal gland* is located in the lateral aspect of the frontal bone in the orbital cavity (Figure 11-2). It is a peanut-sized gland similar to the salivary glands. In each eyelid, a *lacrimal duct* opens onto the eyelid margin, and the *nasolacrimal duct* opens into the *lacrimal sac,* which is buried in the frontal process of the maxillary bone. The *lacrimal puncta* are noted at the edge of the upper and lower eyelids at the *medial* or *inner canthus* and allow the drainage of tears into the *nasolacrimal duct* and the *lacrimal caruncle.* The *lacrimal caruncle* is the elevated area of tissue bordering the upper and lower medial canthus and assists in drainage of tears. Tear production is normally present by 6 weeks of age in the term infant.

The *sclera,* the outermost layer of the exterior structure of the globe or eyeball, is the firm collagenous layer that protects the intraocular structures (see Figure 11-2). The *conjunctiva* is formed by thin mucous membrane lining the anterior surface of the sclera and inner eyelids and acts along with the tear film

TABLE 11-2 PHYSIOLOGICAL VARIATIONS OF THE EYE

Age-Group	Variations
Preterm infant	• 24 weeks: Partially fused eyelids • 24-28 weeks: Eyelids open spontaneously • 28-30 weeks: Eyes have membranous embryonic vascular network over iris to protect lens, producing dull retinal or red light reflex • 36-40 weeks: Membrane over iris normally resolves; persistent membrane may result in anterior cataracts
Newborn	• Macula not fully developed, eyes tend to drift in initial newborn period • Benign scleral hemorrhage often present after birth • Definite ability to follow object not developed until 4 weeks • Lacrimation present at 6 weeks of age
Infancy	• 3-4 months: Fully fixates and follows object • Sucking often stimulates infant to open eyes and focus attention on surroundings • 3-5 months: Color discrimination present • 6 months: Eye color generally established • Infants may have visible sclera above and below cornea • Intermittent convergent strabismus common until 4 months of age
Early childhood	• 2 years of age: Binocular vision and depth perception are developed in healthy eye • Visual acuity should be 20/40 to 20/50 • >3 years of age: Visual acuity should be 20/30 • Accommodation and convergence are smooth and well established
Middle childhood	• Refractive error is common beginning at 9 years of age • Visual concerns about near vision in school-age child often are related to learning differences
Adolescence	• Hormonal changes during early and middle adolescence often cause change in visual acuity

as a protective covering for the cornea. The conjunctiva has two surfaces: the palpebral and bulbar. The *palpebral conjunctiva* lines the inner eyelids, is vascular, and is covered by papillae. The *bulbar conjunctiva* is clear and contains no papillae and very few blood vessels. The *bulbar conjunctiva* covers the sclera up to the *limbus,* the juncture of the sclera and the cornea.

The *cornea,* the most anterior aspect of the external eye, is a lenslike structure that acts as a refractory surface for the eye and connects with the sclera at the limbus. The cornea is transparent and contains no blood vessels. The transparency allows light to be focused on the retina. It derives oxygen

from the aqueous humor and from tears. The *anterior chamber* is directly posterior to the cornea, and the *posterior chamber* is the thin area between the lens and the posterior iris. The anterior and posterior chambers contain *aqueous humor,* a clear nutrient fluid that circulates around the lens and the cornea and provides nutrition and oxygen. *Glaucoma* is increased intraocular pressure resulting from abnormalities in the drainage of the aqueous humor, which damages the optic nerve and may cause blindness.

The *iris* is the pigmented structure containing the sphincter and dilator muscles, connective tissue, and pigmented epithelium. An absence of color in the iris may indicate

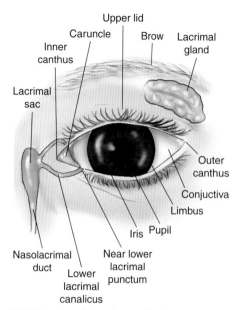

FIGURE 11-2 External eye and lacrimal apparatus.

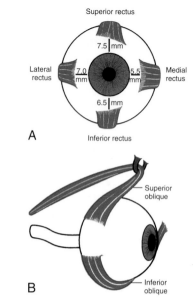

FIGURE 11-3 **A,** Four extraocular recti muscles. **B,** Oblique extraocular muscles. (From Palay DA, Krachmer JH: *Primary care ophthalmology,* ed 2, St. Louis, 2005, Mosby.)

albinism. The center of the iris is controlled by the *ciliary body* and *iris muscles* and forms the aperture, or pupil. The *pupil* constricts or dilates depending on the amount of light entering the eye. The ciliary body produces aqueous humor and controls accommodation. The iris lies behind the anterior chamber and in front of the *crystalline lens* and is protected by a thin clear capsule attached by small filaments to the ciliary body. A *cataract* is an opacity that obscures the crystalline lens.

The upper eyelid is elevated by the *levator muscle,* which inserts into the tarsal plate in the upper eyelid and is innervated by cranial nerve III.

Extraocular Muscles and Internal Eye

The six *ocular muscles,* inserted into the scleral surface, control the movement of the eye (Figure 11-3). The four *rectus* muscles—the *superior, inferior, medial,* and *lateral recti*—originate at the top of the globe deep in the cranium and extend from the anterior to insert at the back of the globe. The medial

rectus muscle is responsible for the movement of the eye toward the midline, and the lateral rectus muscle innervated by cranial nerve VI moves the eye away from the midline. The inferior and superior rectus muscles move the eye upward and downward and also have overlapping functions with the oblique muscles. The two *oblique* muscles—the *superior* and *inferior oblique*—insert at the anterior and posterior globe. The superior oblique tendon passes through the *trochlea,* the small, cartilaginous pulley on the frontal bone. The *superior oblique* muscles are responsible for movement of the eye downward and inward, and the *inferior oblique* moves the eye upward and inward. The superior oblique muscle is innervated by cranial nerve IV, and paralysis of the nerve causes a head tilt or torticollis in children to compensate for the weakened muscle.

The *vitreous body* is the large interior cavity of the globe and contains a clear gel or *vitreous humor.* The *choroid* is the interior layer of the eye between the sclera and the retina and is continuous with the iris and ciliary body. It is highly vascular and nourishes the receptor cells of the retinal epithelium. The outer layer of the *retina* contains photoreceptors, the rods and cones, which are stimulated by light focused by the lens and translate light energy or impulses into neuronal activity. The neurons activate the nerve fiber layer of the retinal epithelium and synaptic activity and transmit through the optic nerve to the brain, which perceives the visual image.

The retinal vessels and optic nerve fibers enter and exit through the *optic cup* and divide into two branches on the surface of the optic disc. The *optic disc,* the anterior aspect of the optic nerve, is pink to orange-red or pale with a yellow cup at its center (Figure 11-4). There are no photoreceptors in the optic disc, which creates a blind spot of 5 degrees in the visual field.[4] The *macula* lies medial to the optic nerve on the *fundus,* the posterior surface of the retina. The *fovea* or *fovea centralis* is a central depression in the macula without vessels and has darker pigmentation than the retina. This is the area where vision is most perfect, and the ciliary body works to accommodate the lens to focus an image on the fovea. The *arteries* on the fundus appear thinner and more orange-red than the *veins,* which are larger and darker (see Figure 11-4). The normal arterial-to-venous ratio (A:V) is approximately 2:3 in the healthy individual. Vascular changes present in the retina often reflect abnormal conditions in the systemic vasculature such as diabetes and hypertension. *Papilledema,* bilateral optic disc edema, is also associated with increased intracranial pressure. *Retinal hemorrhage* is associated with acute traumatic brain injury and inflicted traumatic brain injury. *Retinal hemorrhages* associated with *inflicted traumatic brain injury* in children involve deeper layers of the retina and are found more on the periphery of the retina.[5]

FAMILY, CULTURAL, RACIAL, AND ETHNIC CONSIDERATIONS

Thick epicanthal folds are seen more commonly in infants and young children of Asian and Latino descent. They partially or completely cover the inner canthus at birth and diminish by middle childhood. Asian populations have a genetic predisposition to myopia. In one study, 68% of Asian children were found to be myopic.[3] The pediatric health care provider should focus particular attention to early vision screening in this population of children.

Ethnicity is a risk factor for severe retinopathy of prematurity (ROP). Asian and black infants have a higher risk of developing threshold ROP as compared to white infants.[6]

Retinal pigment or melanin is often found on the scleral surface of Latino and African-American children. The pigmented areas usually become evident in early or middle childhood and persist into adulthood. This is within the range of normal variations of the eye and does not impact visual health. The *retinal light reflex* or "red" light reflex varies in color in darkly pigmented individuals. The *fundus* appears pale yellow or beige because of the increased melanin in the skin, and the optic disc is also often a pale yellow.

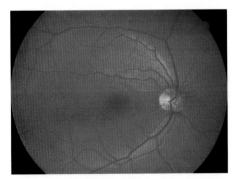

FIGURE 11-4 Normal fundus. (From Palay DA, Krachmer JH: *Primary care ophthalmology,* ed 2, St. Louis, 2005, Mosby.)

SYSTEM-SPECIFIC HISTORY

Detecting vision problems early is critical to the healthy development of the visual system in infants and young children. Obtaining a complete history is key to early identification of visual problems or visual changes in infants, children, and adolescents. The Information Gathering table reviews the pertinent areas of information gathering for each age-group and developmental stage of childhood.

PHYSICAL ASSESSMENT

Equipment

The traditional ophthalmoscope performs all necessary screening in the pediatric population. The PanOptic Ophthalmoscope is the most advanced lens for examining the internal eye structures of infants and children (Figure 11-5). A penlight may be used for screening the corneal light reflex and testing the pupillary reflex. The Snellen E, Tumbling E, Allen vision

INFORMATION GATHERING FOR EYE ASSESSMENT AT KEY DEVELOPMENTAL STAGES

Age-Group	Questions to Ask
Preterm infant	History of oxygen exposure in early neonatal period? History of retinopathy of prematurity? Prolonged phototherapy? History of intraventricular insult? History of maternal substance or alcohol abuse?
Newborn	Significant neonatal or maternal infections? Does infant focus on face of parent when alert? Any eye discharge or swelling? Family history of congenital cataracts or glaucoma? History of maternal substance or alcohol abuse?
Infancy	When did infant begin visually following parent? Does infant blink/react to bright light? Any *rapid* involuntary movement of eyes? Persistent discharge or tearing on one or both sides? Any parental concern about visual development? Significant jaundice in neonatal period? History of maternal infection? Neonatal meningitis? History of abusive head trauma?
Early childhood	Does child sit close to TV? Able to see birds/plane in sky? Any clumsiness/bumping into objects? Holds books close to face? Abnormal head positioning? Appropriate response to visual cues? Frequent eye rubbing? History of frequent stye or hordeolum? Repeated blinking? Difficulty with color recognition? Family history of color vision deficit? History of abusive head trauma?
Middle childhood	History of visual problems? Family history of myopia, strabismus? Is the child squinting? Does child have corrective lenses or refuse to wear them? Date of most recent eye exam? Where is child seated in classroom? Any difficulty reading? Does child learn at grade level? Protective eyewear for sports? Eye pain or strain?
Adolescence	History of eye trauma? Any difficulty with eyestrain when studying? Wears corrective lenses or refuses to wear them? Contact lens wearer? History of corneal abrasion? Date of most recent eye exam? Protective eyewear for sports? History of concussion or head trauma? Driver's license? Restricted license?
Environmental risks	Exposure to eye irritants? Contact with chemical cleaning agents, hazardous chemicals, or smoke?

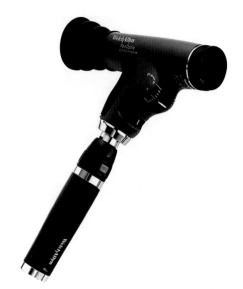

FIGURE 11-5 PanOptic Ophthalmoscope. (Copyright Welch Allyn. Used with permission.)

cards, Blackbird Vision Screening System, and color vision and near vision testing cards may be used in the clinical setting for vision acuity testing for the young child through young adulthood. An eye cover will assist in proper vision testing. Testing of cranial nerves is presented in Chapter 19.

Inspection of the External Eye

Begin the inspection of the eyes with a general inspection of the periorbital region, globe position, and lid margins. Note any asymmetry in the eyelids or eyebrows, and whether the eyelashes are normally distributed. Note the size and shape of the periorbital cavity. The *palpebral fissure* or opening should be on a horizontal plane between the medial and lateral canthus in infants, and slants upward laterally in infants and children of Asian descent or children with Down syndrome. The upper eyelids should appear symmetrical. Inspect the *conjunctiva* for erythema or irritation, and the lid margins for erythema, crusting, lash distribution, and cysts or lesions. The eyelashes should be carefully examined for nits or lice. Observe for *entropion* (eyelashes curl inward) or

ectropion (eyelashes curl outward and lower eyelid appears droopy).

Conditions such as *ptosis,* an eyelid that droops or has an absent or faint lid crease, may be a normal variant or the result of a brachial plexus injury during a difficult delivery. *Ptosis* extending partially over the pupil and causing the infant to tilt the head in an effort to see constitutes an impact on the visual field and requires prompt referral to a pediatric ophthalmologist (Figure 11-6). When closed, the upper eyelid should meet the lower eyelid and completely cover the cornea and sclera.

Inspection of the Upper Eyelid

Inspection of the inside of the upper eyelid may be necessary when a child or adolescent presents with conjunctival irritation, infection, trauma, foreign body, or possible injury or abrasion of the cornea. To evert the upper eyelid for examination in the cooperative child, give the child a toy or bright object and ask the child to look down at the object. Grasp the upper eyelashes at the base and *gently* pull out and up while pushing in and down with a cotton applicator on the upper *tarsal plate* (Figure 11-7). Gently remove the cotton applicator and hold the eyelid

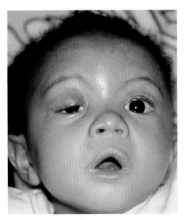

FIGURE 11-6 Congenital ptosis. (From Palay DA, Krachmer JH: *Primary care ophthalmology,* ed 2, St. Louis, 2005, Mosby.)

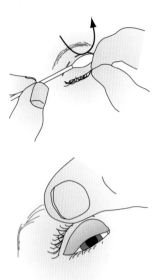

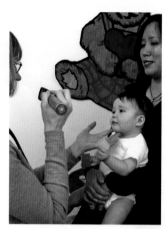

FIGURE 11-8 Position for testing corneal light reflex.

FIGURE 11-7 Examination of the upper eyelid.

while inspecting the *adnexa*. The palpebral conjunctiva should have a pink and glossy appearance and the adnexa should be clear. To return the lid to a normal position, have the child look up as the lid is released. This procedure is well tolerated by middle childhood and in cooperative preschool children. In early childhood, administration of a topical anesthetic, such as proparacaine, may be necessary, or referral to an ophthalmologist may be made if warranted to ensure a thorough assessment. Newborn infants will occasionally have an inverted eyelid, which is within the normal range of variations.

Assessment of Visual Fields and Visual Alignment

The alignment and the position of the *pupil* in the visual field and the clarity of the cornea is determined by the *corneal light reflex,* or *Hirschberg test* (Figure 11-8). It can be performed with a penlight or otoscope light without the speculum. Focus the light source about 12 inches from the infant and note the reflection of the light from the cornea at the center of the pupil. The light should be symmetrical in the center of the pupil. Any asymmetry of the light reflex could indicate ocular misalignment and could impact visual development. Follow the corneal light reflex with testing the muscle balance of the eyes.

Evaluate the six extraocular muscles (EOMs) by having the child follow a penlight or the examiner's finger through the six cardinal fields of gaze in the visual field (Figure 11-9, *A*). This testing evaluates the normal function of oculomotor (cranial nerve III), trochlear (cranial nerve IV), and abducens (cranial nerve VI) nerves (see Figure 11-9, *B-D*). In infancy and early childhood, the examiner should focus the light about 12 inches from the eyes. A cooperative infant should normally be able to follow the light on horizontal and vertical planes by 6 months of age.

The *cover-uncover test* further evaluates ocular alignment and can be performed as early as 6 months of age in an alert infant. The young infant should be assessed on the examination table. The infant or toddler should be seated in the parent's lap. Begin by having the infant or child fixate on a penlight or light of the otoscope, the light of the large aperture on the ophthalmoscope, or a bright object. If the infant is alert but distracted, it is helpful to dim the lights and use a toy. Keep in mind infants will often reach for the toy, but will

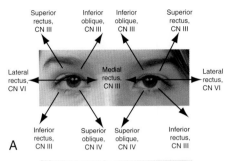

A, Six cardinal fields of gaze labels:

Superior rectus, CN III | Inferior oblique, CN III | Inferior oblique, CN III | Superior rectus, CN III

Lateral rectus, CN VI | Medial rectus, CN III | Lateral rectus, CN VI

Inferior rectus, CN III | Superior oblique, CN IV | Superior oblique, CN IV | Inferior rectus, CN III

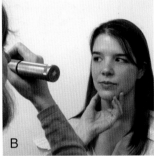

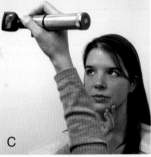

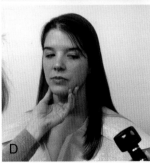

FIGURE 11-9 **A,** Six cardinal fields of gaze with associated cranial nerves. **B,** Testing lateral rectus, CN VI. **C,** Testing superior rectus, CN III. **D,** Testing superior oblique, CN IV. *CN,* Cranial nerve.

often focus on a light. Use the nondominant hand or an occluder brought in laterally over the eye while the infant or child is fixating on the light or bright object. Observe the uncovered eye for fixation on the light or object. Remove the hand or occluder, and note any deviations or movement of the covered or uncovered eye from the central gaze. Any deviation or movement of the eye from the central gaze or focus on refixation on the light by either the covered or uncovered eye may indicate abnormal alignment and should be further evaluated (Figure 11-10). An inward deviation of the eye is referred to as *esotropia* (Figure 11-11); an outward deviation is referred to as *exotropia.* If a *phoria* is present, the covered eye will deviate and refixate when the hand or occluder is removed. This indicates a focusing abnormality and should be referred. A common finding in the young infant is *pseudoesotropia,* a crossed appearance of the eyes caused by the large epicanthal folds covering the sclera (Figure 11-12). As visual acuity develops, the cover-uncover test should be performed with the child fixating on a distant object or wall poster and should continue to be part of the physical examination until 10 years of age.

Conditions of Visual Alignment

Abnormalities in ocular alignment noted on examination may be congenital or acquired and may involve conditions affecting the muscle or nerve. *Congenital esotropia* occurs in the first 6 months and *accommodative esotropia* occurs between 12 months and 7 years of age.

Strabismus is nonalignment of the eyes causing the visual image to fall on the retina at a distance from the fovea. This disrupts binocular vision or visual fusion and keeps the eyes from working simultaneously. The resultant double vision and loss of depth perception from the blurred image impacts normal visual development during the critical period of development in the first 5 to 6 years of life. Young children are often unaware of visual changes

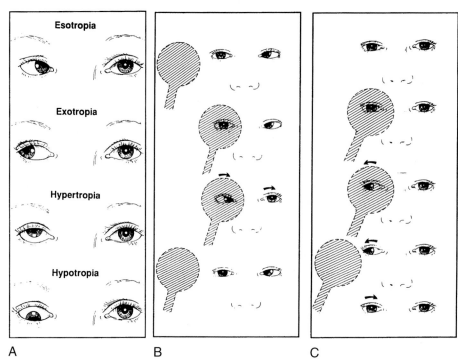

A   B   C

FIGURE 11-10 **A,** Types of strabismus. **B,** Cover-uncover test for tropia. **C,** Cover-uncover test for phoria. (From Magramm I: Amblyopia: etiology, detection, and treatment, *Pediatr Rev* 13[1]:7-14, 1992.)

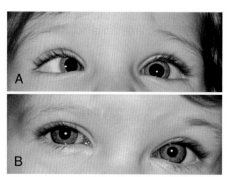

FIGURE 11-11 **A,** Esotropia. **B,** Shortly after corrective muscle surgery. (From Palay DA, Krachmer JH: *Primary care ophthalmology,* ed 2, St. Louis, 2005, Mosby.)

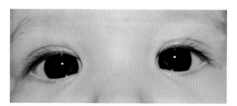

FIGURE 11-12 Pseudoesotropia. (From Palay DA, Krachmer JH: *Primary care ophthalmology,* ed 2, St. Louis, 2005, Mosby.)

or deficits. If strabismus goes undiagnosed, amblyopia develops.

Amblyopia is a monocular loss of vision due to insufficient visual stimulation during the critical period of visual development in the first 6 to 8 years of life. The *cover-uncover test* and the *corneal light reflex* are both required in a complete ophthalmological examination to detect strabismus and amblyopia.

Nystagmus is spontaneous, involuntary movement of one or both eyes and is an indication of poor visual acuity. In the preterm infant, *persistent* or *horizontal nystagmus* can indicate retinopathy of prematurity, intracranial hemorrhage, or tumor. In the term infant, *congenital nystagmus* can be associated with Down syndrome, atrophy of the optic nerve, retinal dystrophy, congenital cataracts, abnormalities of the ocular muscles or nerves, vestibular disturbances, and decreased visual acuity. In the older child or adolescent, drug overdose or chemical toxicity is a possible cause. Slight horizontal nystamus in the lateral fields is normal. Children with amblyopia exhibit nystagmus because of loss of vision in the affected eye. If nystagmus is noted, a thorough neurological examination is warranted as well as an evaluation by a pediatric ophthalmologist.

Assessment of the Internal Eye

The *retinal light reflex* or *red light reflex* determines the clarity of the posterior chamber of the eye, the receptivity to light, and the sensitivity of the *retina* to visual stimulus. To elicit the retinal light reflex, the examiner brings the ophthalmoscope to the eyebrow and positions it obliquely at a 15- to 25-degree angle lateral to the eye about 12 inches from the infant or child. Use the ophthalmoscope on the "0" setting to view the fundus. In dimmed light, bring the retinal light reflex into view in each eye. Inspect for symmetry and brightness, or brilliance, of the retinal light reflex. A lens that is congenitally dislocated or abruptly dislocated because of trauma also appears as a darkened or asymmetrical retinal light reflex. Any asymmetry in size or color or darkness in the uniformity of the retinal light reflex indicates the need for immediate referral to an ophthalmologist.

The *Bruckner test* assesses the retinal light reflex simultaneously in both pupils

---

PEDIATRIC PEARLS

To visualize the retinal or red light reflex in the newborn or early infancy, hold the infant upright, cradling the head, and gently rock the infant. As the head is lowered to the exam table, the eyes usually will open.

---

from a distance of 2 feet to 3 feet from the infant or child. Compare the pupil and iris in both eyes for color, size, shape, movement, and clarity. To inspect for *opacities,* illuminate the cornea by shining the light of the ophthalmoscope obliquely about 15 degrees from the lateral canthus. An alert infant with normal visual development should blink at a bright light directed at the eye.

To test for *visual accommodation* and *pupillary reaction,* shine a bright light momentarily into the eye. As the light approaches the iris, the pupil should begin to dilate. When bringing the light of the large aperture of the ophthalmoscope near the pupil from a distance, the pupils constrict as the light nears.

Conditions of the Internal Eye

Any serious defect of the cornea, aqueous chamber, lens, and vitreous chamber can be detected in the infant and young child by assessing the quality of the retinal light reflex. A *coloboma,* an irregular or teardrop-shaped iris, indicates a deficit in the visual field and requires immediate referral (Figure 11-13).

Leukokoria, a whitish opacity of the pupil visible in dim light or in room light, is highly abnormal and appears as an absent retinal light reflex or a partially darkened reflex if

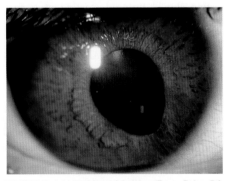

FIGURE 11-13 Iris coloboma. (From Palay DA, Krachmer JH: *Primary care ophthalmology,* ed 2, St. Louis, 2005, Mosby.)

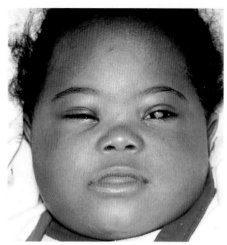

FIGURE 11-14 Leukokoria. (From Palay DA, Krachmer JH: *Primary care ophthalmology*, ed 2, St. Louis, 2005, Mosby.)

the opacity does not cover the entire pupil (Figure 11-14). This finding is usually *unilateral. Congenital cataracts* and *retinoblastoma* are associated with an absent or incomplete retinal light reflex and may have a presenting sign of leukokoria.

Visual Acuity Testing

Visual acuity testing begins at 2 to 3 years of age with the Allen vision cards (Figure 11-15 and Table 11-3). Children should be allowed to practice with a parent or caretaker to familiarize themselves with the figures. Then testing should proceed starting at a near distance, testing each eye separately using an occluder held by the parent. The examiner should then show the Allen vision cards while walking backward and continue testing one eye and then both eyes until the distance is 15 feet to 20 feet for the 3- to 5-year-old child. Allen vision cards test to 20/30 or 15/30 depending on the distance from the child and the figure size of the cards.

The Snellen *Tumbling E test* begins in the prekindergarten age-group and is used until the child knows standard letters with accuracy. It is also used with children and adolescents with low literacy or learning problems. The examiner may ask the child which way the "legs of the table" are pointing. Using this directional approach may be difficult for children with learning disabilities or attention or behavior problems. The Snellen distance acuity chart can be used when the child achieves literacy. Children of school age may become *myopic* (nearsighted) as the eye matures. This condition is most often noted in girls between 9 and 11 years of age and slightly later in boys. *Myopia* increases throughout adolescence and into early adulthood.

Testing the eyes separately to detect a difference in refractive error is extremely important in young children. Occluding the eye properly is the key to accurate testing of visual acuity. *Anisometropia,* a difference in refraction between the eyes, can lead to amblyopia. It is difficult to detect in the young child because the eye initially remains in alignment. Referral is indicated if accurate visual testing yields a >20 difference in refraction between the eyes, for example 20/40 in the left eye and 20/70 in the right eye.

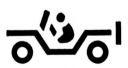

FIGURE 11-15 Allen vision cards. (From Palay DA, Krachmer JH: *Primary care ophthalmology*, ed 2, St. Louis, 2005, Mosby.)

TABLE 11-3 VISUAL ACUITY TESTING

Age-Group	Examination at All Well Visits	Referral Criteria
Preterm infant	Red or retinal light reflex Penlight exam of cornea Evaluate for nystagmus	Criteria for high-risk preterm infants: <33 weeks, <1500 g, oxygen required >48 hours; referral to pediatric ophthalmologist required for evaluation
Newborn	Red or retinal light reflex Penlight exam of cornea Evaluate for nystagmus	Asymmetrical, absent, or white reflexes Cloudiness of cornea Presence of *rapid* involuntary ocular movement
Infancy	Red or retinal light reflex Penlight exam of cornea Evaluate for nystagmus Corneal light reflex Cover/uncover test Fixation to light/follow 90 degrees	Asymmetrical, absent, or white reflexes Objects to occlusion for *cover/uncover test* Strabismus: Any ocular misalignment or deviation of eye from central axis after 3 to 4 months of age
Early childhood	Red or retinal light reflex Corneal light reflex Cover/uncover test Visual acuity: Allen vision cards, Tumbling E, Blackbird Vision Screening System Funduscopic exam	Acuity of 20/50 to 20/40 in one or both eyes with accurate vision testing Difference of >20 between right and left eye Strabismus: Abnormal cover/uncover test
Middle childhood	Red or retinal light reflex Corneal light reflex Cover/uncover test Extraocular muscle testing Visual acuity: Tumbling E, Snellen Funduscopic exam	Acuity of 20/40 in one or both eyes Difference of >20 between right and left eye Strabismus: Abnormal cover/uncover test Abnormal funduscopic exam
Adolescence	Visual acuity: Snellen Tumbling E for low literacy Extraocular muscle testing Funduscopic exam	Refractive error: Acuity of 20/40 in one or both eyes Abnormal funduscopic exam

EVIDENCE-BASED PRACTICE TIP

In all patients with unilateral nasolacrimal duct obstruction (NLDO) and anisometropia, the side with the NLDO had higher hyperopia. Of the 70 infants with risk factors, 44 were later treated for amblyopia: 29 with spectacles alone, 2 with occlusion therapy, 13 with spectacles and occlusion therapy. Six patients required strabismus surgery. In all patients with unilateral NLDO and anisometropia, the side with the NLDO had higher hyperopia.[7]

EVIDENCE-BASED PRACTICE TIP

Vision problems can interfere with the process of reading, but children with dyslexia or related learning problems have the same visual function and ocular health as children without such conditions. Currently, there is inadequate scientific evidence to support the view that subtle eye or visual problems cause or increase the severity of learning problems.[8]

Color Vision Testing

Visual testing for color sensitivity should occur at 4 years of age or before school entry. Children should be tested between 4 and 8 years of age for any history of difficulty with color recognition. Difficulty or confusion when identifying colors may be related to cognitive learning differences and should alert parents and teachers. The incidence of *color vision deficit,* previously referred to as *color blindness,* is 8% in white males and 4% in African-American males. The incidence in females is from 0.4% to 1%. Testing should be completed with the *Hardy-Rand-Rittler (HRR) test.* The HRR test uses a series of symbols rather than numbers, which allows reliable testing to be done on young children. The *Ishihara test,* which uses a series of figures and letters composed of spots of certain colors, can be used on the older child. The child with a color vision deficit does not see letters or figures of a certain color.

Funduscopic Examination

The ophthalmoscopic exam permits the pediatric health care provider to clearly visualize the internal structures of the eye in a child who is able to sit for examination and focus steadily on a distant point. This generally occurs in the prekindergarten or early school years.

Using the lens selector disc, focus the ophthalmoscope on the palm before examining the child to determine the clarity of the image and accommodate for any visual deficit in the examiner. The lens indicator may read "0" or +/− to produce the clearest image depending on the visual acuity of the examiner. Resting the left hand on the child's forehead just above the eyebrow, begin with the ophthalmoscope positioned laterally about 2 inches from the eye to decrease *miosis,* constriction

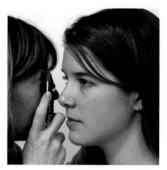

FIGURE 11-16 Positioning ophthalmoscope for exam.

of the pupils (Figure 11-16). The rubber pad on the face of the ophthalmoscope should be resting on the eyebrow of the examiner. Use a distant focal point to attract the child's attention and help him or her fixate. As the examiner moves medially toward the central field of vision, the vessels of the *fundus* should come into view. Once a vessel in the *retina* is in focus, follow along the vessel; where it "branches" will point toward the *optic nerve.* The *optic disc* should come into view in the medial aspect of the fundus. The macula is examined last to minimize miosis. Forcibly opening the eyes of a child results in a frustrated child and an incomplete examination. If examination is immediately necessary but cooperation is not achieved through verbal preparation or proper positioning of the child, then referral to a pediatric ophthalmologist is warranted.

EYE CONDITIONS

Table 11-4 presents the most common and chronic eye conditions seen in infants, children, and adolescents by the pediatric health care practitioner.

TABLE 11-4   EYE CONDITIONS

Condition	Description
Sundowning	Downward deviation of the eyes associated with hydrocephalus, intracranial hemorrhage, other pathological brain conditions, or early sign of cerebral palsy; a sign of increased intracranial pressure when symptoms of lethargy, poor feeding, vomiting, bulging fontanel, or rapidly increasing head circumference are noted
Exophthalmos	Protrusion of the globe, also known as *exophthalmia* or *proptosis,* may be unilateral (e.g., orbital tumor, orbital cellulitis, or a retrobulbar hemorrhage) or bilateral (Graves' disease or *hyperthyroidism*)
Conjunctivitis	Acute inflammation of palpebral and bulbar conjunctiva; etiology includes viral, bacterial, corneal abrasion, allergy, or environment irritation
Blepharitis	An acute or chronic irritation of the eyelid; may be caused by allergic conditions such as seborrhea, bacterial infections (staphylococcal), inflammation of meibomian glands, or parasites
Chalazion	A cyst in the eyelid caused by inflammation of the meibomian gland; differs from a stye or hordeolum because it is usually painless. Also known as *meibomian gland lipogranuloma*
Stye or hordeolum	An infection of the sebaceous glands of Zeis at base of eyelashes; can be external or internal. Internal stye or hordeolum is an infection of the meibomian sebaceous glands lining the inside of the eyelid
Pterygium	Overgrowth of conjunctival tissue extending from the lateral canthus to cornea; begins in childhood with overexposure to sun and constant dust/environmental irritants
Scleral icterus	Yellowish coloration of sclera extending to the cornea; most often first indication of systemic jaundice and liver dysfunction in neonate
Lacrimal duct obstruction	Abnormal tearing pattern; upward pressure on lacrimal sac often yields mucoid discharge; massage of nasolacrimal duct with downward pressure on lacrimal sac may open duct to normal drainage by 6 months of age
Dacryocystitis	Inflammation of nasolacrimal sac; swelling and redness occur around lacrimal sac in area of inner canthus
Retinoblastoma	Solid intraocular tumor; presents as abnormal retinal or red light reflex in newborn or as white pupillary reflex in infant; can be associated with proptosis, protruding eye bulb
Congenital glaucoma	Triad of symptoms in 30% of infants: photophobia (sensitivity to bright light), epiphora (excessive tearing), and blepharospasm (eyelid squeezing); conjunctival injection, ocular enlargement, and visual impairment may occur in some infants

SUMMARY OF EYE EXAMINATION

- Begin by noting the symmetry of the eyes and the size and shape of the periorbital cavity.
- Perform the corneal light reflex to determine the clarity of the cornea as well as the alignment and the position of the pupil in the visual field.
- Evaluate the extraocular muscles in the six cardinal fields of gaze.

- Perform the cover-uncover test for ocular alignment.
- Elicit the retinal light reflex or red light reflex.
- Check for pupillary accommodation.
- Perform age-appropriate visual acuity testing.
- Perform an ophthalmoscopic examination for children and adolescents

Charting
3-Year-Old Child

Eye: Vision with Allen vision cards 20/40 bilaterally. Extraocular movements intact, sclera and conjunctiva clear, corneal reflex intact bilaterally, irides brown, pupils accommodate. Funduscopic examination reveals a symmetrical red or retinal light reflex.

Charting
Well Adolescent

Eye: Sclera and conjunctiva clear, extraocular movements (EOMs) normal (nl), irides brown, PERRLA (*P*upils, *E*qual, *R*ound, *R*eact to *L*ight, and *A*ccommodate), funduscopic examination—without opacities, optic disc visualized, pale yellow, disc margins clear (cl). Vessels nl, arteries/veins (A/V) ratio 2:3.

REFERENCES

1. Chen J, Smith LEH: Retinopathy of prematurity, *Angiogenesis* 10(2):133-140, 2007.
2. Davidson S, Quinn GE: The impact of pediatric vision disorders in adulthood, *Pediatrics* 127(2): 334-339, 2011.
3. Bremond-Gignac D, Copin H, Lapillonne A, et al: Visual development in infants: physiological and pathological mechanisms, *Curr Opin Ophthalmol* 22(Suppl):S1-8, 2011.
4. Wright KW: *Pediatric ophthalmology for primary care*, ed 3, Elk Grove, IL, 2008, American Academy of Pediatrics.
5. Minns RA, Jones PA, Tandom A, et al: Prediction of inflicted brain injury in infants and children using retinal imaging, *Pediatrics* 130(5):1-8, 2012.
6. Aralikatti AK, Mitra A, Denniston AK, et al: Is ethnicity a risk factor for severe retinopathy of prematurity?, *Arch Dis Child Fetal Neonatal Ed* 95(3):F174-176, 2010.
7. Matta NS, Silbert DI: High prevalence of amblyopia risk factors in preverbal children with nasolacrimal duct obstruction, *J AAPOS* 15(4):350-352, 2011.
8. Handler SM, Fierson WM, Section on ophthalmology: learning disabilities, dyslexia, and vision, *Pediatrics* 127(3):e818-856, 2011.

CHAPTER 12

EARS

Patricia Jackson Allen

The ear is a sensory organ that functions as part of the complex sensory system for hearing and vestibular equilibrium. Visual inspection of the ear is only the first step in determining the normal function of this complex organ. The role of the pediatric health care provider is to maintain function of the ear to preserve hearing in the child and adolescent, and to detect any abnormalities early in infancy to promote optimum development of hearing and to support normal development of speech and language.

EMBRYOLOGICAL DEVELOPMENT

External Ear

The ear is located in the temporal bone of the skull and is composed of the inner, middle, and external ear (Figure 12-1). The structures of the ear evolve in the mesoderm, and development of the external ear begins during the sixth week of gestation when the six *hillocks of His* develop from the first and second branchial arches. The individual portions of the *auricle,* or flap of the ear, begin to fuse and assume the classic adult shape by the twelfth week of gestation, and fusion is complete by the twentieth week (Figure 12-2). The normal auricle should be no greater than 10 degrees off vertical plane or slope, and the superior portion should be in line with the outer canthus of the eye (Figure 12-3). Minor malformations of the auricle may be normal variants such as *preauricular skin tags,* a *preauricular sinus* or *Darwin tubercle,* a slight thickening or nodule at the upper portion of the helix (Figure 12-4). Malformations can also be the result of intrauterine position or may be related to genetic syndromes or other alterations in development occurring during the same gestational period.

Inner Ear

Although the external ear formation coincides with the gestational formation of the internal ear structures, they develop separately. The auditory placode and the acousticofacial ganglion are present the fourth week of gestation. Over the next month, the first of the three turns in the cochlea develops. Arrest in development during this phase results in a common bony abnormality of the inner ear associated with congenital sensorineural hearing loss known as *Mondini deformity.* The final 2.5 turns of the cochlea occur by the twelfth week of gestation. The *organ of Corti* develops from the epithelium of the cochlea and is responsible for transmission of sound impulses to the eighth cranial nerve, the *acoustic nerve.* Improper development of the membranous labyrinth of the organ of Corti results in a *Scheibe deformity,* the most common congenital abnormality of the cochlear duct, resulting in sensorineural hearing loss (see later section, Hearing Loss). The semicircular canals first appear in the sixth week of gestation with differentiation of canal structures being complete by the sixteenth week. The sensory cells needed for equilibrium actually attain adult size by the twenty-third week of gestation. Alterations in development during this period due to chromosomal abnormalities or other causes can lead to hearing loss of particular tones.

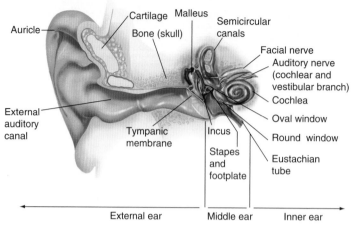

FIGURE 12-1 Anatomy of the middle and inner ear in skull.

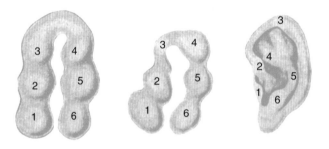

6th Fetal week   12th Fetal week   20th Fetal week

FIGURE 12-2 Auricular development in the fetus. (Adapted from Flint P, Haughey B, Lund V, et al: *Cummings otolaryngology–head and neck surgery*, ed 5, Philadelphia, 2011, Mosby.)

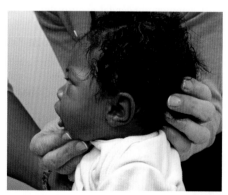

FIGURE 12-3 The normal alignment of the ear.

Middle Ear

Simultaneous with the early development of the inner ear is the formation of the first pharyngeal pouch in the oropharynx. The proximal portion of the pharyngeal pouch develops into the *eustachian tube,* and the distal portion becomes the tympanic cavity and supporting structures. The eustachian tube is 17 to 18 mm long at birth and lies 10 degrees off the horizontal plane. The development of the tympanic cavity with ossicles is not complete until the eighth month of gestation, but the malleus

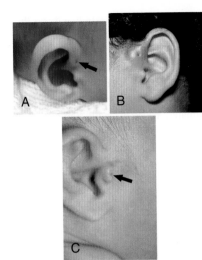

FIGURE 12-4 **A,** Preauricular sinus. **B,** Abscessed preauricular sinus. **C,** Preauricular skin tags. (A, From Department of Otolaryngology, Southampton General Hospital: The preauricular sinus: a review of its aetiology, clinical presentation, and management, *Int J Pediatr Otorhinolaryngol* 69(11):1469-1474, 2005; **B,** From Zitelli BJ, Davis HW: *Atlas of pediatric physical diagnosis,* ed 4, St. Louis, 2002, Mosby; **C,** Adapted from Field et al: *Pediatrics: an illustrated color text,* Edinburgh, 1997, Churchill Livingstone.)

and incus reach adult size and shape by the eighteenth week of gestation and the stapes by the twentieth week of gestation.[1] The *manubrium, malleus,* and *stapes* and their supporting ligaments are formed by the *Meckel* and *Reichert cartilage.* Failure of ligaments to form properly results in a conductive hearing loss[2] (see later section, Hearing Loss). A conductive hearing loss is also seen in children with *osteogenesis imperfecta,* which causes *otosclerosis,* an abnormal destruction and redeposition of the bony structures of the labyrinth.

DEVELOPMENTAL VARIATIONS

Table 12-1 presents variations in the pediatric age-group from the preterm infant to the school-age child.

ANATOMY AND PHYSIOLOGY

External Ear (Pinna)

The external ear is divided into sections: the outer portion is called the *helix,* just medial and parallel to the helix is the *antihelix,* and

---

TABLE 12-1 DEVELOPMENTAL VARIATIONS OF THE EAR

Age-Group	Physiological Variations
Preterm	Vulnerable to hearing loss, particularly before 33 weeks, from noise exposure, hypoxia, ototoxic drugs, hyperbilirubinemia, persistent pulmonary hypertension
Newborn	At birth, tympanic membrane is almost adult size but lies in a more horizontal plane compared to the adult ear, which alters visual assessment Intrauterine positioning may result in disfiguring of the pinna, which will usually resolve after birth with proper positioning because of the elastic quality of the ear cartilage Whitish material including vernix caseosa may be present in external auditory canal Canal narrow and curved making assessment of the middle ear difficult Determining patency of canal is critical
Infancy	Fluid easily trapped in the middle ear due to eustachian tube dysfunction, particularly common in infants with Down syndrome, preterm infants, and any infant with craniofacial abnormalities
Early childhood	External auditory canal ossifies by 2 years of age, straightening the canal and improving visualization of tympanic membrane The pinna is approximately 80% of the adult size in the 4- to 5-year-old
Middle childhood	In a 9-year-old, the pinna and external auditory canal have attained adult size The canal measures 2.5 cm and has become somewhat S-shaped

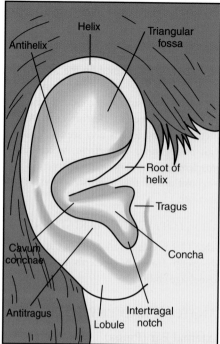

FIGURE 12-5 Anatomy of the external ear of small child labeled with anatomy. (From Zitelli BJ, Davis H: *Atlas of pediatric physical diagnosis*, ed 5, St. Louis, 2008, Mosby.)

the *concha* is the cavity leading to the opening of the external canal (Figure 12-5). A firm protuberance on the anterior portion of the ear just at the entrance to the auditory canal is the *tragus,* and across from the tragus on the border of the antihelix is the *antitragus*. Beneath the

tragus is the soft fold of skin that forms the ear lobe. Although the shape of the auricle varies slightly from person to person, the ears should be comparable bilaterally in size, shape, and position and not significantly varied bilaterally.

The external auditory canal, measuring approximately 2.5 cm in length, connects the outer ear to the middle ear and funnels sound waves to the tympanic membrane. The auricular muscles are innervated by the seventh cranial nerve, or *facial nerve.* The medial portion of the canal is innervated by the fifth cranial nerve, or *trigeminal nerve,* and the posterior canal by the tenth cranial nerve, or *vagus nerve.* The exterior third of the ear canal contains hair follicles, ceruminous glands, and sebaceous glands. The ceruminous gland, a modified apocrine sweat gland, secretes a milky substance that forms cerumen when exposed to the secretions of the sebaceous glands and air. *Cerumen* lubricates the skin, acts as a barrier to foreign objects entering the interior canal, and has protective antibacterial properties to reduce the incidence of skin infection in the external canal. Natural lateral movement of skin in the external canal facilitates drainage of cerumen and other debris from the external ear canal.

Middle Ear

The tympanic membrane is a thin layer of oval-shaped skin attached to the wall of the external canal and is approximately 9 to 10 mm in diameter (Figure 12-6). It is surrounded by a fibrous

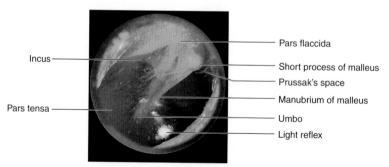

FIGURE 12-6 Normal left tympanic membrane. (From Seidel HM, Ball JW, Dains JE, et al: *Mosby's guide to physical examination,* ed 7, St. Louis, 2011, Mosby.)

band called the *annulus*. The medial surface of the tympanic membrane is attached to the manubrium and lateral process of the malleus. The tympanic membrane has a resonance frequency of 800 to 1600 Hz, approximating the normal speech frequency of 500 to 2000 Hz found in humans. The tympanic membrane is divided into sections: (1) the *pars flaccida* is superior to the lateral process of the malleus, (2) the *pars tensa* comprises the majority of the tympanic membrane inferior to the lateral process of the malleus, and (3) *Prussak's space*, which lies medial to the pars flaccida in the anterior superior quadrant of the tympanic membrane (see Figure 12-6). *Prussak's space* is the most common location of retraction pockets and congenital or acquired *cholesteatoma* (Figure 12-7), an asymptomatic white mass in the middle ear that is thought to arise from the continued growth of the epidermoid layer over the tympanic membrane.[1] Tympanosclerosis, thickening and scarring of the tympanic membrane, is commonly seen after chronic infections of the middle ear (Figure 12-8).

The three *ossicles* of the inner ear, the malleus, incus, and stapes, the smallest bones

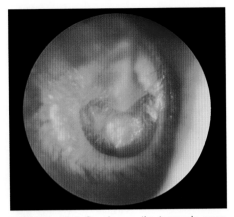

FIGURE 12-8 Scarring on the tympanic membrane. (From Zitelli BJ, Davis H: *Atlas of pediatric physical diagnosis*, ed 5, St. Louis, 2008, Mosby.)

in the body, transmit the movement of the tympanic membrane to the oval window and subsequently to the vestibular and cochlear branches of the eighth cranial nerve, the *acoustic nerve* (Figure 12-9). The head of the *malleus* articulates with the body of the *incus* at the incudomalleolar joint. The long crus or leglike structure of the incus, articulates with the head of the *stapes* at the incudostapedial joint. These joint areas are the most vascular regions of the *ossicles,* and therefore are the most susceptible to trauma or infection. The footplate of the stapes sits upon the oval window of the inner ear at the fibrous stapediovestibular joint. Because of the mechanical function of the three ossicles and the transmission of sound waves from the larger surface area of the tympanic membrane to the smaller surface area of the oval window, there is a net increase of 22 times the sound energy radiating from the tympanic membrane to the oval window.

The eustachian tube opens into the oropharynx just behind the nasal cavity and is the drainage and ventilatory structure for the middle ear. The eustachian tube connects the middle ear with the back of the throat. The middle ear is an air-filled space and when patent has the same air pressure as the outside air pressure.

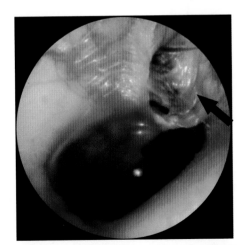

FIGURE 12-7 Cholesteatoma. (Adapted from Flint P, Haughey B, Lund V, et al: *Cummings otolaryngology–head and neck surgery*, ed 5, Philadelphia, 2011, Mosby.)

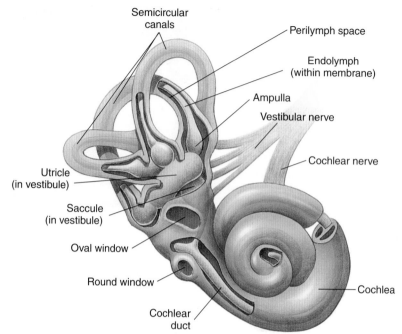

FIGURE 12-9 Anatomy of the inner ear. (From Thibodeau GA, Patton KT: *Anatomy and physiology*, ed 6, St. Louis, 2007, Mosby.)

Normally, swallowing opens the eustachian tube and restores and equalizes the pressure between the middle ear and the outside air pressure. Changes in altitude or ambient pressure, such as occurs on an airplane, can change the middle ear pressure, resulting in pain or discomfort. Repeated swallowing or in infancy sucking on the bottle or breast can often equalize the eustachian tube pressure and reduce the associated pain. In the adult, the eustachian tube averages 35 mm in length. In infancy, it is half that length (around 18 mm), which allows bacteria and viruses to more easily migrate from the oropharynx to the middle ear (Figure 12-10). The musculature of the eustachian tube, which controls function, is innervated by the motor division of the fifth cranial nerve, or trigeminal nerve. In infants and children with cleft palate and other central craniofacial abnormalities such as Down syndrome, structural or functional

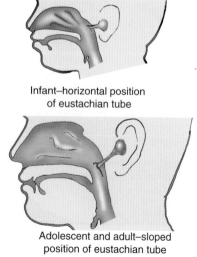

Infant–horizontal position of eustachian tube

Adolescent and adult–sloped position of eustachian tube

FIGURE 12-10 Position of eustachian tube in infant and in adult.

abnormalities of the eustachian tube interfere with normal ventilation and clearance of the middle ear, increasing the incidence of otitis media in these children. Equalization of pressure in the middle ear is critical for normal sound wave vibration of the tympanic membrane.

Muscle maturation, elongation of the eustachian tube, and a more vertical position all contribute to the decreased incidence of otitis media and middle ear effusions in middle childhood, adolescence, and young adulthood.

Inner Ear

The inner ear is the sensory end organ and is directly responsible for hearing and balance. The inner ear contains the *vestibule, semicircular canals,* and *cochlea* and is bathed in fluid that facilitates the transmission of sound waves to the auditory nerve and sensations of balance in the *semicircular canals* (see Figure 12-9). The sound waves pass over approximately 30,000 innervated hair cells in the cochlea, which are the primary receptors, transducers, and conveyers of sound energy to the brain.

PHYSIOLOGICAL VARIATIONS

In recent years, the understanding of genetics and the auditory system have increased significantly. Autosomal recessive genetic sensorineural hearing loss (SNHL) accounts for about 80% of all SNHL in children, and autosomal dominant genetic SNHL accounts for 10%.[1] Some children with hearing loss have identifiable syndromes, such as Usher syndrome, Pendred syndrome, or Jervell and Lange-Nielsen syndrome. Infants with malformed external ear structures require close monitoring. Infants identified with nonsyndromic hearing loss may be missed and are harder to diagnose. Many genetically determined causes of hearing loss do not present at birth and may not be identified through newborn screening. Radiographic imaging such as a CT scan or MRI can identify up to 40% of middle and inner ear abnormalities, but imaging is used cautiously because of the

concern of long-term risks of radiation exposure for infants and young children. Genetic testing is now often the first investigative tool to identify the cause of hearing loss.[3]

Acquired causes of hearing loss are numerous and risk factors must be identified (Box 12-1). Prenatal risk factors include gestational diabetes in the mother, congenital infections (cytomegalovirus, rubella, toxoplasmosis, herpes, syphilis, varicella), exposure to teratogens (alcohol, methyl mercury, thalidomide, cocaine), and ototoxic medications (aminoglycosides, loop diuretics, quinine). Prematurity, birth hypoxia, hyperbilirubinemia, sepsis, and administration of ototoxic medication are risk factors for acquired hearing loss in the perinatal period. Head trauma, infections (mumps, measles, varicella, meningitis, Lyme disease), recurrent otitis media, and excessive noise exposure are risk factors for hearing loss any time they occur.[3]

BOX 12-1   RISK FACTORS FOR HEARING LOSS IN INFANTS AND CHILDREN

- Congenital syndromes (Alport, Jervell, Lange-Nielsen, Usher, Down, Treacher Collins)
- Congenital infections: cytomegalovirus, rubella, toxoplasmosis, herpes, syphilis, and varicella
- Premature birth
- Very low birth weight (VLBW)
- Persistent pulmonary hypertension of the newborn
- History of extracorporeal membrane oxygenation (ECMO) therapy
- History of meningitis
- Exposure to ototoxic drugs (aminoglycosides, platinum-containing chemotherapy) and cranial radiation
- Cholesteatoma
- Chronic or recurrent acute otitis media (AOM) and otitis media with effusion (OME)
- Osteogenesis imperfecta

FAMILY, CULTURAL, RACIAL, AND ETHNIC CONSIDERATIONS

The research literature is inconclusive on the ethnic variations in the prevalence of hearing loss or frequency of otitis media. There is research indicating an increased incidence of otitis media in Native American/Alaska Native children.[4] Other risk factors for otitis media across ethnic groups include children living in low-income households and maternal smoking.[4,5] There is a predisposition or genetic inheritance pattern for both otitis media and sensorineural hearing loss; therefore, family history should be carefully evaluated when gathering a comprehensive health history, and children at risk should have more frequent screening for both otitis media and hearing deficits.

SYSTEM-SPECIFIC HISTORY

The Information Gathering table presents the important information to be gathered for each age-group and developmental stage. Table 12-2 presents the important information for a symptom-focused history for children or adolescents presenting with ear symptoms.

INFORMATION GATHERING FOR EAR ASSESSMENT AT KEY DEVELOPMENTAL STAGES

Age-Group	Questions to Ask
Preterm infant	History of maternal infection? Maternal drug use or maternal diabetes? Antibiotic treatment with aminoglycosides, other ototoxic antibiotic use, salicylates?
Newborn	Newborn hearing screening results? ABO incompatibility? Elevated bilirubin level >20 mg/100 dL of serum? Premature infant? History of anoxia, pulmonary hypertension, ECMO therapy, or meningitis? Any craniofacial abnormalities noted? Family history of hearing deficit, congenital or acquired?
Infancy	Does infant react to sound with startle response or change in activity? Turn head or body toward sound? Does the infant make cooing or babbling noises? Does infant have frequent colds? History of recurrent ear infections or ruptured tympanic membrane? Parental concerns regarding infant hearing or verbalization? Does infant turn head towards parent when name is called?
Early childhood	Do you have any concerns about child's ability to hear or speak? How many words does child use? Does child combine words into meaningful sentences? How clear is child's pronunciation? How many languages are spoken at home or by care providers? Does child play with his ears? Has he ever put small objects in his ears or nose? Has child ever had a hearing test done? Were the results normal? History of ear infection? Was it treated with antibiotics? Does child have frequent colds or respiratory allergies? Does the child attend daycare? If in daycare or preschool, do care providers have any concerns about child's hearing or speech? Has the child had any serious infections or head trauma?

INFORMATION GATHERING FOR EAR ASSESSMENT AT KEY DEVELOPMENTAL STAGES—CONT'D

Age-Group	Questions to Ask
Middle childhood	Does child have frequent colds or respiratory allergies? Has child had any drainage from ears? Frequent ear pain?
	Do you or child's teachers have any concerns about child's hearing or speech?
	Does child have difficulty following directions in school?
	Has child been exposed to unusually loud noises? Does child use headphones to listen to music? Is the volume loud?
	Has child ever complained of ringing in ears, dizziness?
	Does child spend a lot of time playing water sports?
	Previous injury/trauma to head, ears, or mouth?
	History of meningitis?
	History of cancer therapy?
Adolescence	History of frequent colds, nasal allergies, or ear infections?
	Does adolescent use headphones to listen to music? Is the volume loud?
	Has adolescent been exposed to unusually loud music or noises (e.g., rock concerts)?
	Has adolescent ever complained of ringing in ears, dizziness?
	Does adolescent spend a lot of time playing water sports?
	Any recreational activities potentially affecting ear (e.g., swimming, scuba diving, flying, boxing) or work activities (construction work, machinery use)?
Environmental risks	Crowded living conditions?
	Exposure to secondhand smoke?
	Exposure to loud noises?

ECMO, Extracorporeal membrane oxygenation.

TABLE 12-2 SYMPTOM-FOCUSED HISTORY FOR EAR ASSESSMENT

Symptom	Questions to Ask
Ear pain	Onset, duration, and intensity of pain?
	Associated symptoms (e.g., fever, rhinorrhea, cough, ear drainage, hearing loss, vertigo, ringing in ears, swelling or redness around ear, mouth sores, dental pain, sore throat, difficulty sucking or swallowing, vomiting, neck swelling, tenderness)?
	Concurrent illness (e.g., upper respiratory infection, mouth infection, skin infection)?
	Home management of pain (e.g., medications/home remedies): type, how much, how often, how effective?
	Changes in activities of daily living (e.g., loss of sleep, change in appetite, ability to attend daycare, school, or work)? Changes in activity level, talking, or movement of temporo-mandibular joint? Change in interaction with others (e.g., playful, withdrawn, irritable)?
	What makes the pain feel better, worse?
	Others at home, daycare, school, or work with similar symptoms?
	What do you think might be the cause of the pain?
	In infancy: is infant pulling at ear, showing increased irritability, feeding poorly, or waking more frequently at night?

Continued

TABLE 12-2 SYMPTOM-FOCUSED HISTORY FOR EAR ASSESSMENT—CONT'D

Symptom	Questions to Ask
Ear drainage	Onset, duration, and intensity of discharge?
	Associated symptoms (e.g., fever, rhinorrhea, cough, ear pain, hearing loss, vertigo, ringing in ears, swelling or redness around ear, vomiting)?
	Concurrent illness (e.g., upper respiratory infection, mouth infection, skin infection)?
	Changes in activities of daily living (e.g., loss of sleep, change in appetite, ability to attend daycare, school, or work)? Changes in activity level, interaction with others (e.g., playful, withdrawn)?
	Home management of drainage (e.g., medications/home remedies): type, how much, how often, how effective?
	Injury caused by pressure or trauma (e.g., laceration or barotrauma)?
	Others at home, daycare, school, or work with similar symptoms?
	How do you care for/clean your child's ears?
	What do you think might be the cause of the ear drainage?
Hearing difficulty relevant in school-age child and adolescent	Gradual or sudden onset? Progressive?
	Bilateral or unilateral?
	Associated with other symptoms (e.g., ear pain, sense of fullness, drainage, systemic symptoms of illness)?
	Concurrent illness (e.g., otitis media, otitis media with effusion, respiratory allergies)?
	Trauma or exposure to loud noises?
	Changes in activities of daily living (e.g., difficulty hearing in school, at home, watching television, talking on phone)?
	Home management of hearing difficulty (e.g., sitting closer to television or in front of classroom, increasing visual cues for communicating)?
	What conditions make hearing better or worse?
	What do you think might be the cause of the hearing difficulty?
Dizziness or vertigo relevant in school-age child and adolescent	Gradual or sudden onset?
	Associated with other symptoms (e.g., nausea, vomiting, tinnitus, ear pain, ear drainage, hearing loss, systemic symptoms of illness)?
	Concurrent illness (e.g., viral illness, gastroenteritis, respiratory allergies/illness)?
	Use of medications or recreational drugs?
	Changes in activities of daily living (e.g., ability to attend school and work)?
	Home management of dizziness? Others in home with similar symptoms?
	What makes dizziness better or worse?
	What do you think might be the cause of the dizziness?

PHYSICAL ASSESSMENT

Equipment

Equipment for examining the ear includes an otoscope with halogen light and speculum, pneumatic bulb attachment, and gloves if any apparent skin infection or ear drainage is present. Advanced MacroView Otoscopes (see Figure 12-14, *B*) offer improved images of the ear canal and tympanic membrane, and computer-aided software is also available for advanced viewing and education in the clinical setting.

Positioning

Proper positioning of the infant and young child will ensure the least discomfort during the examination, prevent injury to the canal or tympanic membrane during examination, and ensure the health care provider has sufficient opportunity to visualize the canal and tympanic membrane. Letting the young child become familiar with the otoscope by touching the light of the otoscope on the finger or hand often decreases the anxiety of the ear exam (Figure 12-11, *A*). The infant is best positioned lying on the examination table with head securely held on either side by the examiner and the arms restrained by a comforting parent. Older infants who are able to sit securely and young children are best positioned in the parent's lap with the arm and head secured by the parent or examiner (see Figure 12-11, *B*). The curve of the pediatric ear canal can be lessened by pulling the auricle inferiorly and posteriorly (down and back) in the infant and young child, as compared to superiorly and posteriorly (up and back) in middle childhood and adolescence. Be sure not to hold the auricle too firmly causing pain when attempting to straighten the ear canal. Another examination technique that is very useful in the pediatric patient is for the examiner to position the hand above the ear, supporting the ear with the forefingers, and pulling the tragus forward or anteriorly with the thumb or forefinger (see Figure 12-11, *C*). This position effectively opens the external canal in young children to improve visualization of the tympanic membrane. The handle of the otoscope should be held horizontally or vertically when examining children to help stabilize the head and prevent movement of the otoscope during the examination (Figure 12-12).

PEDIATRIC PEARLS

The technique of pulling the tragus forward straightens the auditory canal for ease in examination and causes less discomfort than pulling on the pinna in young children.

External Ear

Inspection

Before examining the ear, inspect the head, face, and neck for any asymmetry or indication of craniofacial abnormality, defect, or infection. The superior portion of the auricle should be equal in height to the outer canthus of the eye and vertical with no more than a 10-degree tilt. An ear that is set lower than an imaginary horizontal line drawn from the outer canthus of the eye or tilted greater than 10 degrees may indicate chromosomal abnormality or congenital abnormalities in other body systems or structures (see Figure 12-3).

Inspect the auricles for size, shape, deformity, placement, discharge, and color. The size and shape of the ears should be similar and may have familial characteristics. In the newborn, the cartilage should have instant recoil, but in the premature infant, the cartilage may appear flattened and have less prominent incurvings of the helix or concha. Grossly misshapen external ears are often associated with anomalies of the middle and inner ear structures and with hearing loss. The placement and angle or tilt of the external ear is discussed earlier. There should be no

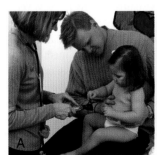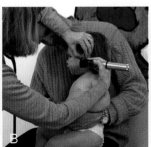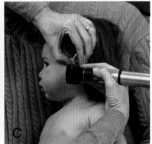

FIGURE 12-11 **A,** Preparing the young child for the ear exam. **B,** Positioning of the toddler for ear exam. **C,** Positioning of tragus forward with hand above the ear.

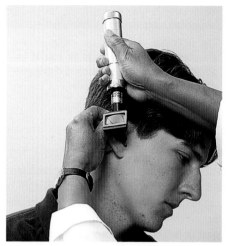

FIGURE 12-12 Holding the otoscope handle in the upright position. (From Wilson S, Giddens J: *Health assessment for nursing practice*, ed 3, St. Louis, 2005, Mosby.)

discharge from the external ear canal, although cerumen may be evident near the opening to the canal. Serous or purulent drainage may indicate a ruptured tympanic membrane, the presence of patent myringotomy tubes, inflammatory response to a foreign object in the ear, or a cholesteatoma. A white cheesy drainage may indicate an infection in the external auditory canal. The color of the auricle should be similar to the facial skin. Redness may indicate inflammation or trauma, and bruising is of particular concern as an indication of trauma possibly associated with head injury or child abuse.

The common normal variations of the auricle include *auricular* or *preauricular sinus, preauricular skin tags,* and *Darwin tubercle* (see Figure 12-4). Occasionally an infection can occur in the preauricular sinus, resulting in inflammation, redness, or discharge from the sinus. Ear piercings should be examined for signs of infection, excessive scar tissue, or trauma.

Palpation

Palpate the auricle for any masses or areas of tenderness. Scar tissue may be palpable around ear piercings but is generally nontender. Sebaceous cysts may occur around the auricle or in the external canal and are often mildly inflamed and tender. If movement of the auricle results in pain, the examiner should suspect *otitis externa,* or other inflammation of the auditory canal. A foul-smelling cheesy discharge is commonly found with otitis externa and often is caused by the bacterium *Pseudomonas.* The mastoid process, posterior to the auricle, should be assessed for swelling, redness, or pain on palpation. *Mastoiditis* is an uncommon but serious complication of otitis media in the developing world. If undiagnosed and untreated, it can lead to meningitis and hearing loss.

External Canal

Inspection

Inspect the external auditory canal for patency, color, discharge, odor, and foreign bodies. The largest speculum that will fit comfortably into the external canal should be used to increase the field of vision. The smallest ear speculum (2.5 mm) is often used for the infant and young child. During the initial newborn examination, patency or atresia of the external auditory canal must be determined. If the canal is not patent or is abnormally narrow or curved, additional abnormalities of the auditory system should be suspected and referral to a specialist for further evaluation should be made immediately. Children with Down syndrome have external canals that are narrower than normal, so the tympanic membrane may be difficult to visualize in early infancy. Vernix caseosa, a whitish cheesy debris, can often be seen in newborn ear canals and can obstruct visualization of the tympanic membrane. It also can be a contributing factor in failed newborn hearing screening or *evoked otoacoustic emission* (OAE) testing in the newborn. Because of the normally curved S shape of the canal, visualization is improved with minimal discomfort if the tragus is pulled forward to visualize the auditory canal and the tympanic membrane. The tympanic membrane of the newborn infant is thicker, grayer, and less translucent than in older children and lies on a more horizontal plane, making visualization more difficult.

Internal Ear

Inspection

Inspect the tympanic membrane for contour (normally concave), intactness (no perforations, tympanostomy or myringotomy tubes), color (normally gray or silver but may be pink or red after crying), translucency (normally translucent without scarring or opacity), and presence of visible landmarks (umbo, handle of malleus, and light reflex) (see Figure 12-6). The light reflex is usually found between the 4 and 6 o'clock positions on the right tympanic membrane and 6 to 8 o'clock on the left tympanic membrane. The examiner should also look for the appearance of fluid bubbles behind the tympanic membrane or a fluid line indicating the eustachian tube is not properly draining the middle ear (Figure 12-13).

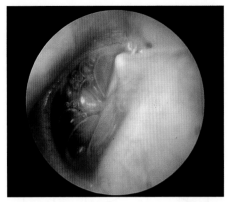

FIGURE 12-13 Middle ear with eustachian tube dysfunction and fluid bubbles. (From Zitelli BJ, Davis H: *Atlas of pediatric physical diagnosis*, ed 5, St. Louis, 2008, Mosby.)

PEDIATRIC PEARLS

Color of the tympanic membrane is less important in diagnosing middle ear infections than the movement and quality of the tympanic membrane. A red or pink tympanic membrane may occur as a result of crying, irritation, or fever and may not be an indication of an acute otitis media.

Mobility of the tympanic membrane, an important indication of middle ear pressure, can be assessed with a pneumatic attachment to the otoscope (Figure 12-14) or by use of a tympanometer. If the middle ear pressure is equalized, the tympanic membrane will move or flutter in response to air pressure from the pneumatic insufflator in the external canal. This can be visualized through the otoscope as movement of the light reflex or recorded on the tympanometer as an equal rise and fall of pressure over the normal pressure setting of zero (Figure 12-15). Decreased or limited

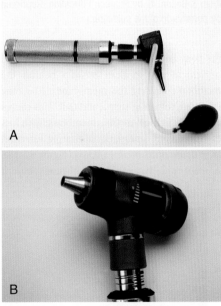

FIGURE 12-14 **A,** Insufflator or pneumatic attachment to otoscope. **B,** Advanced MacroView Otoscope. (From Wilson S, Giddens J: *Health assessment for nursing practice*, ed 5, St. Louis, 2013, Mosby.)

movement indicates either *increased negative pressure* in the middle ear, which is associated with *eustachian tube dysfunction* and *otitis media with effusion* (OME) with the tympanic membrane being retracted and taut and

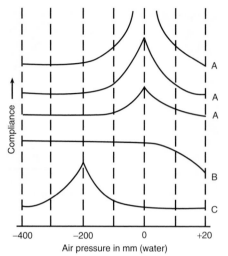

FIGURE 12-15 Tympanometry readings. (From Martin R: *Introduction to audiology,* Boston, 1991, Allyn & Bacon, © by Pearson Education. Reprinted by permission of the publisher.)

the bony landmarks accentuated, or decreased movement due to fluid buildup behind the membrane causing the membrane to become inflamed, convex in shape, and taut. This causes an opacity in the tympanic membrane with loss of visible bony landmarks indicating infection as in *acute otitis media* (AOM) (Figure 12-16). A ruptured tympanic membrane, patent tympanostomy tubes, or cholesteatoma can result in discharge from the middle ear into the external canal. Ear drainage should alert the examiner to these conditions as well as otitis externa.

Ear Cerumen

Parents and caretakers should always be told cerumen is a normal, protective ear secretion. Some infants and children naturally have more wax than other children, particularly children with an oily skin type. Children with allergic skin conditions often have additional cerumen complicating the assessment of ear complaints associated with allergic symptoms or upper respiratory infections. Cerumen has two predominant types. Dry cerumen, which is gray and flaky, is found in 84% of Asians and Native Americans, and wet, honey-colored to dark brown cerumen is found in 97% of whites and 99% of blacks.[1]

Parents should be encouraged to clean the child's ears only with warm soapy water and should not use cotton-tipped applicators to prevent injury to the ear canal or tympanic membrane, and to prevent further impaction of cerumen. School-age children and adolescents should also be instructed to not use cotton-tipped applicators. Removal of cerumen or

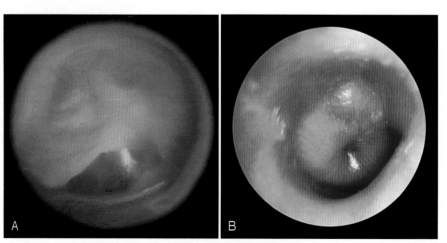

FIGURE 12-16 **A,** Retracted tympanic membrane (TM). **B,** TM with otitis media. (From Lemmi FO, Lemmi CA: *Physical assessment findings multi-user CD-ROM,* St. Louis, 2000, Saunders.)

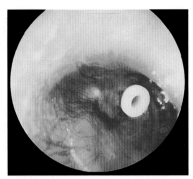

FIGURE 12-17 Tympanostomy or ventilation tubes in serous otitis media. (From Zitelli BJ, Davis H: *Atlas of pediatric physical diagnosis*, ed 5, St. Louis, 2008, Mosby.)

debris from the ear canal may be necessary to visualize the tympanic membrane. If the child can cooperate, a plastic or metal cerumen spoon can be used for removal. An infant or young child must be positioned securely before attempting cerumen removal. If the child cannot cooperate for removal of cerumen when necessary, then irrigating the ear canal with warm water will usually loosen and flush out built-up cerumen. Irrigation should never be attempted if a ruptured tympanic membrane is suspected. Tympanostomy or myringotomy tubes inserted into the pars tensa area of the tympanic membrane for eustachian tube dysfunction are also a contraindication for irrigation of the external auditory canal (Figure 12-17). If the child is asymptomatic, cerumen buildup can be reduced and the canals cleared by daily use of eardrops made of mineral oil and hydrogen peroxide or commercially prepared eardrops for dissolving earwax.

HEARING ASSESSMENT

Hearing impairment in infants and children is a common disability with implications in cognitive, psychosocial, and academic development.[3] Approximately 1 in 1000 neonates has hearing loss identified in the newborn period by universal newborn hearing screening (UNHS).[6] The goal of UNHS is to have all neonates screened for hearing loss before hospital discharge or by 1 month of age to ensure appropriate follow-up is obtained. Newborns who fail the newborn hearing screening and subsequent rescreening should be referred for audiological and medical evaluations to confirm hearing loss by 3 months of age. All infants with hearing loss should begin receiving early intervention services before 6 months of age. Children who receive intervention for hearing loss by 6 months of age usually have normal language development by 5 years of age.[2] The health care provider should not assume if the newborn hearing screening is normal that the growing infant or child's hearing is normal and no further hearing screening is necessary. Ten percent of childhood hearing loss is acquired after birth. It is important to routinely screen for hearing deficits and inquire about any changes noted in the home or school setting when gathering the health history.

The American Academy of Audiology recommends all children and adolescents be screened annually via conventional pure tone audiometry starting at age 3 years.[7] Any child under 3 years of age who has a history indicating high risk for hearing loss or whose parents have concern regarding the child's hearing should be referred to an audiologist or otolaryngologist for testing (see Box 12-1). If significant concerns about hearing are present at any age, generated either from the health history or initial screening, then referral is indicated. Most primary care practices have access to conventional pure tone audiometry, but a variety of other screening tests are available for infants and young children (Table 12-3).

Behavioral audiometry determines the weakest intensity at which a child shows behavioral awareness of the presence of sound. Normal sound fields include 250 Hz to 6000 Hz, but hearing screening is often performed at 25 decibels between 500 Hz and 4000 Hz. Physiological measures of hearing determine the infant's physiological response to stimulation of the auditory system (Table 12-4). Speech audiometry determines the child's response to speech stimuli and tests the clarity of sound received and perceived (Table 12-5).

TABLE 12-3   BEHAVIORAL AUDIOMETRY IN INFANTS AND YOUNG CHILDREN

Test	Age	Method
Conventional audiometry	4 to 5 years	Child is instructed to listen quietly for the test tone and to raise a hand or give a verbal response when it is heard
Bone-conduction testing	5 years	Calibration standards have not been established on infants and children; responses to bone-conducted stimuli may be inferred by head-turn response or as in conventional testing; young children may object to wearing oscillator
Hear test	Infants	Infant reaction to different frequency sounds is observed; elicited with standardized toys (e.g., bell, squeak toy) that make noises at different frequencies
Conditional play audiometry	2 to 5 years	Child performs a repetitive play task (e.g., places block in dish or peg in pegboard) in response to transmitted tone
Visual reinforcement audiometry	Developmental age 6 months to 2 years	Loudspeakers, earphones, or bone-conduction oscillator is used to observe child's ability to hear and localize sound (by turning head or body); visual reward (e.g., lighted toy) provided for accurate responses
Behavioral observation audiometry	Developmental age birth to 5 months	Similar to visual reinforcement audiometry but used for infants or children unable to move head or eyes reliably; any repeatable response to sound may indicate hearing

TABLE 12-4   PHYSIOLOGICAL MEASURES OF HEARING

Screening Test	Response
Auditory brainstem response (ABR)	Measures electrical activity via scalp electrodes in the entire hearing pathway. Headphones or ear probes administer sounds and electrodes on the head measure the waveform response to sound. Can be used for UNHS with pass/fail reading or as diagnostic test. Results can give frequency range and decibel response level information.
Otoacoustic emissions (OAE)	Measures function of the external auditory canal, tympanic membrane, middle ear, and outer hair cells of the cochlear but not the inner hair cells or cochlear nerve. Failure may indicate a nonpatent ear canal, nonaerated middle ear, or lack of normal outer hair cell function needed for auditory nerve function.

UNHS, Universal newborn hearing screening.

TABLE 12-5   SPEECH AUDIOMETRY

Screening Test	Response
Speech detection threshold	Speech stimulus used to determine the ability to hear at varying decibels and frequencies via sound field, earphones, or bone conduction
Speech reception threshold	Word stimulus given and child repeats word or points to picture to indicate word heard
Central auditory processing tests	Tests evaluate school-age children with normal pure tone audiograms to determine speech perception with background noise, sounds in contralateral ear, rapid rate of presentation, or filtering

WEBER AND RINNE HEARING SCREENING TESTS

In older children and adolescents, the *Weber* and *Rinne* tests can be performed as additional screening tests to determine deficits in either conductive hearing or sensorineural hearing, although these tests are rarely used outside of the laboratory or specialty setting. The Weber test is performed by placing a vibrating tuning fork (512 Hz) midline on the skull, making sure the examiner's hand does not touch the prongs of the tuning fork or the child's head. The child/adolescent is then asked if he or she hears the sound of the tuning fork better on one side or the other, or equally well on both sides. If the child/adolescent indicates the sound is heard better on one side, this is called *lateralization* and indicates a conductive hearing deficit in the ear perceived as hearing the tuning fork better.

The Rinne test compares air conduction to bone conduction (Figure 12-18). A vibrating tuning fork is placed on the child's mastoid bone to determine hearing via bone conduction. When the sound is no longer heard, the tuning fork should be moved to a position 1 to 2 cm from the external auditory canal. Sound is then being processed via air conduction in that area. Air conduction should be twice as long as bone conduction. If the bone conduction of sound is heard longer than air conduction, then a conductive hearing loss is present in the affected ear. If the ratio of air conduction to bone conduction is less than 2:1, then a sensorineural hearing loss is present. The Weber and Rinne tests are not reliable on children until school age.

EAR CONDITIONS

Hearing Loss

Before the advent of UNHS, the average age of identification of congenital hearing loss was 2.5 to 3 years. The average age of identification of hearing loss in infants has fallen to 14 months, still too late for ideal early intervention,

because almost half of the infants who fail the UNHS do not receive follow-up testing.[3] In addition, some infants with mild hearing loss will be missed in UNHS, and a proportion of children who pass the UNHS will develop acquired hearing loss. The Joint Committee on Infant Hearing has established guidelines to improved identification of children at risk for late-onset hearing impairment (see Box 12-1).[2]

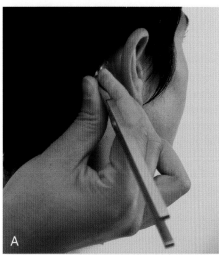

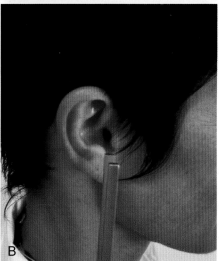

FIGURE 12-18 **A,** Rinne test—bone conduction. **B,** Rinne test—air conduction. (Published in Legent F, Bordure P, Calais C: *Audiologie pratique audiométrie,* ed 3, p. 9. Copyright © 2011 Elsevier Masson SAS. All rights reserved.)

Ongoing regularly scheduled surveillance of developmental milestones, auditory skills, speech and language development, parental concerns regarding hearing, and objective hearing testing are needed to identify children with progressive or acquired hearing loss.[2,7]

Conductive Hearing Loss

Conductive hearing loss is caused by an abnormality in the transmission of sound waves through the ear canal, the tympanic membrane, middle ear space, or middle ear ossicles. The auditory nerve system is intact, but the sound impulses do not reach the nerve. Transient *conductive hearing loss* is common during episodes of otitis media with effusion (OME) or acute otitis media (AOM). Recurrent or chronic bilateral ear effusions during the early years of rapid language, speech, and communication development may impede development. Cholesteatoma, with its associated destruction of the middle ear, is another common cause of *conductive hearing loss,* but this hearing loss will be permanent and progressive unless the cholesteatoma is surgically removed and middle ear reconstructed. Chronic or recurrent ear infections can cause *tympanosclerosis,* visualized as white scarring and thickening of the tympanic membrane (see Figure 12-8), but scarring alone rarely results in measurable hearing loss. Acquired ossicular fixation from chronic diseases of the ear is almost never seen in children, although it is a relatively common cause of acquired hearing loss in older adults. Children with *osteogenesis imperfecta* do develop otosclerosis and must be followed by an ear specialist.

Congenital Conductive Hearing Loss

Congenital conductive hearing loss can occur with Down syndrome or any gestational abnormality of the craniofacial structures. Isolated malformations of the external ear or *microtia,* malformations of the ear canal, can result in *conductive hearing loss.* Congenital stenosis, congenital atresia of the stapes known as *Treacher Collins syndrome,* or congenital fixation of the stapes in the middle ear also result in a *conductive hearing loss.*

Sensorineural Hearing Loss

Sensorineural hearing loss is caused by abnormalities of the cochlea, auditory nerve, or the auditory pathways that traverse the brainstem ending in the auditory cortex of the brain. Sensorineural hearing loss is often congenital and genetically acquired. Genetic predisposition is thought to play a role in 50% of those affected by sensorineural hearing loss. Genetic syndromes that are associated with sensorineural hearing loss are Alport, Jervell and Lange-Nielsen, and Usher syndromes.

Newborns with possible perinatally acquired infections from a variety of pathogens should be screened for sensorineural hearing loss based on their clinical presentation. Any newborn with a history of TORCHS (*t*oxoplasmosis and *o*ther diseases: *r*ubella, *c*ytomegalovirus [CMV] infections, *h*erpes simplex, *s*yphilis) should also be tested and monitored for sensorineural hearing loss. Infants and children with symptomatic congenital cytomegalovirus infection have a 44% chance of developing progressive hearing loss, and asymptomatic infants have a 7.4% chance of developing progressive hearing loss. CMV infection at any age may result in hearing loss.

Premature infants and very low birth weight (VLBW) infants are at increased risk for hearing loss and have a higher incidence of hearing loss than full-term infants. Newborns with a history of persistent pulmonary hypertension or extracorporeal membrane oxygenation (ECMO) therapy have a 20% to 25% incidence of late-onset or progressive hearing loss. Children of any age who develop meningitis must be carefully tested for hearing loss because of both the consequences of the infections and the ototoxic side effects of many antibiotics used to treat meningitis.

Children treated for malignancies with platinum compounds (cisplatin or carboplatin) or who are receiving cranial radiation may develop delayed sensorineural hearing loss and must be followed carefully with audiometry testing.

Mixed Hearing Loss

Hearing loss may also be a combination of conductive hearing deficits and sensorineural hearing deficits. Children with congenital syndromes often have mixed hearing loss.

The management of hearing deficits in children has advanced with new surgical techniques and bone-anchored, bone-conduction hearing aids (Figure 12-19). Cochlear implantation and advances in hearing aids have improved the treatment of hearing loss dramatically, providing some sound to most children with even severe hearing loss.

Otitis Media and Otitis Media with Effusion

Otitis media (OM) is an inflammation within the middle ear that is most often acute but can be chronic, lasting more than 3 months. OM is one of the most common conditions seen in pediatric practice in young children between 6 months and 3 years of age.[3] Children exposed in daycare or crowded living situations are prone to upper respiratory infections that may result in inflammation in the middle ear. Exposure to secondhand smoke has also been shown to increase the risk for OM, whereas breastfeeding

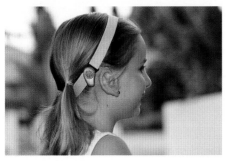

FIGURE 12-19 Example of a bone-anchored hearing aid. (Copyright Oticon Medical. Used with permission.)

has been shown to be protective.[8] There is a genetic component to OM, with a higher incidence of OM in children who have older siblings or parents with a significant history of OM.

Abnormal clearance of middle ear fluid is the cornerstone of OM and OME. Viruses and bacteria from the nasal pharynx enter the middle ear via the eustachian tube opening in the oropharynx. Young children are more prone to OM because of their short, horizontal, less mature eustachian tubes and more frequent upper respiratory tract infections. Children with allergies are more prone to OM because inflammation of the respiratory tract associated with allergies often causes swelling and obstruction of the eustachian tube, trapping fluid. Viruses or bacteria in the middle ear from respiratory infection cause further inflammation and often obstruction. Children with craniofacial defects or immunodeficiencies are at greatest risk for ear infections, and children with placement of nasogatric tubes also have a higher susceptibility.

The majority of OM infections are presumed to be of viral etiology. *Streptococcus pneumoniae, Haemophilus influenzae,* and *Moraxella catarrhalis* are the most common bacterial pathogens found in OM. Expanded immunization schedules covering an increased number of phenotypes of *H. influenzae* and pneumococcal strains have resulted in decreased incidence of OM caused by these organisms.

The presenting symptoms of OM include rapid onset of ear pain or *otalgia,* fever, irritability, and occasionally *otorrhea,* or drainage from the ear. Physical assessment should include careful otoscopy and pneumatic otoscopy to determine inflammation in the middle ear. OM results in opacity and bulging of the tympanic membrane, making bony landmarks difficult to see (see Figure 12-16, *B*). The light reflex becomes diffuse and abnormally positioned on the tympanic membrane. With pneumatic otoscopy, the normal fluttering of the membrane is not present because of the increased fluid pressure in the middle ear. The tympanic membrane is usually erythematous, often with increased vascularity; but these findings can also be present in a child who has been crying, and color should not be used as the primary finding to diagnose OM in young children.

Otitis media with effusion (OME) is actually more common than OM and is defined as middle ear effusion without signs or symptoms of an acute infection.[9] OME presents often with opacity of the tympanic membrane, decreased movement of the tympanic membrane on pneumatic otoscopy or tympanogram, a retracted membrane, and visible air bubbles or a fluid line indicating eustachian tube dysfunction. OME may occur after OM as the acute infection resolves but before air pressure equilibrates, or it may result from eustachian tube dysfunction without acute infection. Chronic OME interferes with sound wave transmission and hearing and is a common cause of conductive hearing loss.

Diagnosing OM or OME with certainty in infants and young children can be a challenge. Positioning and restraining an irritable child, presence of cerumen in a narrow curved ear canal, and difficulty obtaining a proper seal of the ear canal for pneumatic otoscopy or tympanostomy all make certainty of diagnosis difficult. Treatment guidelines and algorithms for OM and OME are well established and take into consideration the child's age, duration of symptoms, and risk factors.[8,9]

SUMMARY OF EXAMINATION

- Before examining the ear, inspect the head, face, and neck for any asymmetry. The superior portion of the auricle should be equal in height to the outer canthus of the eye.
- Inspect the auricles for size, shape, deformity, placement, discharge, and color.
- Inspect the tympanic membrane for contour, intactness, color, translucency, and presence of visible landmarks (umbo, handle of malleus, and light reflex).
- The light reflex is usually found between 4 and 6 o'clock position on the right tympanic membrane and 6 to 8 o'clock on the left tympanic membrane.

- Mobility of the tympanic membrane, an important indication of middle ear pressure, can be assessed with a pneumatic attachment to the otoscope or by use of a tympanometer.
- Ear drainage in the external canal should alert the examiner to otitis externa, a ruptured tympanic membrane, patent tympanostomy tubes, or cholesteatoma.
- Ten percent of childhood hearing loss is acquired after birth. Routinely screen for hearing deficits and begin puretone audiometry at 3 years of age.

Charting
Term Newborn Infant

Ears: Auricle well formed, symmetrical, with normal alignment. External canals patent with small amount of white residue. Tympanic membranes partially visible, gray, opaque, without visible light reflex or bony landmarks. Newborn hearing screening normal.

Charting
Adolescent

Ears: Auricles well formed, symmetrical, with two healed piercings on outer border of helix and one healed piercing center of lobe. No masses, erythema, or tenderness noted. External canals partially blocked with dark brown cerumen. Tympanic membranes pearly gray, concave, light reflex and bony landmarks visible. + movement with insufflation. Audiometry—NL. 500-6000 frequency (Hz) at 25 decibels (dB).

REFERENCES

1. Kliegman R, Stanton B, St. Geme III J, et al: *Nelson textbook of pediatrics*, ed 19, Philadelphia, 2011, Elsevier.
2. American Academy of Pediatrics: Joint Committee on Infant Hearing Practice Guideline: principles and guidelines for early hearing detection and intervention programs, *Pediatrics* 120(4):898-921, 2007.
3. Schoem S, Darrow D: *Pediatric otolaryngology*, Elk Grove, IL, 2012, American Academy of Pediatrics.
4. Daly K, Hoffman H, Kvaerner K, et al: Epidemiology, natural history, and risk factors: panel report from the Ninth International Research Conference on Otitis Media, *Int J Pediatr Otorhinolaryngol* 74(3):231-240, 2010.
5. Smith DF, Boss EF: Racial/ethnic and socioeconomic disparities in the prevalence and treatment of otitis media in children in the United States, *Laryngoscope* 120(11): 2306-2312, 2010.
6. US Preventative Services Task Force: US Preventive Services Task Force recommendation statement: universal screening for hearing loss in newborns, *Pediatrics* 122(1):143-148, 2008.
7. Harlor AD, Jr., Bower C: Hearing assessment in infants and children: recommendations beyond neonatal screening, *Pediatrics* 124(4):1252-1263, 2009.
8. American Academy of Pediatrics: Diagnosis and management of acute otitis meda, *Pediatrics* 131 (3):e964-e999, 2013.
9. American Academy of Family Physicians, American Academy of Otolaryngology-Head and Neck Surgery, American Academy of Pediatrics Subcommittee on Otitis Media With Effusion: Otitis media with effusion, *Pediatrics* 113(5):1412-1429, 2004.

CHAPTER 13

NOSE, MOUTH, AND THROAT

Patricia Jackson Allen

A thorough assessment of the nose, mouth, and throat is an essential part of the pediatric physical examination. Infants and children have frequent upper respiratory and viral infections, and viewing the oropharynx is particularly important when looking for a focus of infection in a febrile child. Also, the oral health of children is key to overall health, and the pediatric health care provider is an important link in providing oral health assessments and prevention of dental caries.

EMBRYOLOGICAL DEVELOPMENT

The facial structures develop in the embryo during the first few weeks of gestation. The tongue, lips, gums, and tooth enamel all evolve from the ectoderm of the primitive mouth, the *stomodeum,* early in the fourth week. The lips are formed during the fourth to eighth weeks of gestation. The primary teeth and salivary glands are formed between the sixth and eighth weeks of fetal life. By the sixth fetal month, the ducts are hollow and begin producing saliva. Calcification of the *primary teeth* begins in the fourth month of fetal life and is complete by the first year of age. Any insult to the sensitive process of tooth formation can result in an anomaly in the color, size, or shape of the primary or permanent dentition.

Early development of the nose begins during the fifth week of gestation, with development of muscle, bone, and cartilage complete by the twelfth week of gestation. The *palate* evolves from fusion of the maxillary prominences during the seventh and eighth weeks of gestation and is completely formed by the twelfth week of gestation during the fusion of the primary and secondary palates. Failure in fusion results in cleft palate. *Cleft palate* is a relatively common congenital anomaly and occurs in 1 in 700 births[1] (Figure 13-1). The incidence varies with race, with Native Americans having a rate of 3.6 in 1000 births, and blacks having the lowest rate of 0.3 in 1000 births.[2] It can be an isolated defect, bilateral cleft, associated with cleft lip, or a component of a syndrome.[2] The etiology is usually unknown, but genetics is thought to be involved in both syndromic and nonsyndromic clefts. Environmental factors may increase the risk of cleft palate; folic acid deficiency, ingestion of some teratogens such as alcohol and phenytoin (Dilantin), and maternal smoking have also been implicated. A *subcutaneous cleft* also can occur during this period with incomplete fusion of the palate; it often goes undetected in the newborn and is associated with persistent abnormal speech patterns.

DEVELOPMENTAL VARIATIONS

Table 13-1 presents the developmental variations to be monitored from infancy to adolescence. Table 13-2 reviews the development of the sinuses from infancy through adolescence.

ANATOMY AND PHYSIOLOGY

External Nose

The nose of the newborn and young infant is generally flattened and malleable (Figure 13-2). In the neonate, the septum is composed of cartilage; ossification occurs during childhood. The nose becomes pyramid-like by adolescence and develops a bony structure. It is divided into four

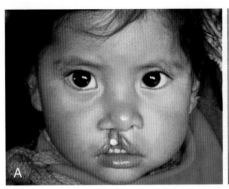
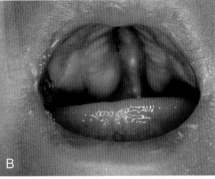

FIGURE 13-1 **A,** Cleft lip. **B,** Posterior cleft soft and hard palates. (**B** from Chaudhry B, Harvey D: *Mosby's color atlas and text of pediatrics & child health,* St. Louis, 2001, Mosby.)

TABLE 13-1   **PHYSIOLOGICAL VARIATIONS OF THE NOSE, MOUTH, AND THROAT**

Age-Group	Physiological Variations
Newborn	Nose cartilage is soft, malleable; deformities in external appearance from intrauterine or birth positioning usually resolve spontaneously; congenital anatomic deformities, obstructive masses, or traumatic obstruction can occlude the nasal passages Natal teeth may be present Epstein pearls—small whitish nodules or cysts—at juncture of hard and soft palates may be visible in first month of life; Bohn nodules, or mucous gland cysts, may be present on gum surface in first 2 to 3 months Rooting, gag, sucking reflexes are present A short tight frenulum or frenulum attached to the inferior tip of the tongue may impede movement of the tongue and breastfeeding
Infancy	Anatomically small airway passages Occlusion of nasal pathways can occur with nasal secretions Deciduous teeth appear between 6 and 24 months Rooting, sucking reflexes wane about 4 to 6 months Drooling increases as salivary gland production increases Anterior permanent teeth begin to calcify at 3 to 12 months Ethmoid and maxillary sinuses present but undeveloped
Early childhood	Tonsils, adenoids enlarge and remain 2+ to 3+ Nasal passages enlarge allowing easier airflow Maxillary and ethmoid sinuses present but sphenoid and frontal sinuses limited in size and function Sinuses not normally assessed in children until middle childhood because of their limited development Swallowing coordination improves; drooling decreases Permanent molars begin to calcify at 18 months to 3 years

Continued

TABLE 13-1 PHYSIOLOGICAL VARIATIONS OF THE NOSE, MOUTH, AND THROAT—CONT'D

Age-Group	Physiological Variations
Middle childhood	Tonsils and adenoids usually begin to atrophy returning to size 1+ to 2+ Horizontal creases on anterior nose may develop in children with nasal rhinitis Deciduous teeth begin to shed; permanent teeth erupt causing change in facial structure, appearance Bridge of nose becomes more prominent Third molar, last permanent tooth, is formed and begins calcifying
Adolescence	All permanent teeth present Bridge of nose formed by bone creating pyramid shape Frontal and sphenoid sinuses completely formed and functioning

TABLE 13-2 DEVELOPMENT OF SINUS CAVITIES

Sinus Cavity	Development
Maxillary	Present at birth; first sinuses to develop significantly; can be seen radiologically at 4 to 5 months of age; opens beneath the middle turbinate into the middle meatus; rapid growth occurs between birth and 4 years of age and 6 to 12 years of age.
Frontal	Last sinuses to develop beginning between 4 and 8 years of age and do not develop fully until late adolescence. Secretions drain into the middle meatus. The walls of the frontal sinus border the orbital and intracranial cavities, increasing the risk for frontal sinus infections spreading directly into these adjacent structures.
Ethmoid	Present at birth, but not developed, grow rapidly during the first 4 years and are fully developed by 12 to 14 years of age; they are first seen radiologically at 1 year of age. Ethmoid sinuses are divided into anterior portion, draining into the middle meatus, and posterior portion, which drains into the superior meatus.
Sphenoid	Undeveloped at birth and do not begin to grow rapidly until 3 to 5 years of age; development complete between 12 and 15 years of age. They lie anterior to the pituitary fossa, and the optic nerve and carotid artery are located on the lateral wall of the sinuses offering a potential route for spread of infection into the central nervous system.

Data from Schoem SR, Darrow DH: *Pediatric otolaryngology,* Elk Grove Village, IL, 2012, American Academy of Pediatrics.

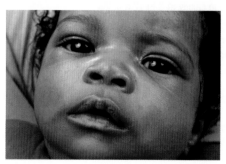

FIGURE 13-2 Flattened nasal bridge in newborn.

sections: the proximal bony portion, often referred to as the *nasal bridge;* the mid cartilaginous vault; the tip, *columella* and *nares;* and the interior *vestibule* (Figure 13-3).

Nasal breathing is the normal breathing pattern, and infants and young children are prone to increased airway resistance because they have anatomically small airway passages. Nasal congestion in the neonate is a common normal finding, and newborn nurseries often discharge infants with a nasal bulb syringe to enable the

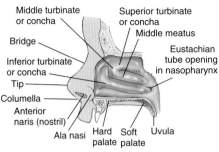

Middle turbinate or concha
Superior turbinate or concha
Middle meatus
Bridge
Eustachian tube opening in nasopharynx
Inferior turbinate or concha
Tip
Columella
Anterior naris (nostril)
Ala nasi
Hard palate
Soft palate
Uvula

FIGURE 13-3 Anatomy of the nose.

gentle removal of secretions from the small narrow nasal passages. In the past, it was thought that newborns are obligatory nasal breathers for the first few months of life. However, research has demonstrated newborns have the ability to switch from nasal to mouth breathing as needed, so they are "preferential" nasal breathers.[2] Respiratory compromise or distress occurs rapidly in the young infant when the nasal passages become occluded. The most common reason for occlusion is mucosal congestion or increased secretions, but congenital anatomical deformities, obstructive masses, or traumatic obstruction can occlude the nasal passages. Nasal resistance may result in 50% of the total airway resistance being largely determined by the size of the airway passages.

Internal Nose

The internal nose, the *vestibule,* is divided by the bony and cartilaginous *nasal septum.* The septum is rarely perfectly straight and a significant deviation of the septum resulting from the birth process or trauma must be assessed to determine whether it interferes with nasal breathing. The perpendicular plate of the nasal septum ossifies by 3 years of age. The anterior portion of the vestibule is lined with vascular squamous epithelium that has tiny hair follicles and secretes mucus. The vast majority of nose bleeds, or *epistaxis,* result from a network of small blood vessels found in the anterior superficial portion of the septal mucosa known as the *Kiesselbach plexus.* The posterior portion is lined with fragile respiratory epithelium. The

lateral walls of the nose are composed of horizontal bony structures known as the *superior, middle,* and *inferior turbinates,* which mature throughout childhood and resemble those of the adult by 12 years of age (see Figure 13-3). They are covered with vascular mucous membranes. Furrows between the bony structures provide recesses to filter air and form a nasal passage, or *meatus.* The posterior *ethmoid sinuses* drain into the superior meatus, and the *paranasal sinuses* drain into the middle meatus. Until approximately 6 years of age, the inferior meatus is nonfunctioning except that it drains the *nasolacrimal duct.* This is why the nose has increased drainage in children, particularly during periods of crying or eye irritation. The space between the posterior portion of the turbinates and the posterior wall of the nasopharynx is called the *choana* and is of little significance in children unless blocked by a congenital abnormality such as *choanal atresia,* a bony or membranous blockage of the naris posterior to the nasal turbinates, resulting in blockage of the airway. It occurs in 1 in 10,000 births.[3]

Cranial nerve I (olfactory) innervates the nasal area. The *olfactory receptor* cells line the upper reaches of the nasal cavity in the olfactory epithelium and innervate the olfactory nerve. Olfactory learning begins in utero and is well developed in the newborn. It assists newborns in recognizing the distinct smell of their mother's breast milk. Nasal congestion or mucus plugging limits airflow up to the receptors and can block the sensation of smell.

Nasopharynx

The *nasopharynx* forms the superior portion of the pharynx. The *eustachian tube* opening is located along the lateral walls of the nasopharynx (see Figure 13-3). Adenoidal tissue is found along the superior posterior wall of the oropharynx and is referred to as the *pharyngeal tonsils.* The inferior border of the nasopharynx is formed by the soft palate. The nasopharynx is surrounded by bone, ensuring patency unless trauma occurs.

Sinuses

The paranasal sinuses consist of paired cavities: maxillary, ethmoid, frontal, and sphenoid sinuses. The maxillary and ethmoid sinuses are present at birth but are small, and the sphenoid and frontal sinuses develop during infancy and early childhood. The sinuses become air-filled cavities lined with ciliated epithelium containing goblet cells and submucosal glands that produce seromucinous secretions and immune mediators as they develop and mature within the sinus cavity. The sinuses reach their final form between 12 and 14 years of age[2] (Figure 13-4; see Table 13-2).

Mouth and Oropharynx

The *oral cavity* is composed of the lips, cheeks, hard and soft palates, teeth, posterior pharynx, tongue, sensory cells for taste, and the mandible that supports the lower gums and teeth (Figure 13-5). The cheeks form the lateral walls lined with *buccal mucosa.* Cheeks may be particularly prominent in young children because of the buccal fat pad. The cheeks and lips are innervated by *cranial nerves V (trigeminal) and VII (facial).* The central nervous system controls the complex mechanisms of the mouth needed for sucking, swallowing, breathing, and vocalization. The *hard palate* is the anterior two thirds of the palate and separates the nasal and oral cavities. The posterior third of the palate is the *soft palate,* which is contiguous with the lateral pharyngeal wall. It provides a slightly mobile barrier between the nasopharynx and oropharynx and is essential for normal articulation and speech intonation.

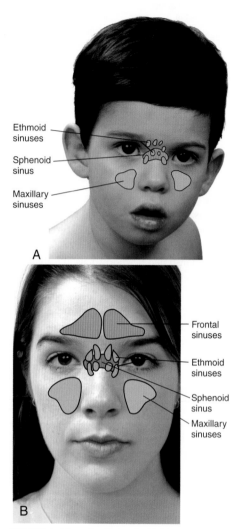

FIGURE 13-4 **A,** Sinus development in childhood. **B,** Sinus development in adolescence.

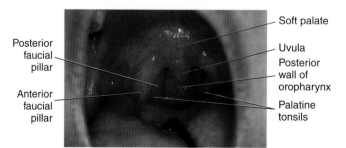

FIGURE 13-5 Anatomy of the posterior oral cavity. (From Fehrenbach M, Herring S: *Illustrated anatomy of the head and neck,* ed 4, St. Louis, 2012, Elsevier.)

TABLE 13-3   TONSILLAR SIZE

Size	Description
1+	Tonsils visible slightly beyond tonsillar pillars
2+	Tonsils visible midway between tonsillar pillars and uvula
3+	Tonsils nearly touching the uvula
4+	Tonsils touching at midline occluding the oropharynx

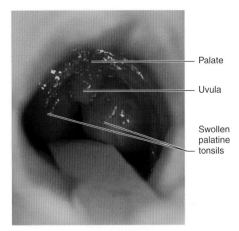

Palate

Uvula

Swollen palatine tonsils

FIGURE 13-6 Enlarged tonsils in child. (From Thibodeau G, Patton K: *The human body in health and disease*, ed 5, St. Louis, 2010, Mosby.)

Tonsils

The *palatine tonsils* form the anterior and posterior tonsillar pillars. Tonsillar size is graded on a scale of 1+ to 4+ (Table 13-3 and Figure 13-6). Additional tonsillar tissues surround the posterior pharynx but are not visible on examination. The *uvula* hangs down from the middle of the soft palate in line with the anterior pillar, or *palatoglossus muscle*. A *bifid uvula,* a cleft with two parts, is an anomaly that results from disruption of the palate development and may indicate a *submucosal cleft palate.* It may also be associated with nasal polyps and is more common in children with cystic fibrosis.

PEDIATRIC PEARLS

In the infant, the palatine tonsils are not normally visible, but by 2 years of age they are usually seen extending medially into the oropharynx. They generally are at their peak size between 2 and 6 years of age and then begin to atrophy or decrease in size along with other lymphatic tissue.

Teeth

The mandibular central incisors are the first to erupt in the majority of infants, followed by the maxillary central incisors then the upper and lower lateral incisors, first molars, cuspids or canine teeth, and then the second molars. Tooth *eruption,* movement of the tooth through alveolar bone and gums, normally occurs between 4 and 12 months of age for the first tooth, and takes place when about two thirds of the root for the tooth is developed. The maxillary incisors usually erupt 1 to 2 months after the mandibular incisors. The eruption of the 20 primary teeth should be complete between 24 and 30 months of age (Figure 13-7, *A*). The timing and sequence of tooth eruption depend on genetic, nutritional, environmental, and systemic factors. Delayed eruption of the primary teeth can occur in premature infants, infants small for gestational age, infants or children with metabolic or chromosomal abnormalities, or children with severe malnutrition. A family pattern of delayed tooth eruption can also occur across generations.

EVIDENCE-BASED PRACTICE TIP

Obstruction of the airway, rather than infection, has become a primary indication for tonsillectomy or adenotonsillectomy in younger children. Infection becomes a more prominent indication as age increases. For children less than 3 years of age, obstruction was the primary indication in 91.8% of procedures and infection in 7.5%. For children 4 years to 10 years of age, 73.2% of procedures were due to obstruction and 25.3% due to infection. For adolescents, 54.2% of the procedures were due to recurrent tonsillar or adenoidal infection.[4]

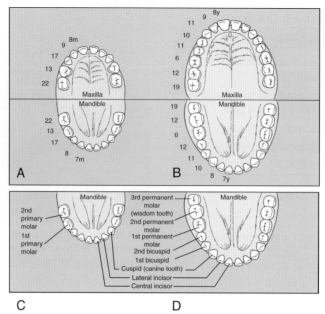

FIGURE 13-7 Ages of tooth eruption. **A,** Primary dentition of maxilla. **B,** Permanent dentition. **C,** Primary dentition of mandible. **D,** Permanent dentition of mandible. (From Zitelli BJ, Davis HW: *Atlas of pediatric physical diagnosis,* ed 4, St. Louis, 2002, Mosby.)

The permanent teeth begin developing in the mandible during the first 6 months of life. The period of *eruption* of the *mixed dentition* occurs between 5 and 13 years of age, beginning with the eruption of the first permanent tooth. *Exfoliation,* or loss of the primary dentition, often begins with the central incisors and follows the eruption pattern. There are 32 permanent teeth (see Figure 13-7, *B*). Low birth weight, infection, and trauma have been associated with delayed eruption of the permanent teeth. Delayed exfoliation of the primary dentition has been associated with Down syndrome, hypothyroidism, osteogenesis imperfecta, and other congenital endocrine disorders. Dental enamel can be eroded, resulting in structurally weakened teeth in some conditions such as chronic gastroesophageal reflux disease, bulimia, and celiac disease.

Dental caries are the most common chronic health condition in childhood.[5] The infectious process of dental decay begins early in infancy when the bacterium *Streptococcus mutans* can be transmitted from parent or caretaker in the first few months of life. Ingestion of a high carbohydrate diet and/or frequent dietary sugars alters the oral bacterial composition, enhancing the development of dental caries in children and adolescents.[6,7]

Tongue

The *tongue* is a mobile muscle, with its anterior two thirds located in the oral cavity and the posterior third located in the oropharynx. The anterior dorsal surface of the tongue is composed of a thick mucous membrane lined with *filiform,* or threadlike, papillae, and the posterior dorsal surface is lined with lymphoid tissue that forms the *lingual tonsil.* The ventral surface of the tongue has a thin mucous membrane with visible vessels and is anchored to the floor of the mouth by the *lingual frenulum* (Figure 13-8). In some infants, the frenulum attaches to the anterior portion or tip of the tongue decreasing tongue mobility, possibly impeding latching onto the nipple for successful breastfeeding. A short frenulum, commonly called "tongue-tie," may also impede speech in the older child. The frenulum may be surgically released during the newborn period, a procedure known as

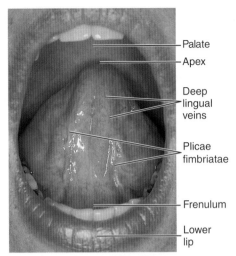

FIGURE 13-8 Ventral surface of the tongue and salivary glands. (From Fehrenbach M, Herring S: *Illustrated anatomy of the head and neck,* ed 4, St. Louis, 2012, Elsevier.)

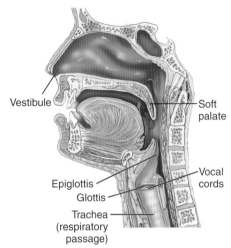

FIGURE 13-9 Sagittal view of mouth and oropharynx.

frenulotomy or frenulectomy, to enhance the latch for breastfeeding. *Cranial nerves IX (glossopharyngeal)* and *X (vagus)* innervate the tongue for sensation and taste, and *cranial nerve XII (hypoglossal)* innervate the tongue for motor function. The sensation of taste is immature at birth and not fully functional until approximately 2 years of age. Infants also have a *tongue-thrust reflex* for the first 4 months of life that aids in breastfeeding or bottle-feeding and to protect them from choking, but it is counterproductive when trying to feed solids by spoon. At the base of the tongue in the oropharynx lies the *epiglottis,* a glistening pink spoon-shaped appendage that helps direct the passage of food into the esophagus and away from the trachea (Figure 13-9). Normally, it is not visible on examination, but in some children it can be seen protruding upward from the posterior oropharynx, almost opposite from the uvula when the tongue is depressed and the child says "ah," which opens the throat area for examination.

Salivary Glands

The *salivary glands* are paired exocrine glands that secrete enzymes that aid in initial digestion. The *parotid glands* are the largest salivary glands and are the glands that become inflamed with *mumps,* or *parotitis.* The *parotid duct,* or *Stensen duct,* empties into the oral cavity opposite the upper second molar. The *submandibular gland* is the second largest gland and is located in the floor of the mouth. The *submandibular ducts,* or *Wharton ducts,* exit into the mouth on either side of the frenulum. The third set of salivary glands is the *sublingual glands,* which release their enzymes through approximately 12 ducts located on the floor of the mouth. The sublingual glands are not visible on examination. Secretions from the salivary glands increase during the first few months of life, which results in increased drooling by 3 to 4 months of age. As infants mature and become more proficient in swallowing and the lower teeth develop to create a dam, the drooling decreases even though the production of saliva increases. Hundreds of additional salivary glands line the mucous membranes of the mouth and oral pharynx in late adolescence, providing additional serous and mucous secretions.

SYSTEM-SPECIFIC HISTORY

The Information Gathering table presents important information to gather for different ages and developmental stages when assessing the nose, mouth, and throat.

INFORMATION GATHERING FOR ASSESSING THE NOSE, MOUTH, AND THROAT AT KEY DEVELOPMENTAL STAGES

Age-Group	Questions to Ask
Preterm and newborn	History of maternal infection, TORCH infections? Maternal drug use? Perinatal exposure to infection? Any difficulty sucking, feeding? Difficulty breathing through nose? Any natal teeth or lesions in mouth?
Infancy	Any nasal discharge? Any difficulty sucking, feeding, introducing solid foods? Any sores, white patches, or bleeding in mouth? Have any teeth erupted? Use of juice in bottle? Is infant on fluoride supplement or is water fluoridated? Plans for weaning from breast or bottle? Does infant habitually put objects in mouth? Use pacifier or suck thumb or fingers?
Early childhood	Does child have difficulty eating solid foods? Use bottle for milk or juice? Frequently puts objects in mouth or nose? Are there any concerns about child's speech? Does child's speech have a nasal or congested resonance? History of frequent nasal congestion, chronic rhinorrhea, or tonsillitis? Does the child snore? Has child had nose injuries? Does child suck a finger or pacifier? Is child in daycare or preschool? Age at first dental visit? Does child brush teeth with parental assistance? History of trauma to mouth or gums?
Middle childhood	Any mouth or nose injuries? History of nasal congestion, chronic rhinorrhea, tonsillitis? Does child snore? Have restless or interrupted sleep pattern? Any known exposure to group A streptococcal infection? Has child had a documented GABHS pharyngitis? Or other respiratory infections? Routine dental care? Does child brush and floss? Has child had any teeth extracted? Tonsils or adenoids removed?
Adolescence	Any injuries to mouth or nose? History of nasal congestion, chronic rhinorrhea, tonsillitis? Does adolescent snore? Exposure to group A streptococcal infection? History of oral sex? Are there any oral piercings? Routine dental care, brushing, flossing? Dental braces or orthodontic appliances? Has adolescent had any teeth extracted or tonsils or adenoids removed? Does adolescent use a dental guard with contact sports? Oral lesions/sores?
Environmental risks	Exposure to household tobacco smoke? Recreational drug or tobacco use or exposure to use? Recreational activities or sports with increased risk of injury to mouth or nose?

GABHS, Group A beta-hemolytic streptococci; *TORCH,* toxoplasmosis, other diseases (syphilis), rubella, cytomegalovirus, herpes simplex virus.

PHYSICAL ASSESSMENT

Equipment

Equipment needed for examination of the nose, mouth, and throat includes an otoscope with halogen light and speculum, tongue depressor, and gloves for palpation of palate and gums if any skin lesions are present.

Positioning

Delay the examination of the mouth and nose in the infant and young child until after the "quiet" parts of the exam and after the ear examination. If the infant or young child cries, attempt to visualize the mouth and oropharynx. Infants and young children are best positioned on the examination table with the arms secured by the sides and head supported to visualize the internal nose and mouth. Securing the arms above the head often increases fear and frustration in the child. Infants and young children are often resistant to the oral and nasal examination, and proper positioning ensures the least discomfort.

Examination of the older infant or young child can also take place while the child is sitting in the parent's lap with the head secured at the forehead and hands secured by the sides (Figure 13-10). The feet may need to be secured between the caretaker's legs if the child is uncooperative. An alternative position for conducting the oral exam and inspection of the teeth is to place the child in the "knee-to-knee" position.[5] In this position, the examiner and parent sit face to face with their knees touching to make a comfortable support for the young infant, and the examiner can look directly into the child's mouth (Figure 13-11). This position is also used for examining the teeth and applying fluoride varnish in the older infant and young child.

External Nose

While the child is comfortable, note any flaring or narrowing of the nares with breathing. If an infant is feeding, watch carefully for indications of nasal obstruction requiring mouth breathing. Note the shape of the nose, any obvious deviation of the bridge or columella, the tip of the nose. An *allergic salute* results in a transverse crease across the nose caused by repeated upward swipes with the hand due to chronic nasal drainage. If there is drainage from the nose, note the color, consistency, and quantity and whether it is unilateral or bilateral. Allergic conditions and upper respiratory infections cause bilateral drainage, whereas foreign objects in the nose can cause unilateral, purulent, malodorous discharge. *Epistaxis,* hemorrhage from the nose, occurs

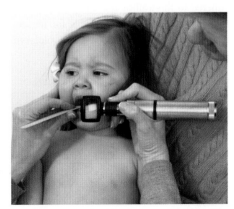

FIGURE 13-10 Position for the oral examination in the infant and young child.

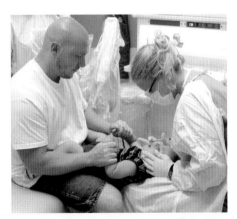

FIGURE 13-11 Knee-to-knee position. (From Dean J, McDonald R, Avery D, et al: *McDonald and Avery dentistry for the child and adolescent,* ed 9, St. Louis, 2010, Elsevier.)

from irritation of the nasal mucosa, often due to cold, dry environmental conditions; nasal allergy; or as a result of trauma. Sinus infections also may cause unilateral drainage. Swelling or discoloration under the eyes, often called *allergic shiners,* may occur with nasal congestion, *sinusitis,* or nasal allergy.

Palpate any areas around the nose that appear discolored or inflamed. If there is a history of facial trauma, palpate the bridge of the nose to determine tenderness or pain. If the child has a recent history of head or facial trauma and clear watery nasal discharge, a cerebrospinal fluid leak must be ruled out. Fractures of the protective facial bones increase the risk of meningitis developing. Children with obvious deviation of the nose should be referred to a craniofacial surgeon for evaluation. Patency of each side of the nose can be determined by gently occluding one naris at a time. In the newborn, this technique assists in diagnosis of choanal atresia.

Internal Nose

To inspect the internal nose, use a penlight or otoscope with halogen light and nasal speculum. Be careful not to touch the sensitive internal nasal septum. A large ear speculum can be inserted 2 to 3 mm into the nares in older children and adolescents for inspection of the nasal cavity but is not recommended in infants and young children, to avoid trauma. An otoscope with halogen light used without a speculum is effective for visualizing the nares in infants and young children who are positioned on the exam table or on the parent's lap (Figure 13-12).

The vestibule of the nose should be assessed for any blockage by foreign body, polyps, nasal secretions, mucous plugs, or dried blood. The mucosal lining should be assessed for consistency of color, abrasions, lesions, and swelling. The color is normally deep pink, and a thin layer of clear mucus gives it a shiny appearance. The septum should be examined for alignment, perforations, abrasions, bleeding, or crusting. It should be relatively straight and

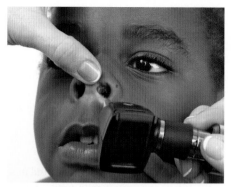

FIGURE 13-12 View of the nasal vestibule and turbinates.

midline in the nose. Significant deviations of the septum may interfere with breathing. The turbinates should be assessed for color and swelling. Pale, swollen mucosa and edema of the turbinates is associated with allergic rhinitis and occlusion of air passage; and inflamed, reddened mucosa and turbinates are associated with respiratory infections. Children with chronic respiratory conditions may develop polyps that appear as shiny sacs extending into the vestibule.

If a foreign body is suspected, attempt to have the child blow out the object while occluding the unaffected side. If this is not successful in dislodging the object, a gentle probe with a curette or tweezers can be attempted but often is unsuccessful if the object has become adhered to the wall or septum. Securely position the child on the exam table for removal of the object or refer to a pediatric otolaryngologist if necessary for removal.

Sinuses

Only the maxillary and frontal sinuses can be assessed by physical examination through inspection and palpation. The facial area over the maxillary and frontal sinuses should be evaluated for swelling and tenderness in school-age children and adolescents. Percuss or apply mild pressure with the thumb or forefinger over the maxillary and frontal sinus area. Evaluate tenderness and increased sensation from side to side, especially if there is a history of prolonged upper respiratory infection (Figure 13-13). It may be difficult for young school-age children to accurately determine increased pain or tenderness caused by sinus inflammation. Computed tomography (CT) scan is the gold standard for sinus imaging but alone cannot diagnose bacterial sinusitis. CT scans are reserved for children who are unresponsive to medical therapy, who develop complications of rhinosinusitis, or who are being considered for surgical intervention.[2]

Mouth

While inspecting the oral cavity, observe for the presence of any unusual odor or lesions. Inspect the lips for color, symmetry, lesions, swelling, dryness, and fissures. The color should be pink at rest and with feeding or crying. Note any asymmetry of movement or drooling that might indicate nerve impairment. Drooling during infancy from 3 to 15 months of age is normal, but drooling later may indicate nerve damage and loss of control of oral secretions. Young infants may have a callus or blister on the lip from vigorous sucking. This is particularly common in breastfed infants in the first few months of life (Figure 13-14). Swelling of the lips may be caused by injury or allergic reaction. Cracked, dry lips can be caused by harsh weather conditions, repeated lip licking or biting, or mouth breathing due to nasal allergy, fever, or dehydration. Sores in the mouth or on the lips may indicate a viral infection such as *coxsackie virus* or *herpes simplex virus* type 1. Halitosis, mouth odor or bad breath, in children may be caused by poor oral hygiene and dental caries, tonsillitis, or sinusitis. Note the frenulum under the inner surface of the upper lip, which extends to the maxillary ridge. It is prominent in the infant and disappears slowly in childhood with growth and development of the maxilla. Trauma to the upper lip and gum in the young child often includes trauma to the frenulum.

Inspect the buccal mucosa and gingivae with a tongue blade or tongue depressor for color, moisture, symmetry, and lesions (Figure 13-15).

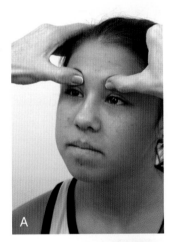

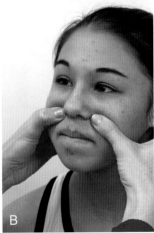

FIGURE 13-13 **A,** Palpation of ethmoid sinuses. **B,** Palpation of the maxillary sinuses.

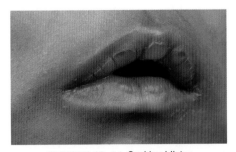

FIGURE 13-14 Sucking blister.

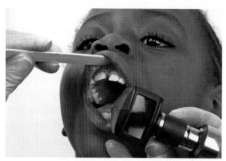

FIGURE 13-15 Inspection of teeth and gums in an older child.

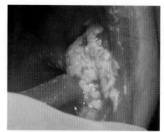

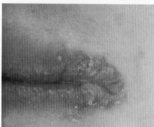

FIGURE 13-16 Candidiasis. (From Zitelli BJ, Davis HW: *Atlas of pediatric physical diagnosis,* ed 4, St. Louis, 2002, Mosby.)

The mucosa normally is shiny, smooth, and moist throughout. The oral mucosa may appear bluish or pale in children with darkly pigmented skin and is pinker in white children. Use a tongue depressor or a gloved finger to move the tongue and lips to ensure all surfaces of the mucosa are inspected. *Epstein pearls,* white pearly papules at the juncture of the hard and soft palates or on the anterior surface of the buccal mucosa, are common in newborns and resolve spontaneously. With a gloved finger, palpate unusual-looking areas for swelling and tenderness of the gum. If the mucosa of the gum appears inflamed or swollen, palpate for erupting teeth or hematomas. An *eruption hematoma,* a bluish blisterlike swelling on the gum, may precede tooth eruption, particularly with the first and second molars.[7] Reddened, swollen, or friable gums can be an indication of poor oral hygiene, infection, or poor nutrition. Anticonvulsants may cause hyperplasia of the gums.

Candidiasis, appearing as bright white superficial lesions on the tongue and buccal mucosa of the cheeks, is often seen in the young infant or child after use of oral antibiotics or with chronic infection (Figure 13-16). The lesions of candidiasis can be differentiated from milk or formula residue by the bright white appearance. *Candidiasis lesions* do not scrape off the mucosa with the side of the tongue depressor. *Petechiae,* pinpoint erythematous lesions, may be present on the soft palate with streptococcal infections or may be indicative of a bleeding disorder.

Teeth

Inspect and note the number, color, size, and shape of the primary and permanent teeth and the pattern of eruption (Figure 13-17). *Natal teeth* are prematurely erupted primary teeth that are present at birth (Figure 13-18). The

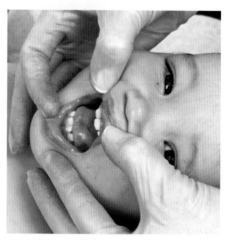

FIGURE 13-17 Inspection of primary teeth.

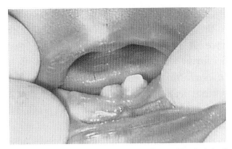

FIGURE 13-18 Natal teeth. (From Hardwick F, Ketchem L: *Oral pathologies in children: pediatric basics,* Fremont, Mich, Winter 1990, Gerber Medical Services, p 53.)

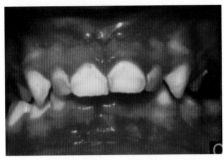

FIGURE 13-19 White spot lesions. (Courtesy Dr. Francisco Ramos-Gomez, University of California at San Francisco School of Dentistry.)

incidence of natal teeth is approximately 1 in 2000 births and is often seen in infants with cleft palate and other chromosomal deletion syndromes.[8] If the teeth are supernumerary, very loose, or cause feeding problems, extraction may be indicated. *Neonatal teeth* erupt in the first month of life, and 90% of neonatal teeth are lower primary teeth, or *mandibular incisors.*[8] Precocious eruption of primary teeth has been associated with precocious puberty. In older children with loose teeth, precaution with surgical procedures and anesthesia is indicated.

Inspection of the teeth in infants and young children includes identifying any presence of plaque on the teeth. Evaluate oral hygiene practices. Check the primary teeth in the infant and young child for *white spot* lesions, or decalcifications, and *brown spot* lesions, or cavitations, indicating the first sign of dental decay. White spot lesions on the anterior surfaces may be a sign of *early childhood caries.* They are caused by early transmission of bacterium from parent or caretaker to child and frequent dietary sugars reducing the pH of oral secretions, resulting in demineralization of the tooth enamel (Figure 13-19). The mandibular incisors in infants are protected by the tongue when sucking, and they are therefore not prone to decay with prolonged bottle-feeding or breastfeeding. Dental care should commence as soon as teeth erupt. Daily oral

hygiene using a damp cloth to gently rub the gums and teeth of the infant can prevent plaque development. Teeth should be brushed at least twice daily with parental supervision.

The American Academy of Pediatric Dentistry recommends establishing a dental home with a comprehensive dental assessment by 12 months of age.[7] Fluoridated drinking water and application of topical fluoride by pediatric health care providers helps to reduce the incidence of early childhood caries.[9] Application of fluoride varnish is particularly important in children living in poverty who have a higher incidence of dental caries.[10] Access to a pediatric dental home and application of dental sealants also improves oral health and reduces the incidence of dental caries.

Maxillary permanent incisors may erupt widely spaced and protruding outward, and mandibular incisors may erupt behind the primary incisors, but align with normal development of the oral cavity unless there is a familial pattern of malocclusion or dental deformities. A slight overlap of the maxillary incisors to the mandibular incisors occurs with normal permanent dentition. Children with significantly misaligned teeth should be referred to a pediatric orthodontist for evaluation and treatment. *Bruxism,* or tooth grinding, which induces moderate wear on the surface of the canines and molars, may be noted on inspection. The peak incidence is during the developmental period of mixed dentition, and it rarely damages the dentition in young children but may be significant in older children or children with special health care needs. Dental hygiene in children with special health care needs is often a challenge because of oral aversion, oral side effects of medications or special diets, and the child's ability/inability to participate in daily oral hygiene.

Tongue

Inspect the tongue, noting color, size, and movement. The dorsal surface should appear slightly rough but moist and pink to pale pink. There may be variation in the papillae, giving the dorsal surface a patterned appearance. *Geographic tongue,* a benign inflammation of the dorsal surface of the tongue, causes pink areas with absent papillae and a surrounding whitish border (Figure 13-20).

The ventral surface appears thin with prominent vessels without hematomas. Connecting the ventral surface of the tongue to the floor of the mouth is the lingual frenulum. The lingual frenulum should allow movement of the tongue past the lips and to the roof of the palate. Movement of the tongue can be assessed through observation while an infant

cries or a child vocalizes. Infants who are able to breastfeed or bottle-feed without difficulty have adequate movement of the tongue, and no further assessment of *cranial nerve XII (hypoglossal)* is needed. Newborns with significant feeding problems should be referred to an otolaryngologist and an occupational therapist trained and experienced in neonatal feeding problems. A significantly shortened lingual frenulum, *ankyloglossia,* is caused by an anterior attachment of the frenulum to the tip of the tongue (Figure 13-21). It may in some cases interfere with adequate latch and sucking in the newborn and impair the infant's ability to breastfeed. Surgical intervention may be indicated in some infants and children. A *frenulotomy* or *frenulectomy* is the surgical procedure in which the lingual frenulum is cut. This surgical procedure is still controversial, particularly in relation to later speech development.

Macroglossia, enlarged tongue, can be congenital or acquired and is associated with hypothyroidism, Down syndrome, and other congenital anomalies. *Pierre Robin* syndrome is associated with a malpositioned tongue, feeding and breathing difficulty, and a high arched or cleft palate. A small jaw, or mandible, can be associated with congenital craniofacial anomalies, genetic conditions, or small for gestational age infant, and may

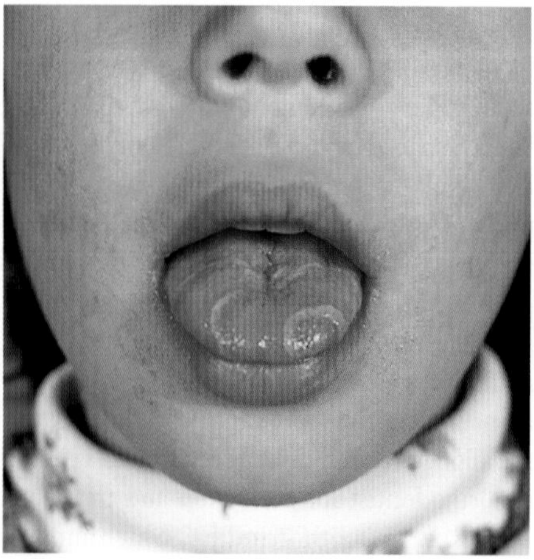

FIGURE 13-20 Geographic tongue. (From Zitelli BJ, Davis HW: *Atlas of pediatric physical diagnosis,* ed 4, St. Louis, 2002, Mosby.)

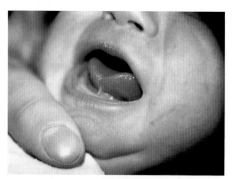

FIGURE 13-21 Ankyloglossia; short lingual frenulum. (From Moore K: *The developing human: clinically oriented embryology,* ed 8, Philadelphia, 2008, Elsevier. Courtesy of Dr. Evelyn Jain, Lakeview Breastfeeding Clinic, Calgary, Alberta, Canada.)

be associated with feeding problems, choking, or gagging.

In the older child and adolescent, ask the child to stick the tongue out past the lips and move the tongue from side to side to test *cranial nerve XII (hypoglossal)*. These maneuvers should be easy to perform without fasciculation of the tongue. The ability to curl the tongue is a hereditary trait in some children. Any lesions, areas of tenderness, or swelling should be palpated to determine the size and depth.

Palate

Inspect the hard palate for patency or lesions. It should appear dome shaped but not deeply indented, lighter in appearance than the skin on the buccal mucosa and soft palate, and have transverse firm ridges. In a newborn infant with jaundice, the hard palate appears yellowish. In darkly pigmented infants and children, it is helpful to inspect the hard palate and sclera to assess for jaundice. The hard palate is contiguous with the soft palate and extends to the anterior pillars and the uvula. The soft palate should appear intact and rise symmetrically along with the uvula when the child vocalizes or says "ah." This movement tests for *cranial nerve X (vagus)*. Movement of the soft palate is necessary for the development of normal speech and articulation.

The hard and soft palates should always be palpated in the newborn to determine whether there is any submucosal cleft not visible on inspection or congenital anomalies associated with cleft palate. A gloved finger can be placed on the infant's palate to determine whether the palate is intact. As the infant sucks, evaluate the strength of the suck reflex and the palate surface. After the newborn period, palpation of the palate is not usually performed unless lesions, swelling, or erythema is noted.

Tonsils

Inspect the palatine tonsils for size, color, exudates, pitting or enlarged crypts, or membranous covering. Tonsils should appear equal in size and position, and should be rated on a scale of 1+ to 4+ during well visits and during periods of illness to evaluate change (see Table 13-3). Some children and adolescents have enlarged tonsils and adenoids that partially block air passage into and out of the oropharynx, requiring them to breathe with their mouth open to enlarge the air passageway. Dry lips are a hallmark of chronically enlarged tonsils in children. During sleep, relaxation of the pharyngeal musculature exacerbates the occlusion of the air passages, resulting in obstruction of airflow and periodic *sleep apnea. Sleep-related breathing disorders*, referring to the duration and quality of sleep, have been associated with nasal allergy, tonsillar hypertrophy related to allergies or recurrent viral or bacterial infections, and childhood obesity. They may impact school performance because of fatigue and inattention, and they have been associated with hyperactivity and behavioral problems.[4] The pediatric health care provider should obtain a health history regarding the child's sleep and the occurrence of snoring. Referral of the child to pediatric pulmonology or pediatric otolaryngology specialists to evaluate the oropharynx and determine the need for sleep studies is often warranted.

> ## EVIDENCE-BASED PRACTICE TIP
>
> Calcification of the dentition and tooth eruption occurs earlier in girls and in African-Americans and Native Americans than in other racial groups.

The tonsils are normally the color of the buccal mucosa or slightly lighter. Tonsils that are larger than normal may indicate chronic respiratory allergies and if reddened indicate infection. Exudate, white or yellow areas of material in the crypts of the tonsils, is often associated with bacterial *tonsillitis* or *infectious mononucleosis*. Unequal size and color may indicate a *peritonsillar abscess*, requiring further diagnostics and hospitalization. Pitting or enlarged crypts of the tonsils is often seen in children with a history of recurrent throat infections or chronic allergies (Figure 13-22).

Vocalization

Vocalization and speech patterns in infants and children should also be assessed. A high-pitched cry in the newborn or young infant may indicate increased intracranial pressure, and a hoarse cry in infants with upper respiratory infection may

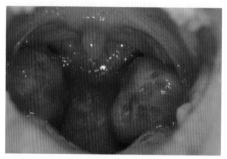

FIGURE 13-22 Large cryptic tonsils. (From Lemmi FO, Lemmi CAE: *Physical assessment findings multiuser CD-ROM*, St. Louis, 2000, Saunders.)

indicate *croup* or *laryngitis.* Prolonged hoarseness in children should be investigated to rule out vocal cord pathology or gastroesophageal reflux disease. Prolonged unintelligible speech may indicate a speech articulation problem, expressive language delay, or a hearing problem and should be promptly evaluated. Intelligible speech is critical for early success in school, and evaluation of speech delay and speech and language therapy should not be delayed in hopes the child will outgrow the problem. See Chapter 3 for further discussion on important developmental milestones for speech and language development and Chapter 12 for hearing assessment.

NOSE, MOUTH, AND THROAT CONDITIONS

Table 13-4 presents abnormal infectious conditions of the mouth and throat in infants, children, and adolescents.

Rhinosinusitis (RS) is one of the most prevalent diseases in childhood. Children average 6 to 8 upper respiratory tract infections per year; the vast majority are caused by viruses

TABLE 13-4   CONDITIONS OF THE MOUTH AND THROAT

Condition	Descriptions
Aphthous ulcers	Round or oval ulcerations with an erythematous halo usually seen on buccal mucosa of cheeks. Exact cause varies. No specific treatment as cause varies. Often resolve spontaneously within one week.
Diphtheria	A thin, tough membrane that becomes grayish-green and covers tonsils and pharynx; rarely seen because of near universal immunization coverage with diphtheria toxin in early childhood.
Epiglottitis	Edema and inflammation of epiglottis resulting in occlusion of trachea and acute respiratory distress; a medical emergency that may require intubation and radiographs for confirmation of diagnosis; avoid exam of oropharynx; incidence has decreased 80% to 90% in children because of *Haemophilus influenzae* vaccine.
Gingivostomatitis	Vesicular lesions of lips, tongue, gingivae, oral mucosa resulting in swollen, painful, friable gums; most common 6 months to 3 years of age preceded by fever, headache, and irritability. May be caused by bacteria or virus, especially herpes simplex type 1 or post coxsackievirus. Treatment focused on symptom management and oral hygiene.

TABLE 13-4 CONDITIONS OF THE MOUTH AND THROAT—CONT'D

Condition	Descriptions
Herpangina (coxsackievirus groups A and B)	Small vesicles on posterior pharynx, tonsils, soft palate that rupture to form ulcers; occurs in young children with onset of sore throat, fever, malaise. Caused by coxsackievirus group A. Treatment focused on symptom management and prevention of dehydration.
Mononucleosis	Enlarged tonsils, general malaise, fatigue, lymphadenopathy, splenomegaly usually caused by Epstein-Barr virus (EBV) but can be caused by other organisms such as cytomegalovirus (CMV); confirmed by monospot test and EBV antibody testing.
Parotitis or mumps	An acute contagious viral illness associated with fever, painful parotid enlargement; organ system involvement includes orchitis, testicular inflammation (in 15% to 25% of cases), deafness (usually unilateral); meningoencephalitis can be seen in 2.5% of cases; about 1500 cases occur annually.
Streptococcal pharyngitis	Group A beta-hemolytic streptococcus: common bacteria in throat characterized by sudden onset of sore throat, fever, headache, exudate on tonsils, tender cervical adenopathy. Treated with penicillin to prevent the possibility of rheumatic carditis because of specificity of the bacteria.

with only 0.5% to 5% progressing to acute sinusitis.[2] Symptoms include nasal congestion, nasal discharge that can be clear, mucoid, thick or thin, low-grade fever, irritability, cough, halitosis, and rarely headache, a cardinal sign of sinusitis in adults. Acute bacterial RS should be suspected when symptoms persist beyond 10 days or if there is purulent rhinorrhea for 3 to 4 consecutive days with fever of 39° C or above. Since RS usually has a viral origin, no antibiotics should be prescribed, and rarely are nasal decongestants indicated. There is no consensus on management of acute bacterial RS in children as compared to adults, with more limited use of antibiotics.

Group A beta-hemolytic streptococci (GABHS) are the most common bacteria associated with pharyngotonsillitis in children and the only "sore throat" treated with antibiotics. "Strep throat," the common term used for GABHS pharyngitis, peaks in winter and spring, and transmission occurs through spread of droplets. History may reveal a contact with similar symptoms or a diagnosed strep throat. Children and adolescents with prior history of GABHS are more susceptible to repeat infection. Signs and symptoms of GABHS pharyngitis are acute in onset and characterized by high fever, cervical lymphadenopathy, sore throat, headache, and abdominal pain, sometimes with nausea and vomiting. Pharyngeal and tonsillar mucosa are typically erythematous with exudate present in 50% to 90% of cases.[2] A throat culture is necessary to accurately diagnose GABHS.

Although symptoms will resolve within a few days without treatment, early treatment with a penicillin (preferred), a cephalosporin, or a macrolide suggest that antibiotic therapy prevents sequelae, including rheumatic fever, and may hasten clinical improvement. The incidence of rheumatic carditis is 0.3% in endemic situations. Acute glomerulonephritis is a sequela of a specific nephritogenic strain of GABHS; 10% to 15% of people infected with this strain of GABHS will develop acute glomerulonephritis regardless of treatment.[2]

SUMMARY OF EXAMINATION

- Newborns have the ability to switch from nasal to mouth breathing as needed, so they are preferential nasal breathers.[2]
- The cheeks and lips are innervated by cranial nerves V (trigeminal) and VII (facial).
- Secretions from the salivary glands increase during the first few months of life, which results in increased drooling by 3 to 4 months of age.
- In the infant, note any flaring or narrowing of the nares with breathing.
- An otoscope with halogen light used without a speculum is effective for visualizing the nares in infants and young children.
- Maxillary and ethmoid sinuses are present at birth but are small, and the sphenoid and frontal sinuses develop during infancy and childhood.
- Percuss or apply mild pressure with the thumb or forefinger over the maxillary and frontal sinus area to evaluate tenderness.
- Inspect the lips for color, symmetry, lesions, swelling, dryness, and fissures.

- Delay the examination of the mouth and nose in the infant and young child until after the "quiet" parts of the exam and after the ear examination.
- Inspect the buccal mucosa and gingivae with a tongue blade or tongue depressor for color, moisture, symmetry, and lesions.
- Tooth *eruption* normally occurs between 4 and 12 months of age for the first tooth, and takes place when about two thirds of the root for a tooth is developed.
- Check the primary teeth in the infant and young child for "white spot" lesions, or decalcifications, and "brown spot" lesions, or cavitations, indicating the first sign of dental decay. Inspect the teeth and gums using a tongue depressor for cavitations and abscesses.
- In the older child and adolescent, ask the child to stick the tongue out past the lips and move the tongue from side to side to test cranial nerve XII (hypoglossal).
- Inspect for tonsillar size and quality. Tonsillar size is graded on a scale of 1+ to 4+.

Charting
Healthy Newborn

Nose, mouth, and throat: Nares patent bilaterally without flaring, clear nasal discharge. Strong suck. Mucous membranes pink, moist without lesions. Soft and hard palate intact. Uvula and tongue midline, nonprotuberant, gag response intact, without natal teeth.

Charting
Adolescent

Nose, mouth, and throat: No nasal discharge, nasal septum midline, turbinates pink, moist. No facial swelling or tenderness over sinuses. Buccal mucous pink and moist without lesions. Gums pink, firm without bleeding. 32 teeth present in good repair without evidence of active decay. Pharynx pink, tonsils 1+ without exudate or pitting, uvula midline, sensitive gag response.

REFERENCES

1. Curtain G, Boekelheide A: Cleft lip and palate. In Allen P, Vessey J, Schapiro N, editors: *Primary care of the child with a chronic condition,* ed 5, St. Louis, 2010, Mosby.

2. Shoem S, Darrow D: *Pediatric otolaryngology,* Elk Grove, IL, 2012, American Academy of Pediatrics.

3. Bluestone CD: *Pediatric otolaryngology,* ed 4, Philadelphia, 2005, Saunders.

4. Parker NP, Walner DL: Trends in the indications for pediatric tonsillectomy or adenotonsillectomy, *Int J Pediatr Otorhinolaryngol,* 75(2):282-285, 2011.

5. Ramos-Gomez FJ, Crystal YO, Ng MW, et al: Pediatric dental care: prevention and management protocols based on caries risk assessment, *J Calif Dent Assoc* 38(10):746-761, 2010.

6. Werner SL, Phillips C, Koroluk LD: Association between childhood obesity and dental caries, *Pediatr Dent* 34(1):23-27, 2012.

7. American Academy of Pediatrics: Preventive oral health intervention for pediatricians. Section on Pediatric Dentistry and Oral Health, *Pediatrics* 122(6):1387-1394, 2008.

8. Zitelli BJ, McIntire SC, Norwalk AJ: *Zitelli and Davis' atlas of pediatric physical diagnosis,* ed 6, Philadelphia, 2013, Mosby.

9. Douglass JM: Fluoride varnish when added to caregiver counseling reduces early childhood caries incidence, *J Evid Based Dent Pract* 11(1):46-48, 2011.

10. da Fonseca MA: The effects of poverty on children's development and oral health, *Pediatr Dent* 34(1):32-38, 2012.

CHAPTER 14

ABDOMEN AND RECTUM

Victoria F. Keeton

The assessment of the abdomen and rectum involves the evaluation of multiple organ systems and functions including the gastrointestinal, renal, vascular, endocrine, immune, and female reproductive systems. The health care provider should always maintain a holistic view of the child, adolescent, and family during the assessment, which may help distinguish clinical symptoms from psychosomatic complaints in the pediatric population and help focus the abdominal examination.

EMBRYOLOGICAL DEVELOPMENT

The primitive gut forms during the fourth week of gestation from the dorsal section of the yolk sac. It begins as a hollow tube arising from the endoderm, which then forms the *foregut, midgut,* and *hindgut.* The *foregut* develops into the esophagus, stomach, upper portion of the duodenum (bile duct entrance), liver, biliary system, and pancreas. It is perfused by the celiac artery. The *midgut* develops into the distal duodenum and the remainder of the small intestine, cecum, appendix, the ascending colon, and most of the proximal portion of the transverse colon and is perfused by the superior mesenteric artery. The hindgut develops into the remaining transverse colon, the descending colon, the sigmoid colon, the rectum, and the superior portion of the anal canal and is perfused by the inferior mesenteric artery.

By the end of the sixth week of gestation, the gut herniates outside of the abdominal cavity, where it rotates 90 degrees counterclockwise and continues to elongate. By the tenth week of gestation, the gut returns to the abdominal cavity and rotates another 180 degrees counterclockwise. With the normal intestinal rotation, the stomach and pancreas rotate into the left upper quadrant and are pressed against the dorsal abdominal wall to fuse into position.

The pancreas arises from ectodermal cells from the most caudal part of the foregut and develops into dorsal and ventral buds. The dorsal bud is larger and becomes the major portion of the pancreas. The dorsal and ventral buds fuse to form the main pancreatic duct. Secretion of insulin begins around the twentieth week of gestation. Up until the fourteenth week, the spleen is only a hematopoietic organ. Between weeks 15 and 18, the spleen then loses its hematopoietic function and transforms into an organ of the immune system.

The liver begins as a bud that develops on the distal part of the foregut and grows into the *septum transversum,* where it divides into two parts. The larger part develops into the right and left lobes of the liver, and the second smaller division of the hepatic bud develops into the biliary system. Hematopoiesis begins at the sixth week of gestation and is responsible for the large size of the liver. It is approximately 10% of the total weight of the fetus. Bile begins to form at 16 weeks of gestation, giving meconium the dark green color.

Development of the kidney begins with a primitive, transitory structure called the *pronephros,* or forekidney, which arises near the segments of the spinal cord. These segments appear early in the fourth week of gestation on either side of the nephrogenic cord. The pronephros itself soon degenerates but leaves behind its ducts for the next kidney formation, the *mesonephros,* or midkidney, to utilize. In the fifth week, the *metanephros,* or hindkidney, begins to develop and becomes the permanent kidney. By the eighth week, the hindkidney begins to produce urine and continues to do so throughout the fetal period.

The adrenal glands develop from the medulla, which originates from the neuroectoderm. At the seventh week of gestation, the medulla attaches to the fetal cortex, which develops from the mesoderm, and by the eighth week, the fetal cortex begins to encapsulate the medulla. The fetal adrenal gland is 20 times larger than the adult adrenal and is large compared to the kidneys. However, the adrenals rapidly decrease in size as the fetal cortex regresses and completely disappear by 4 years of age and are replaced by the adult cortex.

ANATOMY AND PHYSIOLOGY

The abdomen is the area of the torso from the diaphragm to the pelvic floor and is lined by the *peritoneum,* a serous membrane covering the abdominal viscera (Figure 14-1). The membrane of the peritoneum creates a smooth, moist surface that allows the abdominal viscera to glide freely within the confines of the abdominal wall.

The *liver* lies immediately below the right diaphragm and is the largest and heaviest organ in the body. It is composed of the right and left hepatic lobes and is an extremely vascular organ. The liver is perfused by the hepatic artery, which arises from the *abdominal aorta,* and the portal vein, which delivers blood from the spleen, pancreas, and intestines. The liver is responsible for metabolizing carbohydrates, fats, and proteins. It also breaks down toxic substances and drugs; stores vitamins and iron; produces antibodies, bile, prothrombin, and fibrinogen for coagulation; and excretes waste products. The hepatic veins then return blood to the vena cava. Within the inferior surface of the liver lies the *gallbladder,* a saclike organ. The liver excretes bile into the hepatic duct, which is then collected and stored in the gallbladder. Next bile is secreted into the duodenum via the cystic duct and the common bile duct to aid in the digestion of fats.

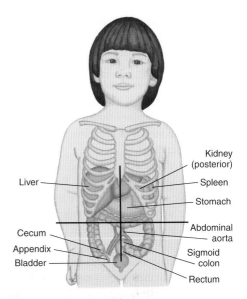

FIGURE 14-1 Abdominal structures. (From James SR, Nelson KA, Ashwill JW: *Nursing care of children,* ed 4, St. Louis, 2013, Elsevier.)

Below the left diaphragm, from posterior to anterior respectively, lie the spleen, pancreas, and stomach. The *spleen* is a concave organ made mostly of lymphoid tissue that lies around the posterior fundus of the stomach. The spleen filters and breaks down red blood cells and produces white blood cells (lymphocytes and monocytes). It also stores blood that can be released into the vascular system during an acute blood loss. The *pancreas* is nestled between the spleen and stomach and crosses the midline over the major vessels. The pancreatic head extends to the duodenum and the tail reaches almost to the spleen. It is responsible for production of enzymes needed for the metabolism of proteins, fats, and carbohydrates; these enzymes are excreted into the duodenum via the pancreatic duct. The pancreas also produces insulin and glucagon, which are secreted directly into the bloodstream to help regulate blood glucose levels. The *stomach* is the most anterior organ in the left upper quadrant of the abdomen. It is connected proximally to the esophagus, which enters through the diaphragm at the *esophageal hiatus.* The stomach receives food from the esophagus through the lower esophageal sphincter. It secretes hydrochloric acid and digestive enzymes used to metabolize proteins and fats. When the stomach is distended, it is stimulated to contract and expel its contents through the pyloric sphincter into the *duodenum,* the first portion of the small intestine.

The *duodenum* is C-shaped and curls around the head of the pancreas. The pancreatic and bile ducts empty into the upper portion of the duodenum. The duodenum then transitions to the *jejunum,* which is responsible for the majority of the absorption of water, proteins, carbohydrates, and vitamins. The *ileum* composes the last and longest part of the small intestine and absorbs bile salts, vitamins C and B_{12}, and chloride. The intestinal contents leave the ileum through the *ileocecal valve* and empty into the *cecum,* located in the right lower quadrant of the abdomen, which is the beginning of the large intestine. The *appendix,* a long, narrow tubular structure, arises from the base of the cecum. The large intestine lies anteriorly over the small intestine, ascends along the right anterior abdominal wall and forms the *ascending colon,* traverses across the abdomen to the splenic flexure forming the *transverse colon,* and descends along the left lateral abdomen wall as the *descending colon* (Figure 14-2). At the level of the iliac crest, the colon becomes the S-shaped *sigmoid* colon. It descends into the pelvic cavity and turns medially to form a loop at the level of the midsacrum. The sigmoid colon connects to the *rectum,* which lies behind the bladder in males and the uterus in females. It stores feces until it is expelled through the *anal canal* and out the *anus,* which is located within a ring of nerves and muscle fibers midway between the tip of the coccyx and the scrotum or vaginal fourchette. The anal canal and anus remain closed involuntarily by way of a ring of smooth muscle, the *internal anal sphincter,* and voluntarily by a ring of skeletal muscle, the *external anal sphincter.*

The *kidneys* lie on either side of the vertebral column in the retroperitoneal space below the liver and spleen. The right kidney tends to be lower than the left because it lies below the right lobe of the liver. Kidneys have a lobulated appearance at birth, which disappears with the development of the glomeruli and tubules in the

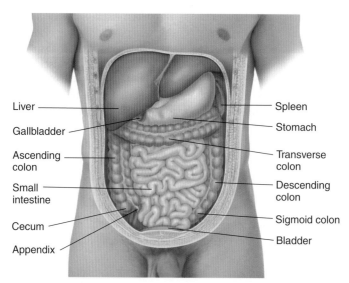

Liver

Gallbladder

Ascending colon

Small intestine

Cecum

Appendix

Spleen

Stomach

Transverse colon

Descending colon

Sigmoid colon

Bladder

FIGURE 14-2 Anatomical structures of the abdominal cavity in an adolescent male. (From Seidel HM, Ball JW, Dains JE, et al: *Mosby's guide to physical examination,* ed 7, St. Louis, 2011, Mosby.)

first year of life. The kidneys are perfused by the renal arteries and filter and reabsorb water, electrolytes, glucose, and some proteins. They regulate blood pressure, electrolytes, and the acid-base composition of blood and other body fluids; actively excrete metabolic waste products; and produce urine. The kidneys are capped by the adrenal glands, pyramid-shaped organs that synthesize, store, and secrete epinephrine and norepinephrine in response to stress. The adrenals also produce the corticosteroids, which affect glucose metabolism, electrolyte and fluid balance, and immune system function.

Urine is excreted from the kidney into the *ureters,* long, thin muscular tubules that transport urine to the bladder. The *ureters* connect to the superior pole of the renal pelvis. They descend posteriorly to the peritoneum and slightly medially in front of the psoas major muscle into the pelvic cavity and implant into the superior posterior wall of the *urinary bladder.* The oblique insertion of the ureters through the bladder wall creates a one-way valvular mechanism that prevents the reflux of urine. The urinary bladder lies anterior to the uterus in females and anterior to the rectum in males. When filled to its capacity, the bladder then contracts and releases urine through the bladder neck and out the *urethra.* The urethra is normally located at the tip of the penis in males and between the clitoris and vagina in females. In nonpregnant females, the reproductive organs lie within the pelvis between the bladder (anterior pelvis) and the rectum (posterior pelvis). They include the *ovaries, uterine* or *fallopian tubes,* and *uterus.* These organs descend into the pelvic cavity during normal growth and development and ascend into the abdominal cavity during pregnancy, or with ovarian cysts or other abnormalities of the female reproductive system.

Finally, a layer of fascia and then muscle cover the anterior abdomen. The *rectus abdominis* muscle extends the entire length of the front of the abdomen and is separated by the *linea alba* in the midline. The *transverse abdominis* and *internal* and *external oblique muscles* cover the

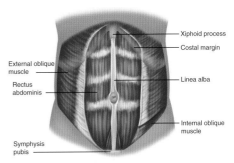

FIGURE 14-3 Abdominal musculature in adolescent.

lateral abdomen. The *umbilicus* lies in the midline usually below the midpoint of the abdomen (Figure 14-3).

PHYSIOLOGICAL VARIATIONS

Many aspects of the development of the organs and structures in the abdomen continue into the first few years of life. The muscle tone of the lower esophageal sphincter is not fully developed until 1 month of age, and may remain slightly weak for the first year. The stomach is round until approximately 2 years of age and then elongates into its adult shape and position by about 7 years of age. Stomach capacity is also smaller in the infant whereas emptying time is faster, which results in the pattern of small and frequent feedings. The small bowel grows from approximately 270 cm at birth to up to 550 cm by 4 years of age. The liver constitutes 5% of the term neonate's body weight, versus 2% in the adult. The kidneys also remain relatively large for the size of the abdomen until adolescence.

SYSTEM-SPECIFIC HISTORY

Information gathering for the assessment of the abdomen should include questions regarding diet, elimination, medications, environmental exposures and a thorough psychosocial history (see Information Gathering table). An assessment of the menstrual cycle in the female and history of sexual activity in adolescents is also essential (see Chapter 17).

INFORMATION GATHERING AT KEY DEVELOPMENTAL STAGES

Age-Group	Topics to Address
Preterm and newborn	Maternal drug use, infection, family history of GI conditions Birth weight and gestational age First meconium and stooling/voiding patterns Amount and type of feedings Spitting up or vomiting Jaundice Any abnormal prenatal ultrasound findings, results of amniocentesis, genetic workup (polyhydramnios, gastric bubble, intestine location, hydronephrosis)
Infancy	Weight gain and growth pattern Amount and type of feedings Food allergies Stooling/voiding patterns Spitting up or vomiting Family history for chronic constipation

Early childhood	Weight gain and growth pattern
	Diet history
	Ingestion of non-nutritive substances (pica)
	Stooling/voiding patterns, including:
	    Toilet training
	    Constipation or stool withholding
	    Enuresis or encopresis
	Rectal bleeding
	Symptoms of UTI (frequency, dysuria, urgency)

Middle childhood	Weight gain and growth pattern
	Nutrition
	Stooling/voiding patterns, including:
	    Constipation or stool withholding
	    Enuresis or encopresis
	Rectal bleeding
	Symptoms of UTI (frequency, dysuria, urgency)
	Abdominal pain
	Recent illnesses
	Psychosocial stressors

Adolescence	Nutrition and BMI Stooling and voiding patterns Abdominal pain Symptoms or history of UTI (Females) Menstrual history and birth control Sexual activity and use of barrier methods Symptoms or history of STI Psychosocial stressors
Environmental risks (all ages)	Water source (exposure to bacteria/parasites) Recent travel to Central America or Asia Recent backpacking or camping Exposure to contaminated foods Environmental lead exposure Family members with chronic abdominal pain or diarrhea Cultural practices for feeding or complementary/alternative healing

BMI, Body mass index; *GI*, gastrointestinal; *STI*, sexually transmitted infection; *UTI*, urinary tract infection.

When a complaint of abdominal pain is reported, the examiner must elicit a detailed history of the pain. Information regarding the character and severity of the pain, onset and duration, location or radiation, position of comfort, things that alleviate or worsen the pain, history of trauma, and any associated symptoms of fever, vomiting, anorexia, constipation, or diarrhea is important in narrowing the scope of the differential diagnosis. A detailed history can help in determining whether the abdominal pain is acute or chronic. Remember that abdominal pain can be referred from an extra-abdominal source or can be a condition associated with systemic disease. For example, abdominal pain is common in children with beta-streptococcal pharyngitis, lower lobe pneumonia, sickle-cell anemia, cystic fibrosis, Henoch-Schönlein purpura, and many other conditions. See Box 14-2 for differential diagnosis of symptoms or conditions related to different abdominal regions.

PHYSICAL ASSESSMENT

Equipment

In performing an abdominal exam in an infant or child, good lighting, warm hands, and a stethoscope may be all the equipment necessary. Diagnostic imaging often plays an important complementary role in the assessment of abdominal complaints.[1] However, a proper

EVIDENCE-BASED PRACTICE TIP

When a child presents with chronic abdominal pain, a primary goal is to determine whether the pain has a functional or organic cause. There are no studies currently indicating that the frequency, severity, or location of pain, or the effects of pain on activities of daily living help to distinguish between functional and organic disorders.[2] Therefore, it is imperative for the health care provider to do a thorough and individualized history and physical examination on any child with chronic abdominal pain to determine other factors that may aid in diagnosis.

physical examination by the health care provider remains essential to determining the best course of action and the level of acuity of the presenting condition. If the assessment reveals abdominal pain accompanied by any red flags or "alarm warnings" (Box 14-1), further evaluation through laboratory analysis and/or diagnostic imaging may be warranted.[2] See later section, Diagnostic Procedures, for further discussion.

Preparation and Positioning

Infants and toddlers can initially sit comfortably on the parent's lap directly facing the examiner. Inspection and auscultation of the abdomen can be done with the child sitting upright. For light and deep palpation, the examiner should be seated in a knee-to-knee position with the

BOX 14-1	RED FLAGS OR "ALARM FINDINGS" DURING THE ABDOMINAL ASSESSMENT

History
Involuntary weight loss
Deceleration of linear growth
Gastrointestinal blood loss
Significant vomiting
Chronic severe diarrhea
Persistent right upper or lower quadrant pain
Unexplained fever
Family history of inflammatory bowel disease

Physical
Localized right upper or lower quadrant
  tenderness
Localized fullness or mass effect
Hepatomegaly
Splenomegaly
Costovertebral angle tenderness
Tenderness over the spine
Perianal abnormalities
Abnormal or unexplained physical findings

Data from American Academy of Pediatrics, North American Society for Pediatric Gastroenterology, Hepatology, and Nutrition: Chronic abdominal pain in children, *Pediatrics* 115(3):e370-381, 2005.

parent and with the child lying with head and torso in the parent's lap and the hips and legs in the examiner's lap (Figure 14-4). The initial examination can occur with the child partially dressed and the diaper can be unfastened or pants and underwear pulled below the groin area. For older children and adolescents, the abdomen should be assessed on the examination table. It is important for the examiner to consistently place the older child or adolescent in the same position when preparing for the abdominal

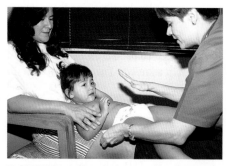

FIGURE 14-4 Knee-to-knee position for examining abdomen in infancy and early childhood. (From James SR, Ashwill JW: *Nursing care of children,* ed 2, St. Louis, 2003, Saunders.)

examination—ideally with the head on the examiner's left and the right side of the child's body in front of the examiner. This will aid in accurate anatomical findings and accurate diagnosis of abdominal symptoms and conditions.

The abdomen is divided into four equal quadrants, with the transverse and midsagittal planes intersecting at the umbilicus (Figure 14-5, *A*). For a child or adolescent who presents with abdominal pain or for other abdominal conditions, use a mapping technique with nine sections to accurately describe findings and for purposes of charting in the medical record (see Figure 14-5, *B*). Keep in mind that the abdomen is a three-dimensional space. Mentally visualizing the anatomical location of the organs and adopting a mapping technique for abdominal assessment is key to an accurate and informative examination. There may be some variation in the anatomical positions of the organs in children and adolescents depending on the body type, respiratory phase at the time of the exam, the amount of contents within the stomach or bladder, and the amount of palpable stool in the abdomen.

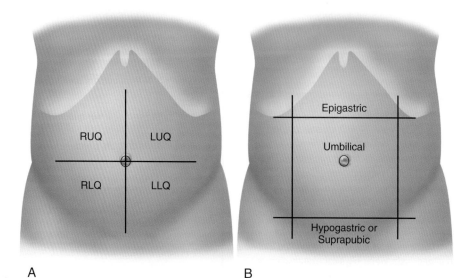

A   B

FIGURE 14-5 **A,** Four quadrants of the abdomen. **B,** Nine regions of the abdomen.

Inspection

Examination of the abdomen begins with the initial inspection of the child or adolescent's facial expression and color, attitude, activity level, and level of comfort to determine any distress. If the child is guarding the abdomen, prefers to keep the legs flexed, or if the abdomen is rigid, this can indicate diffuse peritonitis. Begin the abdominal assessment by extending each leg and note if pain is elicited and the location. Observe whether the child has difficulty walking or climbing onto or off of the exam table. Children with peritoneal irritation often walk cautiously and resist lying on the exam table. Ask the child to hop or jump and note whether these movements elicit pain.

Inspect the abdomen by noting its contour, symmetry, skin texture, color, and integrity. Note any lesions, rashes, pigment variations, piercings, gastrostomy tubes, or scars. Scars can indicate previous abdominal surgery and should always be explored during history taking. View the abdomen from the side and note the shape and anteroposterior dimension. Infants and young children have less developed abdominal musculature so the abdomen is more protuberant and round. Young children to 4 years of age will have a potbellied appearance while supine or standing (Figure 14-6). If the

abdomen is scaphoid at any age, it can indicate malnutrition or displaced abdominal organs as with a diaphragmatic hernia or intestinal atresia in a newborn. If the abdominal contour is distended, it can indicate an intestinal obstruction, a mass, organomegaly, or ascites. Fullness over the symphysis pubis can be seen in a thin child with a full bladder. Asymmetry of the abdomen may indicate a mass, organomegaly, or hollow organ distention, or curvature of the spine.

Observe for any pulsations. It is normal to see pulsations in the epigastric area of a young infant or very thin child. Distended veins in the abdominal integument could indicate vascular compression or obstruction, hypertension, or intestinal obstruction. If an intestinal obstruction is suspected, note any obvious loops of bowel and observe for peristaltic waves on the surface by viewing the abdomen at eye level.

Inspect the umbilicus for any signs of drainage, infection, hernia, or mass. In the initial newborn exam, inspect the cord for the umbilical vessels, two arteries, and a single vein. The arteries are smaller and have a thicker vessel wall. Infants with a two-vessel cord may have congenital anomalies and should be referred for further diagnosis and evaluation. The majority of umbilical cord remnants detach by the tenth day of life but can take up to 3 weeks to slough. Once the cord has detached, the stump should dry and heal within a few days. Occasionally, *umbilical granulomas* or granular tissue at the base of the umbilicus can be present and drain serous or seropurulent fluid or occasionally bleed (Figure 14-7). For persistent umbilical granulomas, cauterization or surgical ligation of the stump may be needed. Any prolonged drainage should be investigated for presence of *urachal remnant* or *cyst*. If stool is noted coming from the umbilicus, an *omphalomesenteric duct remnant* is present, and the infant should be referred immediately to a pediatric surgeon. Any sign of infection in the umbilicus should be aggressively treated in

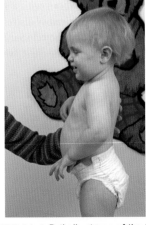

FIGURE 14-6 Potbelly stance of the toddler.

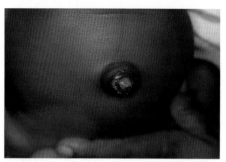

FIGURE 14-7 Umbilical granuloma. (From Clark DA: *Atlas of neonatology,* ed 7, Philadelphia, 2000, Saunders.)

the neonate. *Neonatal omphalitis* is a rapidly progressing, acute, and potentially fatal infection of the abdominal wall caused by a bacterial pathogen. Any infant with purulent discharge or sign of cellulitis should be treated with systemic antibiotics and referred immediately if the infection progresses.

Note any protrusion or mass in the umbilicus. Observe the midline of the abdomen of the infant or young child when reclining or sitting. A wide bulging superior to the umbilicus is likely *diastasis recti abdominis* (Figure 14-8),

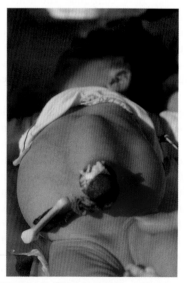

FIGURE 14-8 Diastasis recti. (From Clark DA: *Atlas of neonatology,* ed 7, Philadelphia, 2000, Saunders.)

a common finding in children when the rectus abdominis muscle does not meet in the midline. Diastasis recti abdominis does not create any functional problem during infancy and early childhood and usually diminishes or resolves as the child grows.

Auscultation

Auscultation of the abdomen should be done before palpation or percussion, to prevent any alteration in bowel sounds that may occur from manipulation of the area. Systematically listen to each quadrant or section of the abdomen with a stethoscope. In the infant and young child, auscultate the abdomen when completing the quiet parts of the physical exam (i.e., the cardiac and respiratory assessment). Bowel sounds can be heard within the first few hours of life and indicate peristalsis and movement of contents through the bowels. Normal bowel sounds are heard every 10 to 20 seconds and frequency of bowel sounds may be approximately 5 to 30 in one minute. Hypoactive (more than 30 seconds apart) or absent bowel sounds (none heard within 3 to 5 minutes) may indicate a *paralytic ileus,* or inactivity of the intestines. Hyperactive bowel sounds indicate rapid movement through the intestines, usually associated with diarrhea or a mechanical obstruction. If the child is hypertensive, auscultate for bruits using the bell of the stethoscope to assess for signs of renovascular disease. A newborn with a *scaphoid* abdomen or signs of respiratory distress should be carefully evaluated for bowel sounds or decreased breath sounds in the chest, which may indicate a *diaphragmatic hernia.*

Palpation

Palpation is the most important technique in assessing the abdomen and identifies areas of tenderness, masses, organomegaly, ascites, and signs of inflammation or peritonitis. It should not be omitted even with a child who is having difficulty cooperating with the exam. If the child is supine, gently flex the knees and hips to relax the abdominal wall. Give infants a pacifier or bottle to suck to help relax the abdomen during the exam or distract young children in the parent's lap with a toy or favorite stuffed animal.

Begin with light palpation using the pads of the forefingers to assess the four quadrants of the abdomen. Use a firm therapeutic touch for palpation. Massaging the abdomen should be avoided. Observe the child's facial expression to note any signs of pain, discomfort, or areas of tenderness. During auscultation of the abdomen, the examiner can carefully watch the child's facial expression to identify areas of tenderness while lightly pressing the stethoscope against each section of the abdomen. If areas of tenderness are detected with light palpation, examine those areas last when performing deep palpation.

PEDIATRIC PEARLS

If a child is ticklish during palpation, place his or her hand under your hand with your fingers interlaced and palpate the abdomen together. Distraction with conversation is also effective in eliciting cooperation throughout the exam.

Deep palpation requires a firmer therapeutic touch, and the child may resist palpation because of fear or pain over areas of inflammation. It may be helpful to use two-handed palpation with the nondominant hand to exert pressure over the examining hand when evaluating the abdomen in obese children and adolescents. Tenderness with deep palpation of the right lower quadrant (McBurney's sign) or referred right lower quadrant pain with deep palpation of the left lower quadrant (Rovsing's sign) could be suspicious of *appendicitis* and should be further evaluated and referred. With deep palpation, pain can also be assessed with *rebound tenderness*. To produce *rebound tenderness*, place fingertips at a 90-degree angle against the abdomen and gently but firmly press into the abdomen. Quickly lift the hand off the abdomen and note if any pain is

elicited. The child with *rebound tenderness* will have more pain when the examiner's hand is lifted from the abdomen than with deep palpation. Pain with rebound of the abdomen may be a sign of inflammation or *peritonitis*. *Rigidity* of the abdomen is the involuntary tightening of the abdominal musculature that occurs in response to underlying inflammation in the abdomen. *Peritonitis* may be indicated if pain is worse when the examiner lifts the hand off the abdomen when testing for *rebound tenderness*. *Guarding* is the voluntary contraction of the abdominal wall musculature to prevent pain, and may subside if the child relaxes.

To palpate the liver, place the fingertips at the right midclavicular line a few centimeters below the rib cage at the costal margin. Move the fingers slightly up and inward and feel for a firm nudge by the liver tip on inspiration. Note the distance between the location of the costal margin and liver tip. The liver may be palpable in an infant or toddler 1 to 2 cm below the right costal margin. Hepatomegaly is suspected in any child whose liver is palpable more than 3 cm below the costal margin. In the obese child or adolescent, hepatomegaly is highly suspect for nonalcoholic fatty liver disease (NAFLD) and should prompt further evaluation through laboratory and imaging studies.[3] Other causes of an enlarged liver include infection, tumors, storage disorders, biliary masses, intrahepatic vascular disease, or cardiac disease.

To palpate the spleen, position the fingertips in the left midclavicular line below the costal margin and feel for a firmness on inspiration (Figure 14-9). An alternative technique in infants is to palpate the spleen between the thumb and forefinger of the right hand. The spleen can be felt in about 5% to 10% of children and should be slightly mobile. The spleen must be increased to 2 to 3 times its size to be consistently palpable.[4] If splenomegaly is suspected, an ultrasound can differentiate spleen enlargement from other masses that may arise in the left upper quadrant. Splenomegaly can

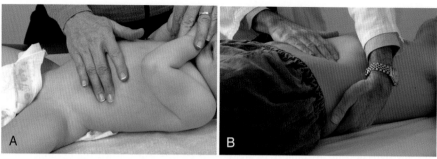

FIGURE 14-9 **A,** Palpating the spleen in the toddler. **B,** Two-handed palpation of the spleen in an adolescent. (**B** from Talley N: *Clinical examination: a systematic guide to physical diagnosis,* ed 6, Sydney, 2010, Churchill Livingstone.)

be caused by infection, inflammation, blood dyscrasias, a mass, or vascular and oncological conditions. If blunt trauma to the abdomen is suspected, avoid deep palpation of the spleen or liver. The spleen is a very vascular organ and should be *gently* palpated. If the liver or spleen is lacerated, a clot that may *tamponade* the laceration could be dislodged and cause further bleeding.

The kidneys can sometimes be palpated in infants. Place the left hand behind the right flank of the infant and using the tips of the right hand, palpate deeply in the right upper quadrant (RUQ), to the right of the midline. The right kidney may be "trapped" between the hands. Repeat the technique, placing the right hand behind the infant's left flank, and use the left fingertips to palpate the left kidney in the left upper quadrant (LUQ). The kidneys should be round, smooth, and firm. A distended bladder may be palpated in the midline above the symphysis pubis, which may indicate a vesico-ureteral or bladder neck obstruction, acute bladder retention, or neurogenic bladder.

Palpate the umbilicus for masses or herniation. The most common umbilical disorder is an *umbilical hernia* in which the intestine protrudes through the abdominal fascia, or *linea alba* (Figure 14-10). The umbilicus appears to protrude especially when the child is crying, stooling, or coughing, but generally can be easily reduced with the examiner applying light pressure with the fingertips to the

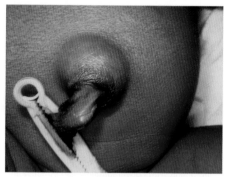

FIGURE 14-10 Umbilical hernia. (From Clark DA: *Atlas of neonatology,* ed 7, Philadelphia, 2000, Saunders.)

umbilicus. Palpate the fascia below the umbilicus with the fingertips to determine the size of the defect. If the opening is larger than the width of two fingers or the child is older than 3 years of age, surgical closure may be necessary. Incarceration of an umbilical hernia is very rare. Most will spontaneously close by the time the child is 3 or 4 years of age. The most common umbilical mass is a *dermoid cyst*. It appears as a firm, skin-covered, nonreducible mass within the umbilicus that may have a slight discoloration and can be lobulated. Other cysts or an *umbilical polyp* should be referred to a pediatric surgeon for evaluation. Diastasis recti abdominis, separation of the abdominal wall musculature, can be noted with light palpation over the midquadrant. An infant between the ages of 3 and 8 weeks of age with projectile, nonbilious vomiting may have *pyloric stenosis.* Examine the infant while the abdomen is relaxed and palpate in the upper abdomen, slightly right of the midline for a firm, olive-shaped mass, which is highly suspicious for a hypertrophic pylorus. If a child presents with constipation, a sausage-shaped mass of stool may be palpated in the lower left quadrant (LLQ) or in the midline below the umbilicus or *rectosigmoid* colon. Palpating stool throughout the abdomen may indicate fecal impaction.

Palpate the groin bilaterally for femoral arterial pulses and presence of lymph nodes (Figure 14-11). Check the groin area for a mass or *inguinal hernia.* Note any persistent bulging in the groin. Palpate to determine size and reducibility. If the inguinal bulge or *hernia* can be reduced, referral is indicated for elective surgery and repair. An irreducible or incarcerated hernia is a surgical emergency. Scars from previous surgical hernia repairs also should be evaluated. An incisional hernia may be present and should be evaluated and referred.

Percussion

Percussion of the abdomen can help identify whether a distended abdomen is caused by air, a mass, or fluid (Figure 14-12). When percussing, place your left or nondominant hand firmly against the abdominal wall so only your middle finger is resting on the skin. Tap on the distal interphalangeal joint of your middle finger two or three times with the tip of your

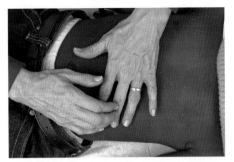

FIGURE 14-12 Percussion of the abdomen.

middle finger of your dominant hand with a relaxed wrist. Air or gas in the abdominal cavity creates a hollow, drumlike sound, or *tympany,* when tapping firmly over the area. Tympany is common in infants and young children because they swallow air when feeding and crying. Percussion also can delineate rough dimensions of solid masses and organs, although in most settings diagnostic imaging is used for accuracy of any abdominal findings. To measure liver size, percuss superiorly between the ribs until no dullness is noted. The upper edge of the liver should be detected at the right midclavicular line near the fifth intercostal space. Mark this point and measure its distance from the lower edge of the liver. The lower edge of the liver should not extend more than 1 to 2 cm below the costal margin. This technique identifies only the anterior surface of the liver and not the anteroposterior dimension. Fluid in the abdomen creates a dull sound when percussing over the area and may indicate the presence of *ascites* in the abdominal cavity.

Rectal Examination

When to perform a rectal exam in a child is a hotly debated topic among health care providers. A rectal exam should be performed if there is concern regarding anal or rectal patency, anal discomfort, constipation or sphincter tone, fissures, hemorrhoids, or rectal polyps. Abdominal pain may be an indication for a rectal exam depending on the child or adolescent health history.

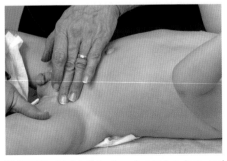

FIGURE 14-11 Palpating femoral pulses and lymph nodes.

If the abdominal exam and health history are unclear or the information obtained from a rectal exam would assist in the diagnosis, explain to the parent and child or adolescent the need for the rectal exam. Keep in mind a rectal exam is physically invasive and many children will no longer cooperate with a physical exam after a rectal exam has been performed. If it is necessary to perform a rectal exam, do so at the very end of the physical examination using the talk-through approach as presented in Chapter 1.

Position the child on the side with knees flexed (fetal position). An infant or toddler can lie supine with the hips and knees flexed. Assess the sacrum for dimples, sinuses, or tufts of hair. Note the location of the anus, which if displaced could predispose a child to issues such as constipation. Inspect the anus for rashes, fissures, skin tags or discoloration. Contraction of the external anal sphincter (anal wink reflex) is a normal response to stroking of the skin in the perineum. Gently insert a gloved, lubricated finger (usually the smallest finger in infants; the index finger in an older child) into the rectal vault and feel for any narrowing. Assess sphincter tones. Feel for any masses or pressure compressing the lumen of the rectum. Note whether there is stool in the rectum and whether it is hard or soft. If an explosive stool is elicited with the rectal exam, it may be a sign of a rectal obstruction such as *Hirschsprung disease*. Gently press toward the right lower quadrant and observe whether it elicits a pain response. This can support a diagnosis of appendicitis. Alternately press in all directions and note any pain. If any stool is retrieved from the exam, perform a guaiac test on the specimen and assess for fecal occult blood in the stool.

DIAGNOSTIC PROCEDURES

A number of diagnostic procedures may be useful to aid in the assessment of abdominal and rectal complaints. Guaiac stool testing or a urine dipstick may be easily performed in the clinic setting or office. Laboratory analyses that could be useful include the evaluation of liver and kidney function, analysis of urine or stool, monitoring of electrolytes, or checking for antibody markers such as for *Helicobacter pylori* or celiac disease. Radiographic procedures such as a KUB (kidneys, ureters, and bladder) x-ray, ultrasound, computed tomography (CT) scan, or magnetic resonance imaging (MRI) can be helpful to locate and measure organs or masses or detect intestinal inflammation, obstruction, or perforation. Endoscopy of the upper or lower GI tract may be useful to visualize anatomy, lesions, and obtain biopsies, or to evaluate for inflammation of the esophagus due to gastroesophageal reflux disease.

ABDOMINAL CONDITIONS

Box 14-2 presents various conditions of the abdomen according to where the signs or symptoms may occur. Keep in mind that many conditions involve diffuse abdominal pain, and that children often have a difficult time localizing pain to a specific region.

BOX 14-2 ABNORMAL CONDITIONS OF THE ABDOMEN

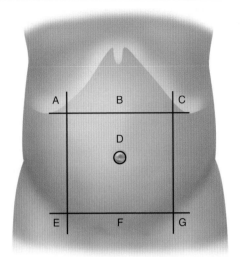

A, Right Upper Quadrant
Hepatitis
Cholecystitis
Liver, renal, or adrenal neoplasm
Hydronephrosis
Pyloric stenosis
Pancreatitis
High fecal impaction
Intussusception

B, Epigastric
Gastroesophageal reflux
Cholecystitis
Hepatitis
Pancreatitis

D, Periumbilical
Acute gastroenteritis
Constipation
Functional abdominal pain
Appendicitis (referred)
Umbilical hernia

C, Left Upper Quadrant
Renal or adrenal neoplasm
Hydronephrosis
Pancreatitis
Splenic mass
Mononucleosis
High fecal impaction

E, Right Lower Quadrant
Appendicitis
Intestinal obstruction
Ovarian torsion or cyst
Mittelschmerz
Dysmenorrhea
Ectopic pregnancy
Mesenteric adenitis
Incarcerated hernia
Lymphoma
Pyelonephritis
Renal neoplasm

F, Suprapubic
Bladder distention
Urinary tract infection
Bladder neoplasm
Ovarian torsion or cyst
Mittelschmerz
Dysmenorrhea
Ectopic pregnancy
Pelvic inflammatory disease

G, Left Lower Quadrant
Constipation
Intestinal obstruction
Hirschsprung disease
Ovarian torsion or cyst
Mittelschmerz
Dysmenorrhea
Ectopic pregnancy
Incarcerated hernia
Lymphoma
Pyelonephritis
Renal neoplasm

Data from Rakel RE, Rakel DP: *Textbook of family medicine,* ed 8, Philadelphia, 2011, Saunders.

SUMMARY OF EXAMINATION

- A thorough and detailed history is an essential part of the abdominal assessment and should include the medical and family health history, nutrition and elimination habits, a psychosocial evaluation, and a review of pain or other presenting symptoms.
- Infants and young children may be more comfortably assessed in the lap of their parent or caregiver.
- Abdominal assessment should be performed using a mapping technique by mentally dividing the abdomen into four quadrants or nine regions
- Begin inspection of the abdomen by observing the child or adolescent's posture, behavior, and activity level; then inspect the abdomen for size, shape, and pulsations.

- Auscultate each quadrant of the abdomen before palpation, and note quality and frequency of bowel sounds.
- Use light palpation to identify areas of tenderness before deep palpation.
- During palpation, note size of organs if palpable, presence of tenderness or pain on palpation, any guarding or rigidity in the abdomen, and the size and quality of any masses.
- Perform percussion to identify the presence of air or gas and to estimate the size of solid organs or masses.
- A rectal examination should only be performed when applicable and, if so, should be done at the end of the physical exam.

Charting
1-Month-Old Term Infant

Abdomen: Abdomen symmetrical, soft, round, nontender without masses or organomegaly. Liver palpated 2 cm below right costal margin. Normal bowel sounds over all quadrants. Umbilicus clean, dry without hernia, mass, inflammation, or discharge. Epigastric pulsations noted. Percussion tones tympanic.

Charting
12-Year-Old Female with Abdominal Pain

Abdomen: Abdomen symmetrical, flat, tender with guarding throughout and rebound tenderness noted in RLQ. Bowel sounds hypoactive especially in the lower quadrants. No masses or organomegaly.

REFERENCES

1. Scammell S, Lansdale N, Sprigg A, et al: Ultrasonography aids decision-making in children with abdominal pain, *Ann R Coll Surg Engl* 93(5):405-409, 2011.
2. American Academy of Pediatrics Subcommittee on Chronic Abdominal Pain, North American Society for Pediatric Gastroenterology, Hepatology, and Nutrition: Chronic abdominal pain in children, *Pediatrics* 115(3):e370-381, 2005.
3. Vajro P, Lenta S, Socha P, et al: Diagnosis of nonalcoholic fatty liver disease in children and adolescents: position paper of the ESPGHAN Hepatology Committee, *J Pediatr Gastroenterol Nutr* 54(5): 700-713, 2012.
4. Kliegman RM, Stanton BF, St. Geme III JW, et al: *Nelson textbook of pediatrics*, ed 19, Philadelphia, 2011, Elsevier.

CHAPTER 15

MALE GENITALIA

Angel K. Chen

The pediatric physical examination is not complete without a thorough evaluation of the developing genitalia. Routine surveillance of the genitourinary system is equally important in all patient encounters, and when assessment of the genitalia is performed routinely abnormalities can be identified and promptly treated. Many parents, children, and adolescents are concerned and anxious about the genitalia, yet may not feel comfortable expressing those concerns initially. A review of systems in the health history and the routine genital exam offer an opportunity for the parent, child, and/or adolescent to voice concerns, and for the health care provider to offer reassurance and education on normal development. The provider has a role in fostering dialogue between the parent and child regarding reproductive health. Establishing this dialogue early with families forms the basis for healthy discussions on reproductive health during puberty and in the developing adolescent.

EMBRYOLOGICAL DEVELOPMENT

The differentiation of the sexual organs begins as early as the third week of embryonic development, dictated by the sex chromosomes at the time of fertilization.[1] The *mesoderm* is the embryonic layer that becomes smooth and striated muscle tissue, connective tissue, blood vessels, bone marrow, skeletal tissue, and the reproductive and excretory organs. As proliferation of the embryonic layers continues, maturation of the external genitalia in the fetus is established by the twelfth week.[1] The sex-determining region of the Y chromosome (*SRY* gene) activates the differentiation of the

embryonic gonad into a testis, without which the gonad would become an ovary. The anti-müllerian hormone (AMH) prevents development of the uterus and fallopian tubes, whereas testosterone stimulates the wolffian ducts to develop into the male reproductive structures, including the *epididymis, vas deferens,* and *seminal vesicles.* Testosterone is also the precursor to dihydrotestosterone (DHT), which stimulates the formation of the male *urethra, prostate,* and *external genitalia.*[1]

Urine production begins between the ninth and twelfth weeks and is excreted into the amniotic cavity through the *urethral meatus.* During development, the fetus continues the production and excretion of urine, which forms the amniotic fluid. Between the seventeenth and twentieth weeks, the *testes,* which develop in the abdominal cavity, begin to descend along the inguinal canal into the scrotum, bringing the arteries, veins, lymphatics, and nerves that are encased within the cremaster muscle and spermatic cord.[1] The inguinal canal closes after testicular descent. Incomplete or abnormal embryonic development of the inguinal canal predisposes the newborn to the formation of hydroceles or hernias. Preterm infants are at increased risk for these conditions. At birth, the infant's genitourinary system is functionally immature with limited bladder capacity, inability to concentrate urine sufficiently and frequent voiding.

Growth of the fetus and differentiation of the sexual organs can be affected by placental function, the hormonal environment during pregnancy, maternal nutrition, maternal infection, and genetic factors or chromosomal abnormalities. A fetal insult from intrinsic or extrinsic factors during the eighth or ninth week of gestation may lead to major abnormalities of the developing external genitalia. The impact of endocrine-disrupting chemicals on the development of the endocrine and genitourinary system is reviewed in Chapter 5.

ANATOMY AND PHYSIOLOGY

Penis

The *penis* consists of the shaft, glans, corona, meatus, and prepuce. The *shaft* is composed of erectile tissue called *corpora cavernosa* (two lateral columns) and *corpus spongiosum* (ventral column). The anterior portion of the corpus spongiosum forms the *glans penis,* the border or edge of which is called the *corona.* The urethra is within the corpus spongiosum, and the orifice, or *urethral meatus,* is the slit-like opening just ventral to the tip of the penis (Figure 15-1).

The *prepuce,* or *foreskin,* is the fold of skin at the tip of the penis that covers the glans penis in the uncircumcised male and forms the secondary fold of skin from the urethral meatus to the coronal region of the penis called the *frenulum.* The skin of the penis is thin, does not contain subcutaneous fat, and is loosely tied to the deeper layer of the dermis and fascia. Often, the skin of the shaft is more darkly pigmented, particularly in children or adolescents with darker pigmentation or darker skin. The skin of the *glans penis* does not contain hair follicles, but does have small glands and papillae that form in the epithelial cells to produce *smegma,* the white oily material made up of desquamated epithelial cells trapped under the foreskin, which is normal and often mistaken as pathological[2] (Figure 15-2). The foreskin is generally nonretractable at birth, because of adherence of the inner epithelial lining of the foreskin and glans.[2,3] Desquamation of the tissue layers continues until the separation of the prepuce and glans penis is complete secondary to intermittent erections and keratinization of the inner epithelium, generally by 5 to 6 years of age. Partial adhesions of the foreskin to the prepuce may produce smegma along the coronal region, which often persists throughout childhood.

Scrotum and Testes

The *scrotum* is made up of a thin layer of skin that forms *rugae* (folds) and contains the *testes.*

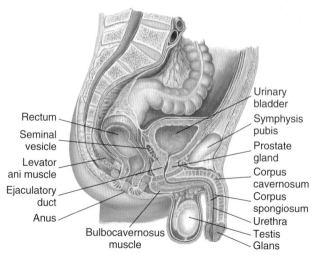

FIGURE 15-1 Internal and external genitalia. (From Seidel HM et al: *Mosby's guide to physical examination,* ed 7, St. Louis, 2011, Mosby.)

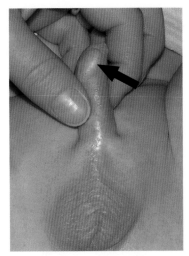

FIGURE 15-2 Smegma. (From Godbole P: General paediatric urology, *Surgery (Oxford)* 26(5):223-227, 2008.)

The *epididymis* is the thin palpable structure along the lateral edge of the posterior side of the testes. Sperm production occurs within the *seminiferous tubules* in the testes, which connect to the *epididymis*. The *vas deferens* is the cordlike structure that is continuous with the base of the epididymis and stores sperm. The *spermatic cord* extends from the testes to the *inguinal ring* and is felt only on deep palpation of the *testicular sac*. The right spermatic cord is shorter in some males, which causes the right testis to hang higher than the left.

The male accessory organs include the *seminal vesicles,* which lay deep in the abdominal cavity alongside the vas deferens and secrete liquid into the *semen* as it passes from the testes. The opening of the seminal vesicles joins the vas deferens to form *ejaculatory ducts* and drains to the posterior urethra. The *Cowper glands,* or bulbourethral glands, lie along the urethra in the male genitalia. These are exocrine glands that produce a viscous secretion that lubricates the urethra for the passage of sperm. It also neutralizes the acidic urethral secretions that could otherwise damage the spermatozoa in the *semen.* The *prostate gland* is the small, firm mass that lies within the pelvic cavity. It first becomes palpable on manual examination in the adolescent male. The prostate gland surrounds the posterior urethra and secrets an alkaline secretion during ejaculation to promote fertilization. The smooth muscle within the prostate gland assists with urinary elimination. An enlarged prostate gland may cause urinary obstruction.

PHYSIOLOGICAL VARIATIONS

Table 15-1 presents the physiological variations of the male genitalia in the pediatric age-group from infancy to early childhood.

TABLE 15-1 PHYSIOLOGICAL VARIATIONS OF THE MALE GENITALIA

Age-Group	Variation
Preterm infant	Rugae absent on scrotum in low birth weight infant Testes undescended in ~20% of infants weighing <2500 g*
Newborn	Rugae present from 37 weeks' gestation Note and evaluate any discoloration of scrotum at birth Testis: volume 1 to 2 ml Length of penis in term infant: 2.5 to 3.5 cm; size should be palpated during exam Shaft may appear short or retracted in infants with significant suprapubic fat pad
Infancy/ early childhood	Foreskin partially retractable over glans penis Testes present in scrotal sac Initial sexual arousal and erection occur with normal sexual exploration or exposure of genitalia

*Data from Thureen PJ, Hall D, Deacon J, Hernandez JA: *Assessment and care of the well newborn,* ed 2, Philadelphia, 2005, Saunders.

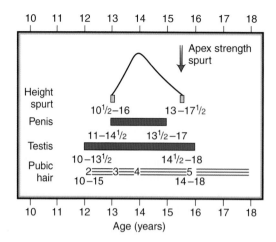

FIGURE 15-3 Pubertal changes. (From Marshall WA, Tanner JM: Variations in the pattern of pubertal changes in boys, *Arch Dis Child* 45:13-23, 1970.)

Physiological Changes in Puberty

Puberty has a gradual onset and although it is marked by a growth spurt, it may be difficult to ascertain when the first changes in the male begin in the transition to secondary sexual characteristics (Figure 15-3). In males, sexual development, or true gonadal activation, begins with an increase in size of the testicles, which is often difficult to determine. Testicular volume should be evaluated and is the most accurate measurement of the progression of puberty in the developing male. In some boys, this begins around 10 years of age and is complete in about 3 years, with the normal range extending to 5 years.[4] The sexual maturity rating (SMR) scale, also known as Tanner stages, helps to classify physical pubertal maturation[4] (Figure 15-4 and Table 15-2). Genital development and pubic hair may develop at different rates. Ejaculation usually occurs at SMR 3 during the midpoint of sexual development. Fertility is established by SMR 4, although sperm are present in some quantity with ejaculation during SMR 3.

In male adolescents, it is the tempo of growth and maturation that is distinctly different than that in females. At mid-puberty, with rising testosterone concentrations, most of the rapid linear growth occurs. Recent studies have provided evidence of earlier onset puberty in

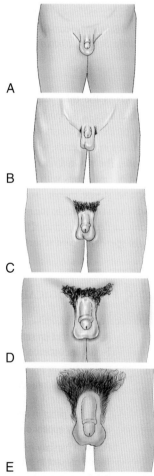

FIGURE 15-4 Sexual maturity rating (SMR) or Tanner staging.

TABLE 15-2 DEVELOPMENTAL CHANGES IN PUBERTY

| Tanner Stage/Sexual Maturity Rating (SMR) | Developmental Changes | | | |
	Pubic Hair	Penis	Scrotum	Testicular Volume
Tanner stage 1 SMR 1	None	Unchanged from early childhood	Unchanged from early childhood	<1.5 mL
Tanner stage 2 SMR 2	Small amount of light, downy hair along base of penis	Unchanged or slightly enlarged	Enlarged and reddened pigmentation; skin taut and thinner; increased rugation	1.6-6 mL
Tanner stage 3 SMR 3	Moderate amount of curly, pigmented coarse pubic hair extending laterally over symphysis pubis	↑ Length and circumference	Further enlargement	6-12 mL
Tanner stage 4 SMR 4	Abundant adultlike quality	Glans penis broader and larger; penis ↑ length and circumference	Further enlargement and darker pigmentation	12-20 mL
Tanner stage 5 SMR 5	Extends to medial surface of the thighs	Adult size	Adult size	>20 mL

Data from Neinstein LS: *Handbook of adolescent care,* Philadelphia, 2009, Lippincott Williams & Wilkins.

males, particularly in African-Americans.[4] The trend is an overall earlier start of puberty but prolonged progression to genital maturity.

FAMILY, CULTURAL, RACIAL, AND ETHNIC CONSIDERATIONS

Understanding and respecting cultural differences is an important part of the role of the health care provider, particularly in relation to the assessment of the genitourinary system. Identifying which family members may be a part of the discussion and/or be present during the examination of the genitalia and how to approach the exam are the first steps in developing a trusting relationship with the family. Parental and family attitudes about sexuality vary widely both within cultures and among cultures. Sexual awakening first occurs in the young child with the discovery of the genitalia as a sensual organ. This initial experience and the parental attitude toward normal fondling and exploration may set the stage for either normal sexual development in a child or a feeling of shamefulness and an attitude in the child that fosters abnormal functioning throughout life. Often, cultural attitudes concerning sexuality and reproduction form the basis of conflict between the parent and young child or maturing adolescent. Mediating this difference between the adolescent and the parent may be the most important and challenging role for the health care provider. Additionally, documentation in the health care record provides opportunity to communicate these attitudes to the next provider to ensure consistent delivery of care.

System-Specific History

Important information for the assessment of the male genitalia at key developmental stages and ages is presented in the Information Gathering table below.

Information Gathering for Male Genitalia Assessment at Key Developmental Stages

Age-Group	Questions to Ask
For all age groups	Gestational and birth history History of maternal hormone ingestion during pregnancy Maternal alcohol and/or drug use Maternal exposure to hazardous chemicals and/or pesticides Family history of GU abnormalities Current medication Circumcision status Scrotal or inguinal mass; $+/-$ pain Voiding history (include voiding frequency, voiding stream, ballooning of foreskin [if applicable]) Elimination history (frequency and consistency)
Preterm, newborn, and infant	History of maternal infection History of significant neonatal infections Presence of testes in scrotum at birth
Early childhood, middle childhood	Toilet training process Additional voiding history (history of urinary frequency, postponing behavior, daytime and/or nighttime wetting, difficulty or pain on urination) History of balanitis and/or (documented) urinary tract infections Physiological phimosis

Adolescence	Family history of delayed puberty
	Onset of growth spurt and puberty
	Painful erection
	History of balanitis and/or (documented) urinary tract infections
	Testicular pain/swelling
	Penile discharge
	Sexual debut:
	    With males, females, or both
	    Number of partners
	    Types of sexual activity (vaginal, oral, and/or anal intercourse)
	    Condom use
	    STI exposure/testing/results
	History of coerced sexual contact (molestation/rape)
	Inability to achieve erection and/or to ejaculate

GU, Genitourinary; *STI,* sexually transmitted infection.

PHYSICAL ASSESSMENT

Preparation

Although there is a tendency toward skipping assessment of the genitalia in the course of performing the physical examination, the provider should be mindful that it is a critical part of evaluating a growing and developing body. If performed regularly by the provider during pediatric well visits, the genital examination then becomes simply an expected part of the routine physical assessment at all ages, including through adolescence. Reticence on the part of the child, adolescent, parent, or even the provider is not a reason for omitting the examination of the genitalia. The provider should proceed as with the rest of the physical examination, maintaining a matter-of-fact approach and using a purposeful technique that is not traumatic for the child or adolescent.

Before the start of the genitourinary exam, the provider should discuss the rationale for performing this exam as well as what to expect during the exam. Anticipatory guidance is of utmost importance for all age groups beyond the infant and young child. Parents of adolescents should be prepared to leave the exam room for the physical examination of the genitalia after bringing up any concerns during the health history. This gives the provider an opportunity to discuss with the adolescent the consent to confidential reproductive health services and the limits to confidentiality, which differ from state to state (see Chapter 4).

PEDIATRIC PEARLS

In early childhood, the provider should emphasize that the exam is only to be done when a parent or guardian is present but not with strangers or other adolescents or adults. In middle childhood, the genital exam is a chance to reinforce normal development, and the exam prepares the child for what to expect as an adolescent. In adolescence, the exam is a chance to be alone with the provider to discuss questions and/or concerns about their genitalia and development.

As with all parts of the physical examination in pediatrics, it is important to *talk through* the assessment of the male genitalia and reassure the adolescent of normal findings as well as discuss any concerns when completing the examination. This is also an opportunity to discuss normal growth and development, hygiene issues, and anticipatory guidance. With the adolescent male, the talk-through exam provides opportunity to establish rapport, and validates feelings and concerns during and after the examination. There is often a hidden agenda with adolescents around issues of normalcy or reproduction. The health care provider must be ready to discuss any issues involving reproductive health in a supportive and professional manner.

Positioning

During the first 4 to 6 months of life, infants are best positioned on the examination table for assessment of the male genitalia. Beyond early infancy, the child may be lying on the parent's lap in a knee-to-knee position with the provider, or continue to be examined on the exam table. The young child may be lying down or sitting in the tailor position (cross-legged) on the exam table (Figure 15-5). The middle-age child may be examined lying supine on the exam table or standing to enhance gravity of the testicles, as in the adolescent and young adult male. It is important to have draping available and only expose the child as long as needed for inspection, palpation, and/or education. Lengthy discussions can be done once the child is dressed. Respecting the need for privacy, particularly in the young child and the developing adolescent, establishes a good patient-provider relationship.

Inspection and Palpation

Assessment of the male genitalia includes inspection and palpation of the penis, foreskin, urethral meatus, scrotum, testes, rectal sphincter, and perineal skin status. Always inform the child or adolescent before beginning inspection and palpation. *Physiological phimosis,*

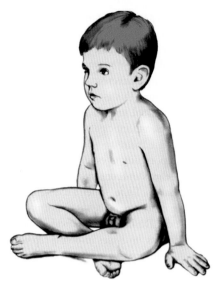

FIGURE 15-5 Young child sitting tailor style (cross-legged) in preparation for testicular exam.

when the foreskin cannot be retracted over the glans penis, is normal before 6 years of age (Figure 15-6). Forcible retraction of the foreskin may cause trauma, with increased risk for infection and/or scarring, leading to pathologic phimosis (see Table 15-4). Good hygiene of the penis and foreskin can decrease the risk of developing infection or adhesions of the

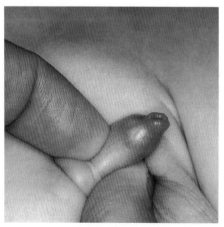

FIGURE 15-6 Physiological phimosis. (From Gearhart J, Rink R, Mouriquand P: *Pediatric urology*, ed 2, Philadelphia, 2010, Saunders.)

foreskin to the glans penis and should be reviewed regularly at well-child visits during childhood.

EVIDENCE-BASED PRACTICE TIP

Do not forcibly retract the foreskin. If indicated, treat with steroid ointment (betamethasone 0.05% or triamcinolone 0.1% ointment), applied 3 times/day to retracted foreskin for 4 to 6 weeks (see Figure 15-6). Surgical intervention is rarely indicated in physiological phimosis.[5,6]

EVIDENCE-BASED PRACTICE TIP

Care of the uncircumcised penis: Rinse penis and foreskin with water and soap during bathing. Always return foreskin over glans following retraction. For older boys, instruct the child to gently retract the foreskin during voiding. Refer parents to the American Academy of Pediatrics website (http://www.healthychildren.org/English/ages-stages/baby/bathing-skin-care/Pages/Caring-For-Your-Sons-Penis.aspx) for more information on caring for a child's penis.

In the newborn, the urethral meatus is normally on the tip of the glans penis. In middle childhood and adolescence, the urethral meatus is a slitlike opening on the ventral side of the glans penis. Examination in the adolescent male includes an inspection for erythema or discharge (Figure 15-7).

Inspection of the scrotum includes assessing the fullness of the scrotum, color, median raphe, and rugae, as well as determining SMR or Tanner stage. Before palpation of the scrotum in the infant and prepubertal male, the provider should place a hand firmly above the inguinal canal, near the superior anterior iliac crest, milk down the testis along the inguinal canal, and trap the testis in the scrotum with the thumb and index finger of the opposite hand to prevent retraction of the testes (Figure 15-8). The *cremasteric reflex* causes retraction of the testes into the inguinal

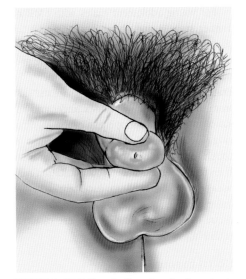

FIGURE 15-7 Examination of urethral meatus in adolescent.

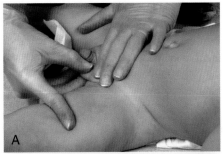

A

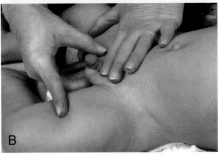

B

FIGURE 15-9 Palpation of scrotal sac.

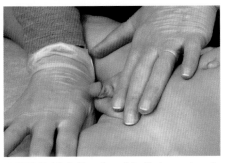

FIGURE 15-8 Trapping of testis in scrotum for examination.

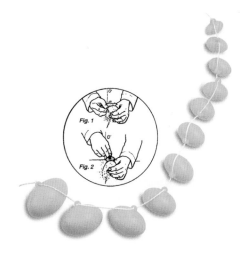

FIGURE 15-10 Orchidometer to evaluate testicular size. (Courtesy Accurate Surgical & Scientific Instruments Corp, Westbury, NY.)

canal/abdominal cavity and can be activated by cold, touch, or emotion, particularly in infancy and early childhood. *Retractile testis,* a testis that may retract on exam but be normally positioned in the scrotum, may confuse the findings of the exam, prompting unnecessary referral in a normal male child. Isolate the testis between the thumb and forefinger, and roll within the pads of the fingers to assess for testicular size, shape, consistency, and any point tenderness (Figure 15-9). Compare the testes bilaterally for any significant difference in size. An *orchidometer* may be used to screen testicular size in the growing and

developing male (Figure 15-10), although scrotal ultrasound is used as a more accurate measurement of testicular volume. If the testis is not palpable in the scrotum in the young child, often a positional change to sitting with legs crossed (tailor style) will facilitate relaxation of the cremasteric muscle and allow for the testes to descend to the scrotal sac (see Figure 15-5). Careful inspection and palpation of the inguinal, suprapubic, scrotal, and perineal region may reveal an *ectopic* testis.[7]

In the adolescent male, the examiner should palpate for the epididymis on the posterior surface. It can be felt on the lateral surface of the testes as smooth, discreet, and slightly irregular. The vas deferens can be palpated from the testes to the inguinal ring. Any testicular nodules should be referred for further evaluation to rule out malignancy. The adolescent male should be educated about testicular self-examination along with a return demonstration. Although there is a lack of evidence for routine screening with clinical examinations or testicular self-exams in reducing mortality from testicular cancer, "most testicular carcinomas are detected by patients themselves . . . unintentionally or through self-examination."[9]

For young adolescent males with SMR or Tanner stage 3 and above, another essential part of the genitourinary exam is the inguinal hernia exam. This is a routine part of the pre-participation sports physical assessment. To examine the inguinal ring, invaginate the skin from the scrotal sac with index finger and advance into the slitlike opening of the inguinal ring (Figure 15-11). Ask him to bear down or cough so any protrusion/masses may be noted. If an inguinal mass is noted, auscultation may occasionally be used to ascertain whether bowel sounds are present, although this technique has been replaced by the use of ultrasound in most instances.

Rectal Examination

Rectal examination in the infant and young child is indicated to assess tone, chronic constipation, rectal bleeding, fissures, hemorrhoids or other gastrointestinal concerns, and history of sexual abuse when indicated. The rectal examination is performed with the child supine with the legs flexed. Inspect the anal area for location of the anus, fissures, rectal tears, hemorrhoids, any lesions, or inflammation. A discoloration around the anus may indicate heavy metal toxins.

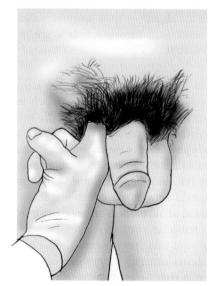

FIGURE 15-11 Examination for inguinal hernia.

Note any sacral sinus, tufts of hair, or dimpling on the buttock. Use the index finger, gloved and lubricated with a small amount of gel. Press the pad of the finger against the anus. The anal sphincter should relax and allow the small digit to slip into the anal canal. Digital exploration of the rectal vault requires a gentle approach. Test any stool obtained on exam for blood using office fecal occult blood testing materials. This is not performed routinely unless symptoms or history warrant the examination.

In the adolescent male, digital manipulation is performed with the adolescent positioned on his left side with knees flexed or standing with hips flexed and upper body supported with hands on the examining table. The index finger, gloved and lubricated, is used for the exam, as previously described. Rotate the finger and palpate the anterior rectal wall to feel the prostate gland, which in the adolescent and young adult male should be firm and smooth and measure about 2 to 3 cm (Figure 15-12). The rectal exam in the adolescent requires careful explanation of the purpose of the exam beforehand to avoid inflicting physical or psychological trauma.

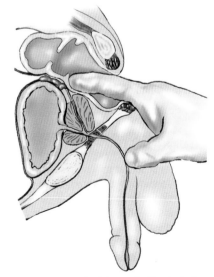

FIGURE 15-12 Rectal examination technique in adolescent.

CIRCUMCISION

Circumcision is the excision of the *foreskin*. In the newborn, the procedure is a matter of parental choice in consultation with the health care provider, taking into consideration the cultural, religious, and ethnic traditions along with medical factors. The American Academy of Pediatrics (AAP) formed a multidisciplinary task force that reviewed the recent data and concluded that the health benefits of newborn circumcision "outweigh the risks of the procedure," and thus families should have *access* to circumcision should they choose to have it done.[10] Benefits of circumcision may include decrease in risk of urinary tract infections, which is most beneficial in high-risk males, as well as potential decrease in risk of transmission of some sexually transmitted infections, including HIV, and development of penile carcinoma.[7,10-12] However, with proper hygiene and care of foreskin, some uncircumcised males can also decrease their risk to that equivalent to their circumcised male counterparts; therefore, evidence is lacking for recommendation of routine newborn circumcision.[7,10-12] Parents should be given accurate and unbiased information and be provided opportunity to discuss and make decisions. Newborns who are circumcised require procedural analgesia for pain control, and the risks of analgesia should be reviewed with parents.

SEXUAL ABUSE

A complete physical examination, including thorough evaluation of the genitourinary system, is warranted with any indication or revelation of sexual misconduct on history taken either from parent or child or adolescent. Although in 95% of sexual assault cases there is no apparent visible physical evidence, children and adolescents who are known or suspected victims of sexual assault require careful evaluation for any evidence that may be present.[13] The history must be obtained in a safe and private environment, while using open-ended and nonleading, developmentally appropriate questions. Examination of the oral cavity as well as the genitals and anus requires careful inspection. Penis and scrotum should be evaluated for bruising or signs of external trauma, redness, swelling, or discharge. The anus and rectum should be inspected for hemorrhoids, warts, rectal dilatation, rectal fissures, or fistulas that would indicate trauma incurred as a result of intercourse. A digital exam should be performed with a gloved, lubricated finger to evaluate the sphincter tone and the rectal vault. A complete explanation of findings to the child or adolescent and family, referral to Child Protective Services (CPS), consultation with child abuse experts, referral to additional resources, and follow-up are indicated.

DISORDER OF SEXUAL DIFFERENTIATION

The first step in diagnosing the infant or child with disorder of sexual differentiation (DSD), including those with disorder of chromosomal sex, disorders of gonadal sex, or disorder of phenotypic sex including ambiguous genitalia, starts with obtaining a detailed history. Family history of previous spontaneous abortion, stillbirth, or any neonatal death of a male sibling that could be related should be noted; family history of excess androgen and congenital adrenal hyperplasia or an autosomal recessive genotype should also be carefully reviewed. Then a careful inspection of any dysmorphic features and examination of the abdominal and genital area is performed.[7] The key finding of the genital exam is the presence or absence of gonadal or testicular tissue palpable in the scrotum, labioscrotal folds, or inguinal canal[7,14] (Figure 15-13). Palpable gonads lead to the high probability that the infant is an XY male because ovaries do not descend.[7] Document size of penis, location of meatus, and any hyperpigmentation of the labioscrotal folds.

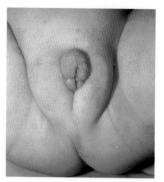

FIGURE 15-13 Ambiguous genitalia. (From Zitelli BJ, Davis, HW: *Atlas of pediatric physical diagnosis,* ed 4, St. Louis, 2002, Mosby.)

Research continues to define new and multigenetic factors involved in the development of DSD, but there is still insufficient information to develop practice guidelines.[15] Acute conditions warrant immediate management. Genetic karotyping and additional laboratory tests are required to make a sex determination, and immediate referral to a multidisciplinary team, including neonatologist, pediatrician/pediatric nurse practitioner, pediatric endocrinologist, pediatric urologist, geneticist, psychologist, social worker, and ethicist, is indicated.[16]

MALE GENITAL CONDITIONS

Table 15-3 summarizes findings that require a referral to a pediatric urologist, and Table 15-4 presents abnormal conditions of the male genitalia in the infant, child, and adolescent.

EVIDENCE-BASED PRACTICE TIP

Acute onset of scrotal pain is presumed to be testicular torsion until proven otherwise and is a true urological emergency. Ischemia longer than 8 hours will attribute to testicular atrophy; thus, the best course of action is to restore testicular blood flow through manual detorsion (temporary relief) or surgical exploration.[17]

TABLE 15-3 ABNORMAL FINDINGS OF MALE GENITALIA

Area	Abnormal Findings and Referral Criteria
Penis	Abnormal position of urethral meatus, ventral or dorsal to tip of penis Abnormal curvature of penis Micropenis: associated with syndromes and organ abnormalities Abnormal discharge, erythema (redness), swelling Thickened/scarred foreskin Foreskin unable to be retracted (>6 years of age) Foreskin unable to return to cover glans (see paraphimosis) **(urological emergency)**
Scrotum	Painful or red/swollen testicle/scrotum **(urological emergency)** Undescended or absent testes Communicative hydrocele (changes in size) Hydroceles that prevents assessment of testes (via manual exam or transillumination) Hernia Onset of puberty before 8 years of age Delayed or absent pubertal development Presence of skin lesions, vesicles, chancre, or lice
Inguinal region	Inguinal mass or hernia Tender lymph nodes
Anus/rectum	Abnormal distance from scrotum to anus Abnormal rectal patency Rectal polyps, hemorrhoids (adolescents)

TABLE 15-4 MALE GENITAL CONDITIONS

Condition	Image	Description
Adhesions (penile)	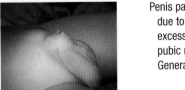	Remnants of fused layer between glans and prepuce. May have smegma trapped underneath. Resolves by adolescent years.
Balanoposthitis/ balanitis		Superficial infection of the penis/foreskin. Redness, swelling, and extreme tenderness of prepuce and glans penis; yellowish discharge may be present. Reoccurrences may cause scarring and/or pathological phimosis.
Buried penis		Penis partially concealed beneath the scrotum due to post-circumcision healing, or due to excessive skin or an excessive fat pad in pubic region. May lead to urinary obstruction. Generally the penile size is normal.

Continued

TABLE 15-4   MALE GENITAL CONDITIONS—CONT'D

Condition	Image	Description
Chordee		Ventral (downward) curvature of penis due to fibrotic tissue; occurs as an isolated condition or often with hypospadias.
Epididymitis	Inflammation of the epididymis	Inflammation and swelling of epididymis from infection or trauma, often preceded by urethritis, generally associated with sexual activity; accompanied by gradual pain in scrotum, inguinal area, or abdomen; generally occurs unilaterally. Exam shows point tenderness on epididymis, (+) cremasteric reflex, and (+) Prehn sign (pain relief with elevation of scrotum).
Epispadias		Abnormal placement of the urethral meatus on dorsal surface of penis.
Hernia		Inguinal mass or protrusion of tissue or bowel through muscle wall due to patent processus vaginalis, and intensifies with straining or crying. The mass may be firm and reducible with gentle pressure, or hard and immobile, which requires immediate referral because of the potential for *incarcerated hernia*.
Hydrocele	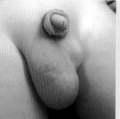	Enlargement of the scrotum due to peritoneal fluid between parietal and visceral layers of tunica vaginalis, which surrounds testis. Scrotum may be taut or firm but nontender on palpation. Transillumination will be clear and may reveal testes in the scrotal sac. *Noncommunicating:* no connection to the perineum; fluid is nonreducible. Resolves spontaneously. *Communicating:* patent processus vaginalis (similar to hernia) and thus fluid is reducible with gentle pressure. Refer to pediatric urology.

TABLE 15-4   MALE GENITAL CONDITIONS—CONT'D

Condition	Image	Description
Hypospadias	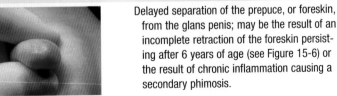	Congenital defect in incomplete development of anterior urethra, corpora cavernosa, and foreskin, which results in abnormal placement of the urethral meatus on the ventral surface of the penis; meatus may be on glans, penile shaft, or penoscrotal junction/perineum. Generally lack of foreskin on ventral side, and excessive foreskin on dorsal side of glans penis.
Meatal stenosis		Recurrent inflammation of meatus from prolonged exposure to moist environment; prolonged urethral catheterization or trauma. May also result from friction with diaper or underwear.
Paraphimosis		***Urological emergency!*** Foreskin trapped behind glans penis due to prolonged retraction and swelling/edema from restricted blood flow. Medical therapy requires manual compression around the shaft of the penis to reduce swelling followed by reduction of the foreskin by manual downward pressure of the foreskin over the glans penis. May require surgical intervention/circumcision.
Penile torsion		Congenital condition with counterclockwise rotation of the penile shaft, involving glans penis with or without corporal bodies. Often associated with other penile abnormalities (penile chordee or hypospadias).
Phimosis		Delayed separation of the prepuce, or foreskin, from the glans penis; may be the result of an incomplete retraction of the foreskin persisting after 6 years of age (see Figure 15-6) or the result of chronic inflammation causing a secondary phimosis.

Continued

TABLE 15-4   MALE GENITAL CONDITIONS—CONT'D

Condition	Image	Description
Testicular torsion	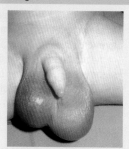	*Urological emergency!* Twisting of testicle on its spermatic cord; causes **sudden onset of unilateral scrotal/testicular pain,** swelling and tenderness of the scrotal sac, venous obstruction, edema, and organ compromise, which leads to **testicular infarction.** Exam shows (−) cremasteric reflex and (−) *Prehn sign* (pain relief with elevation of the scrotum). Testicular lie is horizontal. Occurs in 12- to 18-year-olds; peak at 15 to 16 years. May occur in the newborn period and present as an ecchymotic, nontender testis caused by necrosis of the testis in utero. Immediate referral to pediatric urology is indicated.
Testicular tumor	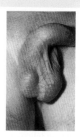	Exam shows firm, circumscribed, painless area of induration within the testis; (−) transillumination. Generally malignant with germ cell origin. The incidence of testicular cancer is quite low (2.3 to 10 in 100,000) but most common in young males 15 to 35 years of age, and 4.5 times more common in whites than in African-Americans.[4] The risk of testicular tumor is 10 to 40 times more in teens with history of cryptorchidism.
Undescended testis/ cryptorchidism	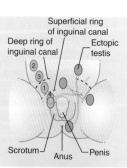	Testis is palpable but cannot be milked into the scrotal sac; may be found along the normal descending pathway, along inguinal ring, or be *retractile* (normal), or *ectopic;* referral for evaluation by 9 months of age (see Table 15-3). *Impalpable testis* is generally found intraabdominally. Bilateral *impalpable testes* in a term male raises concerns about disorder of sexual differentiation/virilizing adrenal hyperplasia.
Varicocele	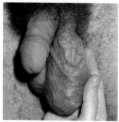	Dilation of internal spermatic vein at venous plexus within spermatic cord; presents as soft mass on spermatic cord ("bag of worms") with or without associated pain; most common on left side and more prominent with straining/standing.

In the undescended testis/cryptorchidism image labels: Superficial ring of inguinal canal, Deep ring of inguinal canal, Ectopic testis, Scrotum, Anus, Penis

TABLE 15-4   MALE GENITAL CONDITIONS—CONT'D

Condition	Image	Description
Webbed penis	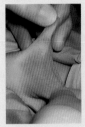	Congenital condition involving a web of skin obscuring the penoscrotal angle in an otherwise normal sized penis. The penis may be concealed by a pubic fat pad or scrotum, or trapped due to phimosis.

Adhesion image is from Ponsky LE, Ross JH, Knipper N, et al: Penile adhesions after neonatal circumcision, *J Urol* 164(2): 495-496.

Balanitis image is from Godbole P: General paediatric urology, *Surgery (Oxford)* 26(5):223-227, 2008.

Buried penis image is from Chin T, Tsai H, Liu C, et al: Modifications of preputial unfurling to reduce postoperative edema in buried penis, *J Pediatr Urol* 1(5):327-329, 2005.

Chordee, hydrocele, and testicular torsion images are from Kliegman R, Stanton B, St. Geme J, et al: *Nelson textbook of pediatrics,* ed 19, Philadelphia, 2012, Saunders.

Epididymitis image is from Zitelli B, Davis H: *Atlas of pediatric physical diagnosis,* ed 5, Philadelphia, 2008, Mosby.

Epispadias image is from Frimberger D: Diagnosis and management of epispadias, *Semin Pediatr Surg* 20(2):85-90, 2011.

Hernia image is from Taeusch HW, Ballard R, Gleason C: *Avery's diseases of the newborn,* ed 8, Philadelphia, 2005, Saunders.

Hypospadias, meatal stenosis, and webbed penis images are from Gearhart J, Rink R, Mouriquand P: *Pediatric urology,* ed 2, Philadelphia, 2010, Saunders.

Paraphimosis image is from Johnson P: Childhood circumcision, *Surgery (Oxford)* 23(9):338-340, 2005.

Penile torsion image is from Wein A, Kavoussi L, Novick A, et al: *Campbell-Walsh urology,* ed 9, Philadelphia, 2007, Saunders.

Phimosis image is from Patel ST, Woodward MN, Williams M, et al: Graft-versus-host disease and phimosis, *J Pediatr Urol* 4(2):165-166, 2008.

Testicular tumor image is from Wolfe J: *400 Self-assessment picture tests in clinical medicine,* 1984. By permission of Mosby International.

Undescended testes image is from de Bruyn R: *Pediatric ultrasound: how, why, and when,* ed 2, Philadelphia, 2011, Churchill Livingstone.

Variocele image is from Swartz MH: *Textbook of physical diagnosis,* ed 5, Philadelphia, 2006, Saunders.

SUMMARY OF EXAMINATION

- Routine examination of the genitourinary system is expected at all routine well visits. It is an opportunity to discuss age-appropriate normal growth and development, provide anticipatory guidance, and identify any abnormality or pathology early in development. Be familiar with the wide variations of "normal."

- Be mindful and respectful of cultural variations in discussion of the genitourinary development and examination. Ask permission to discuss and examine.

- Prepare the child/adolescent by discussing what the exam will entail, and provide proper draping as appropriate; be mindful of exposing child/adolescent longer than necessary. Talk through the exam and provide reassurance of normal development.

- Adolescents will be given the opportunity to have the exam performed without parents in the room, and informed consent/confidentiality policy will be discussed.

- Obtain a thorough history including gestational history, birth history, family history, and voiding/elimination history (see Information Gathering table).

- Assess penis and note foreskin status, penile size, curvature, and meatal location.

- Physiological phimosis is expected until about 6 years of age. Avoid forceful retraction of foreskin. Discuss care of the uncircumcised penis with the family. Refer to pediatric urology if pathological phimosis is unresponsive to steroid ointment trial.
- Assess scrotum and testes. Determine if palpable testes are descended, retractile, undescended, or ectopic. Assess testicular size, shape, and consistency and note the presence of any masses or pain. Refer to pediatric urology if testes are undescended by 9 months of age or impalpable at any age.
- Perform a detailed scrotal and testicular examination for any scrotal mass or pain.
- Evaluate rectum, anus, and lumbar sacral region for dimples or tufts of hair.
- Report and follow up on any suspicion of sexual abuse from history or physical exam.

Charting
Term Infant at 1 Month of Age

External genitalia: nl uncircumcised male, foreskin partially retractable revealing meatus at tip of penis, ∅ discharge noted, nl urinary stream, testes ↓↓×2 of nl size/shape/consistency, ∅ hernia/hydrocele, back nl w/o pits/dimples, rectal sphincter nl.

nl, Normal; ↓↓, descended bilaterally.

Charting
Healthy 12-Year-Old Male

External genitalia: nl Tanner stage 2 circumcised male, urethral meatus at tip, ∅ discharge noted, normal scrotum with testes ↓↓×2 of nl size/shape/consistency, ∅ masses palpated, (−) inguinal hernia exam, back nl w/o pits/dimples, rectal sphincter nl.

nl, Normal; ↓↓, descended bilaterally.

REFERENCES

1. Porth CM, Matfin G: *Pathophysiology: concepts of altered health status,* ed 8, Philadelphia, 2010, Lippincott.
2. McGregor TB, Pike JG, Leonard MP: Pathologic and physiologic phimosis: approach to the phimotic foreskin, *Can Fam Physician* 53(3):445-448, 2007.
3. Hornor G: Genitourinary assessment: an integral part of a complete physical examination, *J Pediatr Health Care* 21(3):162-170, 2007.
4. Neinstein LS, Gordon CM, Katzman DK, et al: *Handbook of adolescent health care,* Philadelphia, 2008, Lippincott.
5. Palmer LS, Palmer JS: The efficacy of topical betamethasone for treating phimosis: a comparison of two treatment regimens, *Urology* 72(1):68-71, 2008.
6. Reddy S, Jain V, Dubey M, et al: Local steroid therapy as the first-line treatment for boys with symptomatic phimosis–a long-term prospective study, *Acta Paediatr* 101(3):e130–e133, 2012.
7. Baskin LS, Kogan BA: *Handbook of pediatric urology,* ed 2, Philadelphia, 2005, Lippincott.
8. Tasian GE, Yiee JH, Copp HL: Imaging use and cryptorchidism: determinants of practice patterns, *J Urol* 185(5):1882-1887, 2011.
9. Hagan JF, Shaw JS, Duncan PM: *Bright futures: guidelines for health supervision of infants, children, and adolescents,* ed 3, Elk Grove, IL, 2008, American Academy of Pediatrics.
10. AAP: Circumcision policy statement. American Academy of Pediatrics. Task Force on Circumcision, *Pediatrics* 130(3):585-586, 2012.
11. Singh-Grewal D, Macdessi J, Craig J: Circumcision for the prevention of urinary tract infection in boys: a systematic review of randomised trials and observational studies, *Arch Dis Child* 90(8):853-858, 2005.

12. Alanis MC, Lucidi RS: Neonatal circumcision: a review of the world's oldest and most controversial operation, *Obstet Gynecol Surv* 59(5):379-395, 2004.

13. Hornor G: Medical evaluation for child sexual abuse: what the PNP needs to know, *J Pediatric Health Care* 25(4):250-256; quiz 257-260, 2011.

14. Douglas G, Axelrad ME, Brandt ML, et al: Guidelines for evaluating and managing children born with disorders of sexual development, *Pediatr Ann* 41(4):e1-, 2012.

15. Houk CP, Lee PA: Update on disorders of sex development, *Curr Opin Endocrinol Diabetes Obes* 19(1):28-32, 2012.

16. Moran ME, Karkazis K: Developing a multidisciplinary team for disorders of sex development: planning, implementation, and operation tools for care providers, *Adv Urol* 2012. 604135, 2012.

17. Leslie JA, Cain MP: Pediatric urologic emergencies and urgencies, *Pediatr Clin North Am* 53(3): 513-527, 2006.

CHAPTER 16

MALE AND FEMALE BREAST

Erica Bisgyer Monasterio; Naomi A. Schapiro

M ale and female breast development is similar until puberty; therefore, the examination of both boys and girls will be reviewed in this chapter along with pubertal changes expected for both genders. The primary intention of the breast exam in children and adolescents is to recognize normal variants, monitor development, and to identify nonmalignant pathology. Making assessment of the breast part of the routine physical examination in preadolescents gives the parent or caregiver and child an opportunity to voice any concerns and fosters a dialogue about reproductive health. It is important to respect privacy in performing the examination of the breast in all children and adolescents. Current evidence and recommendations related to the efficacy of breast examination focus on the detection of breast cancer, which is an exceedingly rare diagnosis in adolescents; therefore, child and adolescent breast exam recommendations are based on expert practice rather than evidence.[1]

EMBRYOLOGICAL DEVELOPMENT

A mammary ridge forms from the ectodermal layer on day 20 of embryonic life and extends from the forelimb to the hind limb. In the sixth week of fetal life, the nipple and areola form over a bud of breast tissue that is composed of the primary mammary ducts and a loose fibrous tissue or stroma. Fifteen to twenty-five secondary buds then develop and bifurcate into tubules, forming the basis of the duct system.[2] Each duct, as it develops, opens separately into the nipple.

PHYSIOLOGICAL VARIATIONS

At birth, the breasts of both male and female infants may be swollen because of the maternal estrogen effect (Figure 16-1). An unusual but normal finding in the newborn is the secretion of a milklike substance, also known as "witch's milk," for 1 to 2 weeks[3] (Figure 16-2). Male and female breasts are similar until puberty, consisting of a small amount of breast tissue. Occasionally, a prepubertal male or female develops an enlargement of one or both breasts, which involves a soft, mobile, subareolar nodule of uniform consistency.[2] Generally, the nipple and areola are not developed or pigmented with such an enlargement, and no associated signs of puberty are present. This condition usually regresses spontaneously within weeks to months, and in the absence of other secondary sexual characteristics, a biopsy is not indicated.[2] If other signs of puberty appear, then these changes could be the first sign of *precocious puberty,* in which case referral and further diagnostic workup are indicated.

Supernumerary nipples may arise from the mammary ridge and be present at birth (Figure 16-3, *A*). They are often raised, generally require no treatment, and become imperceptible over time. There is a weak association between supernumerary nipples and renal and cardiovascular abnormalities in white newborns.[3] In females, supernumerary nipples will on rare occasion develop a small amount of breast tissue during puberty (see *polymastia* in Table 16-2; see Figure 16-3, *B*). The adolescent may elect to have cosmetic surgery for removal of the supernumerary breast tissue.

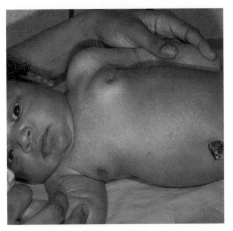

FIGURE 16-1 Estrogen effect in the newborn. (From Shah BR, Laude TA: *Atlas of pediatric clinical diagnosis,* Philadelphia, 2000, Saunders.)

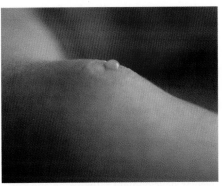

FIGURE 16-2 Witch's milk. (From Clark DA: *Atlas of neonatology,* ed 7, Philadelphia, 2000, Saunders.)

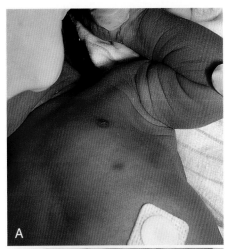

A

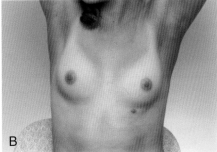

B

FIGURE 16-3 **A,** Supernumerary nipple. **B,** Supernumerary nipple located in the inframammary fold of the left breast of an adolescent female. (**A** from Eichenfield L, Frieden IJ, Zaenglein AL: *Neonatal dermatology,* ed 2, Philadelphia, 2009, Saunders; **B** from van Aalst JA, Sadove M: Treatment of pediatric breast problems, *Clin Plast Surg* 32(1):65-78, 2005.)

Widespread nipples are defined as a nipple spread of greater than 25% of the chest circumference and may be associated with congenital disorders such as Turner syndrome.[3]

Physiological Variations in the Male Breast

At puberty, the ductal and periductal mesenchymal breast tissue of boys proliferates under the influence of estrogens, with later involution as testicular androgens rise to adult levels.[2] Male estradiol levels triple during puberty, and

androgens ultimately increase 30 times. If peak estrogen levels occur before androgen levels, the result is *gynecomastia,* a benign increase in glandular and stromal breast tissue in pubertal males (Figure 16-4). Most circulating estrogens are produced outside of the testes, and an increase in fatty tissue, as in obesity, may lead to an increase in estrogen levels and a higher incidence of *gynecomastia* (Box 16-1).

At 14 years of age, 64% of adolescent males have some degree of gynecomastia, with only 4% of adolescent males having severe gynecomastia

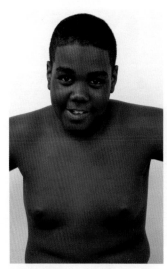

FIGURE 16-4 Gynecomastia.

BOX 16-1   CLASSIFICATIONS OF GYNECOMASTIA

- **Type I:** One or more subareolar nodules, freely movable
- **Type II:** Breast nodules beneath areola but also extending beyond the areolar perimeter
- **Type III:** Resembles female breast development stage 3 (see Table 16-1)

Data from Neinstein LS: *Adolescent health care: a practical guide,* ed 4, Philadelphia, 2002, Lippincott Williams & Wilkins.

---

that persists into adulthood.[2] Approximately 50% of males experience the onset of gynecomastia at Tanner stage 2 of male genital development, another 20% at Tanner stage 1, 20% at Tanner stage 3 of male genital development, and 10% beginning at Tanner stage 4 (see Chapter 15). In general, adolescent males can be reassured that most cases of *physiological gynecomastia* will resolve spontaneously within 6 months, although it can persist up to 2 years after attaining sexual maturity.[4] Treatment alternatives for persistent *gynecomastia,* including pharmacological and surgical options, may be appropriate to discuss with youth and families when this condition does not resolve or is particularly distressing.

Gynecomastia, although a normal variant, is also present in relation to hormone imbalances due to thyrotoxicosis, cirrhosis, adrenal and testicular neoplasm, primary hypogonadism, chromosome abnormalities such as Klinefelter syndrome, and severe malnutrition.[2] In addition, prescription drugs such as cimetidine, ketoconazole, metronidazole, isoniazid, digoxin, spironolactone, phenothiazines, and some illicit drugs (e.g., marijuana, anabolic steroids, amphetamines, and opiates) can cause gynecomastia.[4]

Physiological Variations in the Female Breast

Thelarche, or the beginning of female breast development, is usually the first sign of puberty in girls and occurs between 8 and 13 years of age, on average at the age of 11.2 years[1] (Table 16-1 and Figure 16-5). Full breast development at Tanner stage 5 signals the end of puberty in females. Breast development during puberty involves both multiple hormones and the binding of hormones to breast tissue. Estrogen, especially estradiol, influences ductal development, whereas progesterone influences additional lobular alveolar development.[2] Thyroxine and corticosteroids are also involved.

Breast development, an initial sign of secondary sexual development in girls, is readily apparent to family members and peers, often eliciting unwanted comments as to presence or absence and size of breast tissue. Breast development is a common issue for teasing, bullying, and sexual harassment in middle school. The health care provider should be mindful that sexual harassment is a major issue for teens, often jeopardizing a teen's mental health and school performance. If the preteen or young adolescent seems particularly concerned or uncomfortable with the health history about breast development or the breast examination, gentle exploration of the issue by

TABLE 16-1 FEMALE BREAST DEVELOPMENT SEXUAL MATURITY RATING

Tanner Stage/Sexual Maturity Rating (SMR)	Breast Findings	Areola and Nipple Findings
Tanner stage 1	Prepubertal; no glandular tissue	Conforms to general chest line
Tanner stage 2	Breast bud; small amount of glandular tissue	Areola widens
Tanner stage 3	Larger and more elevation; extends beyond areolar parameter	Areola continues to enlarge but remains in contour with breast
Tanner stage 4	Larger and more elevation	Areola and papilla form a mound projecting from breast contour (half of teens; in some cases persists into adulthood)
Tanner stage 5	Adult size (variable)	Areola part of breast contour, nipple projecting above areola

Data from Neinstein LS: *Adolescent health care: a practical guide,* ed 5, Philadelphia, 2008, Lippincott Williams & Wilkins.

the provider, including queries as to teasing or bullying, or unwanted attention from family members, should be explored.

Premature thelarche is defined as breast development without other signs of puberty, and it commonly occurs in girls younger than 2 years of age. The breast buds of premature thelarche are 2 to 4 cm with little or no change in the areola or nipple. The serum estradiol may be slightly elevated in some infants and children with premature thelarche. In most girls, breast development regresses by 2 years

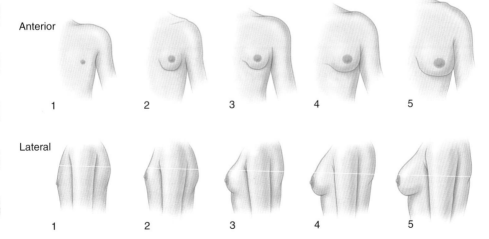

FIGURE 16-5 Normal female breast development, from Tanner stage 1 (prepubertal) to Tanner stage 5 (adult breast). (From Herring J: *Tachdjian's pediatric orthopaedics,* ed 4, Philadelphia, 2008, Saunders.)

of age without other signs of precocious puberty.[5] (See Chapter 5 for a discussion on endocrine-disrupting chemicals.)

ANATOMY AND PHYSIOLOGY

Mature female breast tissue at Tanner stage 5 extends from the second or third rib to the sixth or seventh rib, and from the sternal margin to the midaxillary area with the nipple located centrally, surrounded by the areola. The breast is composed of glandular and fibrous tissue and subcutaneous and retromammary fat (Figure 16-6). Fifteen to twenty lobes radiate around the nipple, and each lobe is divided into 20 to 40 lobules of milk-producing acini cells that empty into lactiferous ducts.[2] These cells are small and inconspicuous in the nonpregnant, nonlactating woman. A layer of subcutaneous fibrous tissue provides support for the breast, as do the suspensory ligaments. The muscles forming the floor of the breast are pectoralis major, pectoralis minor, serratus anterior, latissimus dorsi, subscapularis, external oblique, and rectus abdominis. Vascular supply comes from the internal mammary artery and the lateral thoracic artery. The lymph system drains to the anterior axillary, subscapular, and supraclavicular nodes.

FAMILY, CULTURAL, RACIAL, AND ETHNIC CONSIDERATIONS

African-American girls begin puberty about 1 to 1.5 years earlier than white girls and begin menstrual periods 8.5 months earlier.[6] Breast development occurs at an average age of 9.5 years in African-American girls and at an average of 10.3 years of age in white girls.[7]

SYSTEM-SPECIFIC HISTORY

The Information Gathering table reviews the important information to be gathered for male and female breast assessment at key developmental stages, and for adolescent females presenting with breast symptoms or concerns.

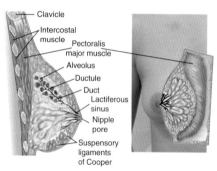

Clavicle
Intercostal muscle
Pectoralis major muscle
Alveolus
Ductule
Duct
Lactiferous sinus
Nipple pore
Suspensory ligaments of Cooper

FIGURE 16-6 Anatomy of the breast.

INFORMATION GATHERING FOR MALE AND FEMALE BREAST ASSESSMENT AT KEY DEVELOPMENTAL STAGES

Age-Group	Questions to Ask
Preadolescent girls and boys	Breast tenderness or breast buds noted? At what age did breast development begin? Any pain in breast? Other signs of puberty noted? Axillary or pubic hair? Concern about breast development?
Female adolescents	Any concerns about breast health or breast development? Last menstrual period? Contraceptive use? Breast tenderness or pain noted? Relationship of breast discomfort or pain to menstrual cycle? Previous pregnancy? Any discharge from nipple? Any lump noted in breast or axilla? Redness or irritation on skin?

PHYSICAL ASSESSMENT

Inspection and Palpation

Prepubertal Breast

Prepubertal breasts are easily inspected and palpated while examining the chest to assess cardiovascular and respiratory status. The health care provider should note any masses or pain, nipple discharge, or signs of premature thelarche, or breast development.

Adolescent Male

Pubertal breasts are inspected with the male adolescent supine with his hands behind his head. Place the pads of the three middle fingers at the margins of the breast. Palpate the breast bilaterally for the presence of adipose tissue or breast buds if evaluating for gynecomastia. Note any nodular tissue or firm rubbery masses. In conditions such as a *lipoma* or *dermoid cyst,* the mass is usually noted to one side of the areola.

Adolescent Female

There is controversy about the age at which health care providers should perform routine breast exams in women. The American Cancer Society (ACS) and the American Congress of Obstetricians and Gynecologists (ACOG) recommend including clinical breast examination (CBE) as part of a routine physical exam every 1 to 3 years for women age 20 to 39 years and annually after age 40 years.[8] The U.S. Preventive Services Task Force recommends CBE starting at age 40 years and paired with mammography.[8] Though malignancies in adolescents are rare, routine examination in early to middle female adolescents provides an opportunity for reassurance and education about normal breast findings and variations of normal. For teens whose close female relatives (mother, maternal aunts) have had premenopausal breast cancer, the breast examination can be an important forum for discussing breast cancer risk and protective factors.

Breast Examination

In a full young adult breast exam, the breasts are initially inspected with the patient sitting, disrobed to the waist, in the following positions: arms extended overhead, hands pressed against hips or against each other, and leaning forward from the waist (Figure 16-7, *A, B*). These three positions are most helpful if examining for a lump or mass.[2] The provider will have to weigh the benefits of full breast inspection in young adult women who are at low risk for breast cancer against the aversion most teens or young adults have to being undressed in front of a provider.

Although the breasts can be palpated with the adolescent sitting and supine, the preferred position for the adolescent is supine, with one arm under her head. With the adolescent supine, the breasts are in a more stable position, and touching of the breast with the nondominant hand of the examiner can be minimized.[2] For purposes of examination, the

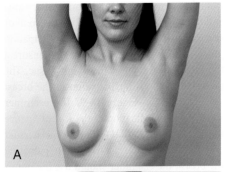
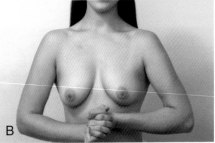

FIGURE 16-7 Inspection of the breast. **A,** Arms extended overhead. **B,** Hands pressed together.

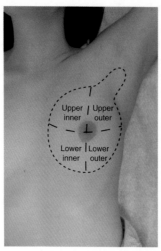

FIGURE 16-8 Quadrants of the left breast, tail of Spence.

breast is divided into four quadrants and a tail that extends into the axilla (Figure 16-8).

The breasts should be palpated with the pads (not tips) of the middle three fingers with the fingers palpating over the breast tissue from the sternal margin to the midaxillary area and from the second or third rib to the sixth or seventh rib at the base of the breast. Palpation proceeds stepwise with the fingers to ensure a thorough assessment of the breast tissue. The preferred methods for palpation of the breast are illustrated in Figure 16-9. The examiner should include palpation of the *tail of Spence* in the axilla in addition to the supraclavicular and infraclavicular regions. When palpating the breast, the examiner should use the domi-nant hand and stabilize the breast, if necessary, with the nondominant hand. Place the pads of the middle fingers at the margins of the breast to begin palpation, and note any masses, pain, nipple discharge, or signs of premature breast development. If firm rubbery tissue or a nodu-lar mass is noted, fine palpation is required for accurate sizing and to distinguish among fatty tissue, cysts, and other nodular masses.

It is important to incorporate patient edu-cation into the breast examination for the young female adult. During the examination, ask permission to guide the adolescent's hand onto her breast, pointing out landmarks and normal findings in the developing breast such as the thicker ridge of breast tissue often found in the inferior aspect of the breast and the nodularity of normal adolescent breast tissue especially in the upper outer quadrant. Also, have the adolescent feel the ribs underneath the medial border of the breast, as this normal finding is often mistaken by adolescents for a breast lump.

PEDIATRIC PEARLS

Asymmetrical breasts are common in early de-velopment in adolescent females.

Breast Self-Exam

Teaching *breast self-exam* (BSE) has become an issue of controversy in the clinical literature. BSE may assist the adolescent in accepting her

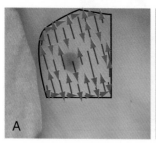
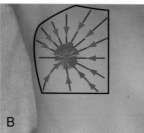
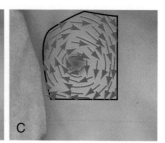

FIGURE 16-9 Methods of breast palpation. **A,** Palpation strip method. **B,** Palpation wedge method. **C,** Palpation circle method.

body, increase comfort with the breast examination, and provide an opportunity to reinforce or correct information the adolescent may have received from health classes, teen magazines, or female relatives about breast health. However, the U.S. Preventive Services Task Force (USPSTF) recommends *against* teaching BSE for adolescents or women of any age.[8] The American Cancer Society's recommendations for detection of early breast cancer include BSE as an option for women starting in their 20s, advising clinicians to inform women of the benefits and risks of BSE. Both the ACS and ACOG recommend teaching *breast self-awareness* to women age 20 years and older. This includes assisting women to become familiar with their breasts' normal feel and appearance, focusing on the importance of self-detection and early assessment of symptoms.[9]

BREAST CONDITIONS

The following are variations of normal that occur with stages of breast development:

- **Physiological swelling and tenderness:** Breast lobules undergo proliferative changes due to the normal menstrual cycle leading to pain and discomfort, swelling, and distinct masses that recede after menses.
- **Asymmetry:** In most women, one breast is slightly larger than the other, and this difference may be accentuated by asymmetrical breast development during puberty, which usually corrects by adulthood.
- **Proliferative breast changes:** Formerly called *fibrocystic disease,* many authorities now consider increased nodularity to be a variation of normal, occurring in more than 50% of women of reproductive age. Adolescents often have painless lumps, which may become tender 1 week before menses. Areas of nodularity may be a few millimeters to 1 cm in diameter.
- **Cysts:** Usually associated with few symptoms, cysts are well-circumscribed, small, and freely movable masses, commonly under 1 cm in adolescents.
- **Montgomery tubercles:** These tubercles arise from sebaceous glands associated with a lactiferous duct. They present as small, soft papules around the areola, with occasional thin, clear to brown discharge, and possibly a small lump under the areola. The condition usually resolves without intervention.

Breast cancer in adolescents is extremely rare. Malignant lesions comprise only 0.9% of all surgically excised lesions in the adolescent and young adult age group. Breast variations and benign tumors are presented in Table 16-2.

TABLE 16-2 CONDITIONS OF THE MALE AND FEMALE BREAST	
Condition	**Description**
Polymastia	Breast tissue that develops around supernumerary nipples; although clinically insignificant, this tissue may become uncomfortably engorged postpartum
Fibroadenoma	Most common benign breast tumor excised during adolescence; firm, rubbery, mobile, nontender; ranges in size from <1 cm to 10 cm; usually discovered by the adolescent
Amastia	Absence of breast tissue. *Athelia,* absence of nipple; often connected to a chest wall defect or more extensive congenital anomalies
Breast atrophy	Most commonly caused by significant loss of fat and glandular tissue as a result of eating disorders, but also may occur in premature ovarian failure, androgen excess (tumors or ingested steroids), and chronic diseases that lead to significant weight loss

Continued

TABLE 16-2 Conditions of the Male and Female Breast—cont'd

Condition	Description
Macromastia	Exceptionally large breasts (Figure 16-10); definition of "normal" breast size is difficult to determine, but this condition is associated with obesity and a strong familial incidence; 80% of cases begin in adolescence with teens complaining of psychological effects as compared to the more common complaints of breast, shoulder, and back pain among adults
Virginal or juvenile hypertrophy	May be an abnormal response of the breast to normal estrogen levels; occurs perimenarchally; breasts may enlarge to as much as 30 to 50 lb
Nipple discharge	• Multicolored or sticky discharge may be caused by duct ectasia • Serous or serosanguineous discharge may be caused by intraductal papilloma, benign changes, duct ectasia, or rarely cancer • Milky discharge (galactorrhea) may be the result of hormonal imbalance, pregnancy, or past abortion; medications or illicit drugs such as marijuana; pituitary tumors; or it may result from stimulation by sexual partners • Purulent discharge due to mastitis • Watery discharge due to papilloma or cancer

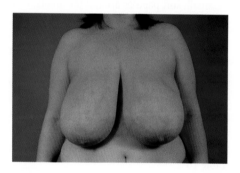

FIGURE 16-10 Profound macromastia. (From Hammond D: *Atlas of aesthetic breast surgery*, London, 2009, Saunders.)

SUMMARY OF EXAMINATION

• Prepubertal breast examination in both male and female children is focused on the identification of normal variants and nonmalignant pathology and monitoring development.

• Focus on the developing breast may be embarrassing and uncomfortable for pubertal children and early adolescents.

• Pubertal gynecomastia is common in approximately 50% of developing male adolescents and may be a source of concern for youths and families.

• Thelarche is the first sign of puberty in developing female adolescents.

• Breast development is often a common issue for teasing, bullying, and sexual harassment in middle school.

• There is insufficient evidence to formulate recommendations for BSE and CBE in adolescents and young adults.

• Young adult females may benefit from patient teaching on breast self-awareness, which includes the normal feel and appearance of the breasts, focusing on the importance of self-detection, and early assessment of symptoms.

Charting

9-Year-Old Female

Chest: Symmetrical, lungs clear to auscultation bilaterally, breast bud noted under R areola, warm and tender to touch, nonerythematous, L breast nl without swelling or tenderness.

Charting

14-Year-Old Male

Chest: Symmetrical, lungs clear to auscultation bilaterally, breast buds noted under L and R areola, warm and tender on palpation.

REFERENCES

1. DiVasta AD, Weldon C, Labow BI: The breast: examination and lesions. In Emans SJ and Laufer, MR, editors: *Pediatric and adolescent gynecology,* ed 6, Philadelphia, 2012, Lippincott Williams & Wilkins
2. Neinstein LS: Breast. In Neinstein LS, editor: *Adolescent health care: a practical guide,* ed 5, Philadelphia, 2008, Lippincott Williams & Wilkins.
3. Thureen PJ, Hall D, Deacon J, et al: *Assessment and care of the well newborn,* ed 2, Philadelphia, 2005, Saunders.
4. Braunstein GD: Clinical practice. Gynecomastia, *N Engl J Med* 357(12):1229-1237, 2007.
5. Mansfield MJ: Precocious puberty. In Emans SJ and Laufer, MR, editors: *Pediatric and adolescent gynecology,* ed 6, Philadelphia, 2012, Lippincott Williams & Wilkins.
6. Slyper AH: The pubertal timing controversy in the USA, and a review of possible causative factors for the advance in timing of onset of puberty, *Clin Endocrinol (Oxf)* 65(1):1-8, 2006.
7. Butts SF, Seifer DB: Racial and ethnic differences in reproductive potential across the life cycle, *Fertil Steril* 93(3):681-690, 2010.
8. U.S. Preventive Services Task Force: Screening for breast cancer: U.S. Preventive Services Task Force recommendation statement, *Ann Intern Med* 151:716–726 W-236, 2009.
9. Hauk L: American College of Obstetricians and Gynecologists updates breast cancer screening guidelines, *Am Fam Physician* 85(6):654-655, 2012.

CHAPTER 17

FEMALE GENITALIA

Erica Bisgyer Monasterio; Naomi A. Schapiro

The female genital examination is a recommended yet an under-performed part of the routine physical for pediatric and adolescent girls. Routine performance of the female genital exam allows the health care provider to build skills and familiarity with normal variants in the genitourinary system, and establish a baseline from which to monitor individual development and provide information and reassurance to children, youth, and parents or caregivers. Many health care providers, however, are underprepared to recognize normal genital findings in the prepubescent girl and are unfamiliar with common variations.[1]

With knowledge of normal development of the female reproductive anatomy, the health care provider can incorporate the routine examination of the genitalia into well-child care. The review of systems and genital exam offer an opportunity to foster a dialogue between parent and child concerning reproductive health. For religious and cultural reasons or personal preference, parents, children, and adolescents may be more likely to request female providers for the breast and female genital exam. In nonemergent situations, it is important to honor this request, either within the practice setting or by referral, and to respect privacy and confidentiality in performing the examination and discussing findings.

EMBRYOLOGICAL DEVELOPMENT

At 5 to 6 weeks of gestation, fetal gonads are bipotential, capable of differentiating into either a testis or an ovary. Both male and female embryos have one pair of primary sex organs, or gonads, and two pairs of ducts, *wolffian* ducts and *müllerian* ducts. During the sixth week, the primordial germ cells migrate into the primary sex cords and begin to differentiate. Leydig and Sertoli cells appear in male embryos, producing testosterone and antimüllerian hormone. In female embryos, the gonads do not produce testosterone, and the gonads develop into ovaries. The wolffian ducts deteriorate, and the müllerian ducts develop into the uterus, upper vaginal tract, and fallopian tubes. The external genitalia differentiate at between 8 and 12 weeks of gestation (Figure 17-1). Active mitosis continues and thousands of germ cells, *oocytes,* are produced. A newborn female may have 2 million primary oocytes at birth. However, after birth, no further oogonia occurs.

DEVELOPMENTAL AND PHYSIOLOGICAL VARIATIONS

In preterm neonates, the *labia majora* may not cover the *labia minora,* and the *clitoris* will be prominent. Term newborns will have enlarged labia majora, which usually cover other external structures, a relatively large clitoris, and labia minora with dull pink epithelium, because of maternal estrogen effects (Figure 17-2). A creamy white or slightly blood-tinged discharge is normal for up to 10 days after birth. The *hymen* is relatively thicker, pink-white, and redundant and may remain so up until 2 to 4 years of age (Figure 17-3).

Disorders of sexual differentiation (DSD) have their genesis in early fetal development and result from developmental variations in one or more of the three components of sex

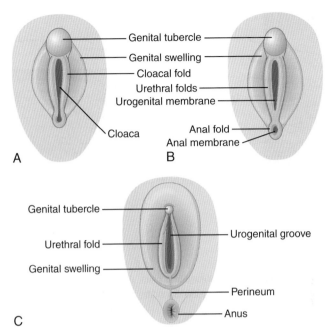

FIGURE 17-1 Development of the external genitalia. **A,** Early development before completion of the urorectal septum. **B,** Separation of the anus from the urogenital sinus lined by the urethral folds. **C,** Development of the genital swelling. (From Crum C, Nucci M, Lee K: *Diagnostic gynecologic and obstetric pathology,* ed 2, Philadelphia, 2012, Saunders.)

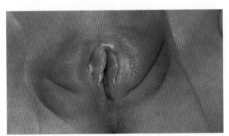

FIGURE 17-2 Newborn with estrogen effect. (From Zitelli BJ, Davis HW: *Atlas of pediatric physical diagnosis,* ed 4, St. Louis, 2002, Mosby. Courtesy Ian Holzman, MD, Mt. Sinai Medical Center, New York, NY.)

determination and differentiation: chromosomal sex, gonadal sex, and/or phenotypic sex. Manifestations of some types of DSD are evident at birth in the newborn with ambiguous genitalia[2]; other types may only become evident in early adolescence with variations in secondary sexual development (see Chapter 15 for further discussion).

In the absence of congenital anomalies, all female infants are born with a hymen, which can present in a variety of configurations. Commonly, the hymen is *fimbriated, annular,* or *crescentic* (Figure 17-4). Annular hymens are more common at birth, whereas crescentic hymens are more common in girls over 3 years of age. Figure 17-5 illustrates hymen types that are rare—*septate, cribriform,* and *imperforate.* Table 17-1 presents congenital anomalies in development of the female genitalia.

ANATOMY AND PHYSIOLOGY

After the newborn period and before menarche, the clitoris is about 3 mm in length and 3 mm in transverse diameter. Hymens in prepubertal girls are thinner, redder, and more sensitive to touch. With the onset of puberty, the hymen often shows an estrogen effect that makes it pinker and more

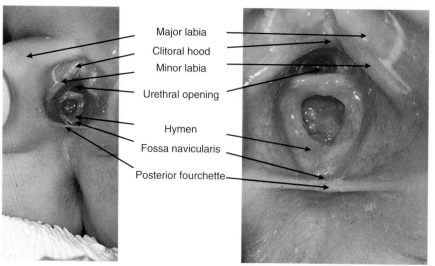

Major labia

Clitoral hood

Minor labia

Urethral opening

Hymen

Fossa navicularis

Posterior fourchette

FIGURE 17-3 External genitalia of the prepubertal child. (From Baren J, Rothrock S, Brennan J, et al: *Pediatric emergency medicine,* Philadelphia, 2008, Saunders.)

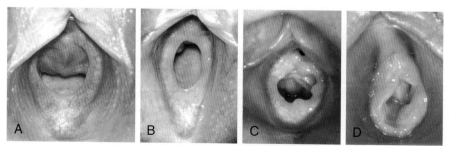

FIGURE 17-4 Variations in normal hymens. **A,** Crescentic. **B,** Annular. **C,** Fimbriated. **D,** Redundant. (From McCann JJ, Kerns DL: *The anatomy of child and adolescent sexual abuse: a CD-ROM atlas/reference,* St. Louis, 1999, Intercorp Inc.)

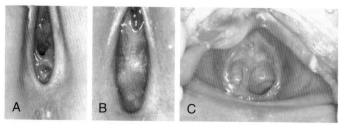

FIGURE 17-5 Abnormal hymens. **A,** Cribriform. **B,** Imperforate. **C,** Septate. (**A** and **B** from McCann JJ, Kerns DL: *The anatomy of child and adolescent sexual abuse: a CD-ROM atlas/reference,* St. Louis, 1999, Intercorp Inc; **C** from Lahoti SL, McClain N, Girardet R et al: Evaluating the child for sexual abuse, *Am Fam Physician* 63[5]:883-892, 2001.)

TABLE 17-1	CONGENITAL ANOMALIES IN THE DEVELOPMENT OF FEMALE GENITALIA	
Condition	**Description**
Ambiguous genitalia	Partially fused labia, enlarged clitoris; hypospadias, bilateral cryptorchidism in an apparent male are signs of a possible intersex condition (see Chapter 15)
Hydrocolpos	Vaginal secretions collecting behind an imperforate hymen at birth may appear as small cystic mass between labia
Vaginal agenesis	Congenital absence of or hypoplasia of fallopian tubes, uterine corpus, uterine cervix, and proximal portion of vagina; occurring in approximately 1 in 5000 births; in approximately 10% of these births, there is a rudimentary or functional uterus Commonly diagnosed at puberty when child presents with primary amenorrhea; however, can be recognized at birth; should be diagnosed before onset of puberty

redundant before the other secondary sexual characteristics appear. The prepubertal *vagina* is rigid, nonelastic, and thin-walled, lined by columnar epithelium, which normally appears redder than the squamous epithelium lining the vagina of pubertal adolescents and adult women.

Adrenarche, the development of pubic and axillary hair, occurs at approximately the same time as *thelarche,* the development of the breast. The mean age of adrenarche in girls is 9 to 10 years of age, but may occur as early as 7 to 8 years of age, particularly in African-American girls (Figure 17-6).

P_1–Tanner 1 (preadolescent). No growth of pubic hair

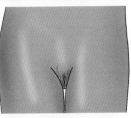

P_2–Tanner 2. Initial, scarcely pigmented straight hair, especially along medial border of the labia

P_3–Tanner 3. Sparse, dark, visibly pigmented, curly public hair on labia.

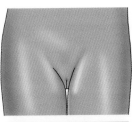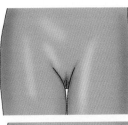

P_4–Tanner 4. Hair coarse and curly, abundant but less than adult.

P_5–Tanner 5. Lateral speading; type and triangle spread of adult hair to medial surface of thighs.

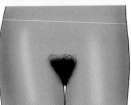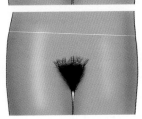

P_6–Tanner 6. Further extension laterally, upward, or dispersed (occurs in only 10% of women).

FIGURE 17-6 Sexual maturity rating in females.

TABLE 17-2 SEXUAL MATURITY RATING (SMR)

Sexual Maturity Rating (SMR)/Tanner Stage	Pubic Hair Development	Genital Changes Due to Estrogenization*
1	No growth of pubic hair	Thicker, more elastic labia minora and hymen, change from columnar (red) to squamous (pink) epithelium in vagina (SMR 1-2)
2	Downy, scarcely pigmented straight hair, especially along medial border of labia majora	Physiological leukorrhea (SMR 2-3)
3	Sparse, visibly pigmented curly (coarse and straight in Asian and American Indian girls) pubic hair on labia	Physiological leukorrhea (SMR 2-3) Onset of menses (SMR 3-4)
4	Hair coarse, curly (coarse and straight in Asian and Native American girls), abundant, but less so than adult; no extension onto medial thighs	Onset of menses (SMR 3-4)
5	Lateral spreading, triangle distribution with some spread onto medial thighs	

Data from Neinstein LS et al editors: *Adolescent health care: a practical guide*, ed 5, Philadelphia, 2008, Lippincott Williams & Wilkins; Jenny C: Sexually transmitted diseases and child abuse, *Pediatr Ann* 21(8):497-503, 1992; Emans SJ and Laufer, MR, editors: *Pediatric and adolescent gynecology*, ed 6, Philadelphia, 2012, Lippincott Williams & Wilkins.
*Not part of classic SMR, but important to note in exam findings and for anticipatory guidance.

Table 17-2 correlates development and *sexual maturity rating* (SMR), also known as *Tanner stages,* which includes breast development and pubic hair distribution in girls. The external genitalia and internal structures—labia majora, labia minora, hymen, vagina, ovaries, uterus—are developing under the influence of increasing estrogens, but they are not included as part of the SMR. Table 17-3 presents pubertal changes of the vagina.

FAMILY, CULTURAL, RACIAL, AND ETHNIC CONSIDERATIONS

Development and amount of pubic and general body hair varies greatly with race/ethnicity. Young women of Asian or Native American descent tend to have less body hair than young women of European or African descent, and pubic hair development may not correlate well with sexual maturity. Many young women remove pubic hair through shaving or waxing, which may make the determination of SMR based on pubic hair distribution challenging.

Female circumcision, or *female genital mutilation,* is prevalent in many parts of the world, particularly sub-Saharan Africa and some Asian countries, and is considered a rite of passage and a prerequisite for marriage in some cultures.[3] The procedure is not legal in the United States or Canada, but immigrant

TABLE 17-3   PUBERTAL CHANGES OF THE VAGINA

Vaginal Changes	Prepubertal Girls	Pubertal Adolescents
Vaginal pH	6.5-7.5 (alkaline)	<4.5
Vaginal mucosa	Columnar epithelium (red)	Stratified squamous epithelium (pink); presence of columnar epithelium on ectocervix, surrounding the os
Vaginal mucous glands, discharge	Absent	Present; physiological leukorrhea usually begins at SMR 2-3
Normal vaginal flora	Gram-positive cocci and anaerobic gram-negative bacteria; gonorrhea and chlamydia focally infect vagina	Lactobacilli; yeast part of normal flora; gonorrhea and chlamydia commonly infect cervix
Vaginal length	4-5 cm	11-12 cm
External genitalia	Thin labia, rigid, nonelastic, thin-walled vagina	Thicker labia; thicker, more elastic, wavy, or redundant hymen; more elastic vagina

Data from Jenny C: Sexually transmitted diseases and child abuse, *Pediatr Ann* 21(8):497-503, 1992.

girls and adolescents may have had the procedure performed previously in their country of origin.[4] Complications include infection, hemorrhage, tetanus, difficulty in urination, sexual dysfunction, and infertility.[5] There is evidence the acceptability of female genital mutilation decreases over time in immigrant communities.

SYSTEM-SPECIFIC HISTORY

The Information Gathering table reviews information gathering on preadolescent and adolescent menstrual history and adolescent sexual history. For approach to adolescent information gathering and obtaining sensitive health information, see Chapter 4.

INFORMATION GATHERING FOR FEMALE GENITALIA AT KEY DEVELOPMENTAL STAGES

Age-Group	Questions to Ask
Preadolescent and adolescent	*Menstrual history:* Age at menarche, regularity of cycles, any spotting or bleeding between cycles, dysmenorrhea, family history of menstrual problems? *For primary amenorrhea:* Age of thelarche and adrenarche, presence or absence of secondary sex characteristics? *For secondary amenorrhea:* Any weight loss attempts, including restriction, binging, purging? Significant physical or emotional stress?
Adolescent	*Sexual history:* Any prior sexual activity, including number and gender of partners, types of activity, use of contraception and/or barrier protection? Coerced or unwanted sexual activity? History of prior examinations, prior infections? Use of over-the-counter medications and cosmetic products or douches? Shaving, waxing or use of depilatories for pubic and thigh hair?

Physical Assessment

Examination of the Newborn

Inspection and Palpation

In the newborn, assess presence and size of the clitoris, patency of the vaginal orifice, presence and location of urethra, and distance between the posterior fourchette and the anus. The labia majora should be palpated for the presence of gonads or hernias, even in a normal-appearing female. Any palpable gonads are likely to be testes, because ovaries rarely descend below the inguinal ring. Reassurance of a normal vaginal examination or prompt communication of any abnormal or concerning physical findings is an important part of building a trust relationship between the parent or caregiver and pediatric health care provider.

Examination of Prepubertal Girls

Positioning

Most young children can be examined in the *frog-leg position:* supine, with knees apart and feet touching in the midline (Figure 17-7). For an apprehensive young child, the parent or caretaker can sit in a chair or on the examination table in a semireclined position (feet in or out of stirrups) with the child's legs straddling her thighs. Older children can be placed in adjustable stirrups. In cases of suspected trauma or abuse, a foreign body in the vagina,

or other suspected structural abnormalities, *knee-chest position* can be used in a child older than 2 years of age (Figure 17-8). Have the child rest her chest on the exam table and support her weight on bent knees, which are positioned 6 to 8 inches apart. Her buttocks will be held up in the air and her back and abdomen will fall downward. In this position, using a penlight or an otoscope head for magnification and light, the examiner can visualize the lower vagina, and in prepubertal girls often the upper vagina. Lateral separation of the labia will be required to visualize the hymen (Figure 17-9).

Touching the hymen in prepubertal girls causes pain. Discharge for wet mounts, potassium hydroxide (KOH) exams, Gram stains, or culture should be collected with a small Dacron-tipped swab moistened with saline.

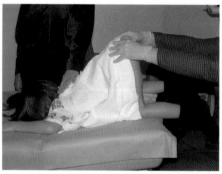

FIGURE 17-8 Knee-chest positioning. (From Gall JA, Boos SC, Payne-James JJ et al: *Forensic medicine,* London, 2003, Churchill Livingstone.)

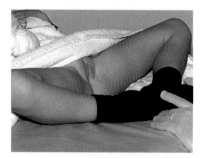

FIGURE 17-7 Frog-leg positioning. (From McCann JJ, Kerns DL: *The anatomy of child and adolescent sexual abuse: a CD-ROM atlas/reference,* St. Louis, 1999, Intercorp Inc.)

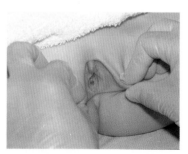

FIGURE 17-9 Anterior labial retraction. (From Gall JA, Boos SC, Payne-James JJ et al: *Forensic medicine,* London, 2003, Churchill Livingstone.)

The child can be asked to take a deep breath for distraction and to open the hymen. If the examiner avoids touching the hymen, this procedure can be painless. Rarely, in cases of suspected abnormalities, a rectoabdominal examination may be performed following inspection of the vaginal area by placing the gloved and lubricated index finger or little finger of one hand into the rectum and placing the other hand on the abdomen. The cervix and uterus may be felt as a "button," and ovaries are not palpable. As the examiner withdraws the finger, the vagina can be gently milked to elicit discharge, a foreign body, or in rare cases, a polypoid tumor.

Young preschool girls are curious about their bodies and often explore the vaginal area. It is not uncommon for young girls to insert foreign objects into the vagina—crayons, beads, coins, batteries, small parts of toys, and other small objects—into their vagina. It is also common for toilet tissue to ball up and enter the vagina. Foreign bodies can remain in the vagina for an extended period and cause inflammation and vaginal discharge, often foul smelling, or bleeding. A foreign body should always be considered when a young preschool girl presents with vaginal or urinary symptoms. If the examiner sees a foreign body, it may be removed by using a moistened cotton swab or by gently irrigating the vagina with normal saline, or consider referral for removal under anesthesia.

There is no indication for a speculum exam in the prepubertal child. Any invasive exams or procedures should be performed under anesthesia.

Examination of the Adolescent

There are currently few indications for a pelvic exam in an adolescent. Regardless of history of sexual activity, only the symptomatic young woman may be a potential candidate for a pelvic exam until age 21 when a Papanicolaou (Pap) smear is indicated.[6] In the case of *primary amenorrhea* or absence of the onset of menstrual periods, abnormal vaginal bleeding, abnormal vaginal discharge or lower abdominal pain, a pelvic exam and/or ultrasound imaging may be appropriate.[7]

Table 17-4 reviews current indications for pelvic exams and alternatives to the recommended exam for adolescents who refuse or are unable to tolerate the pelvic examination.

TABLE 17-4   INDICATIONS FOR PELVIC EXAMS AND ALTERNATIVES

Indications	Recommended Exam	Alternatives
Sexually active adolescent, asymptomatic, ≤age 21 years	Pelvic exam and Pap smear at age 21, then every 3 years. Urine or high vaginal specimen for gonorrhea and chlamydia screen using NAAT technology annually	Pap smear not indicated <21 years. Urine or high vaginal specimen for gonorrhea and chlamydia screen using NAAT technology annually
Adolescent at age 21, asymptomatic, no history of sexual activity	Pelvic exam and Pap smear	
Sexually active adolescent, asymptomatic, desires start of hormonal contraception	Urine or high vaginal swab for NAAT STI screen, urine β-hCG if indicated, history, weight and BP check	May defer STI screen and urine β-hCG if menstruating at time of visit, schedule for STI screening after menses
Adolescent desires start of hormonal contraception, no history of sexual activity	History, urine β-hCG, weight and BP check	

Continued

TABLE 17-4   INDICATIONS FOR PELVIC EXAMS AND ALTERNATIVES—CONT'D

Indications	Recommended Exam	Alternatives
Vaginal discharge without abdominal pain, no history of sexual activity	Vaginal swab for wet mount, KOH prep, STI screen if indicated by microscopic exam	Teen may insert vaginal swab, place in test tube with saline; wet mount, KOH prep
Vaginal discharge without abdominal pain, sexually active adolescent	Urine or high vaginal swab for NAAT STI screen, vaginal swab for wet mount, KOH prep; if wet mount findings consistent with STI, perform pelvic exam, Pap smear if due	Teen may insert vaginal swabs for STI screen and wet mounts
Adolescent with lower abdominal/pelvic pain; no history of sexual activity	Urine β-hCG, bimanual exam, speculum exam if indicated by history or presence of discharge or bleeding; ultrasound if results unclear	Urinalysis, urine β-hCG, urgent ultrasound
Sexually active adolescent with lower abdominal/pelvic pain	Pelvic exam, including speculum exam and bimanual, wet mount/KOH prep, and STI screening	Full exam essential; however, adolescent should not be examined against her will Abdominal exam and U/S imaging may be substituted in patient unable to tolerate pelvic exam

Data from Moyer VA: Screening for cervical cancer: U.S. Preventive Services Task Force recommendation statement, *Ann Intern Med* 156(12):880-891, W312, 2012; Emans SJ: Office evaluation of the child and adolescent. In Emans SJ, Laufer, MR, editors: *Pediatric and adolescent gynecology*, ed 6, Philadelphia, 2012, Lippincott Williams & Wilkins; Blake DR, Duggan A, Quinn T et al: Evaluation of vaginal infections in adolescent women: can it be done without a speculum? *Pediatrics* 102(4 Pt 1):939-944, 1998; Ricciardi R: First pelvic examination in the adolescent, *Nurse Pract Forum* 11(3):161-169, 2000; Shafer MA: Annual pelvic examination in the sexually active adolescent female: what are we doing and why are we doing it? *J Adolesc Health* 23(2):68-73, 1998.

β-hCG, Beta human chorionic gonadotropin; *BP*, blood pressure; *KOH*, potassium hydroxide; *NAAT*, nucleic acid amplification test; *STI*, sexually transmitted infection; *U/S*, ultrasound.

The following description of the pelvic examination should be considered a supplement to careful supervision and mentoring of the novice examiner by the more experienced health care provider. Proper clean technique is more easily demonstrated, and specific procedures for collecting specimens for the *Papanicolaou smear* and testing of sexually transmitted infections (STIs) vary among clinics and laboratories.

EVIDENCE-BASED PRACTICE TIP

Cervical cancer screening (Pap smear) should not begin until age 21 years, regardless of age of onset of sexual activity in immunocompetent young women.[6]

Preparing for the Exam

Explain the pelvic exam carefully, using a plastic pelvic model, diagram, or internet module and video (see http://www.sexualityandu.ca/sexual-health/going-to-doctor/first-pelvic-exam) that enables the adolescent to gain a concrete understanding of the examination process. It is useful to show the adolescent the speculum and specimen collection implements in advance to dispel any anxiety or fear of the unknown. Some examiners provide the adolescent with a mirror, if desired, to observe the examination in progress. The adolescent should be encouraged to empty her bladder before the exam. If any specimens are needed, such as for urine pregnancy test, urinalysis, or urine for STI screening tests, they can be collected at this time. The adolescent should be informed that she can change her mind about the exam at any point, and the exam should never be forced or coerced. Some adolescents may want to have a parent, friend, or partner present for the pelvic examination to provide support. With sufficient preparation and explanations, most adolescents are able to tolerate the examination well. However, adolescents who have been sexually abused, have suffered other trauma, or who are particularly anxious may be helped by specific visualization and relaxation techniques.[8]

Positioning

Adjust stirrups appropriately for the leg length. The adolescent can leave socks on to make the stirrups more comfortable. Ask the youth to move her buttocks forward to the very edge of the exam table, while the feet are in the stirrups. Although many adolescents are uncomfortable with this position, it is necessary for proper visualization and manipulation of the speculum. Avoid touching or pulling the teen, encourage her to move on her own. Most adolescents prefer to have a sheet draped over their abdomen and thighs, but the drape should be positioned so that the examiner can maintain eye contact with the adolescent. The knees should be abducted as far as possible. In order to have the teen's active participation, encourage her to push her knees apart as if she were doing an exercise in stretching in order to avoid any references that could remind her of unwanted sexual activity. The adolescent should be encouraged to take slow, even breaths, to avoid tensing her abdominal muscles, and to keep her buttocks down on the exam table.

Inspection

Note the condition of the clitoris, urethra, labia majora, labia minora, hymen, and introitus (Figure 17-10). Inspect for swelling or lesions such as inflamed pubic hair follicles; *condyloma,* or venereal warts; any clitoral hypertrophy; presence or absence of estrogenization; and any inflammation or discharge. The external

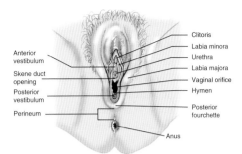

FIGURE 17-10 **External female genitalia.**

structures can be visualized more completely if the examiner gently separates the labia majora.

Palpation

Palpation of the *Skene glands* and *Bartholin glands* is usually avoided in the adolescent, unless the adolescent presents with a complaint of pain or swelling in the labial or vaginal area or the examiner notes abnormalities upon inspection (Figure 17-11).

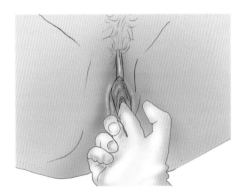

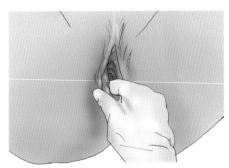

FIGURE 17-11 **Examination of the Skene and Bartholin glands.**

Speculum Exam

Choosing the Speculum

The correct size speculum should be selected, and the speculum warmed, if possible, before insertion. Although many clinics use plastic specula (Figure 17-12), the range of available sizes is limited and the option to use metal specula is more desirable if the capacity to clean and sterilize them is available.

- A Huffman (Huffman-Graves) speculum, (½ × 4½ inches) should be used if the hymenal opening is small, as in virginal teens.
- A pediatric or child speculum (⅝-⅞ × 3 inches) should not be used in the postpubertal adolescent because of the excessive width and inadequate length.
- A Pedersen speculum (⅞ × 4½ inches) and rarely a Graves speculum (1¾ × 3¾ inches) are used for a sexually active teen.
- *Light source:* Some plastic specula have a built-in light source. Otherwise, angle the light over the examiner's shoulder to illuminate

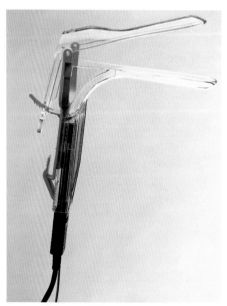

FIGURE 17-12 A vaginal speculum. (From Harkreader H, Hogan MA, Thobaben M: *Fundamentals of nursing: caring and clinical judgment*, ed 3, St. Louis, 2008, Saunders.)

the introitus. Warn the patient the light may feel warm. If the lamp needs readjustment after speculum insertion, remember to change gloves before touching the neck of the light.

- *Inserting the speculum:* The examiner should develop an approach that works for them to maintain clean technique. Some examiners double glove, others change gloves after inspection of the external genitalia and insertion of the speculum. Using the fingers of one hand to separate the labia, one finger, lubricated with water or a scant amount of lubricating jelly, can be inserted into the introitus, pressing down on the posterior fourchette to facilitate easy insertion of the speculum. The examiner should use the other hand to gently insert the speculum, angled toward the sacrum, with slight downward pressure to avoid irritating the urethra. Be careful not to pinch the labia minora or to catch pubic hair in the speculum bills. Figure 17-13 illustrates the steps of speculum insertion.
- Avoid putting pressure on the hymen in virginal teens.
- An alternate method of speculum insertion is to use the second and middle fingers to separate the labia, then press in gently on either side of the lower introitus to relax the fourchette tissues without direct pressure.
- Have the teen take in a deep breath or perform a *Valsalva maneuver* to help relax the introitus to insert the speculum.
- To locate the cervix, use a slight side-to-side motion; if the cervix does not come into view, it may cause less discomfort to withdraw the speculum and use one finger to locate the cervix than to move the speculum excessively.
- Once the speculum is in place and the cervix is in view, secure the speculum in the open position, and remove the first glove on the hand that separated the labia (if double-gloved) or change the glove on the hand that contacted the labia/introitus; then proceed with specimen collection.

into the endometrial canal, is round in a *nulliparous* woman, but may be slitlike in a *parous* adolescent. Physiological variations of the cervix include *nabothian cysts,* which are small, white or yellow, raised, round areas on the cervix; and an *ectropion cervix,* a visible ring of redder, glossy columnar epithelium protruding out and surrounding the os of the cervix. Table 17-5 presents abnormal findings of the female genitalia.

Specimen Collection

The recommended order of specimen collection is to start with the Pap smear then follow with the collection of specimens for STI screening. It may be reasonable to collect STI specimens first in some adolescents if there is a copious amount of discharge or purulent discharge from the cervical os, because the exudate needs to be removed before specimen collection for the Pap smear.

- Use a spatula and cytobrush for Pap smear collection. Follow laboratory instructions for either a traditional Pap smear or the newer liquid cytology, in which the cells are collected and placed in a liquid medium. Be sure to sample the squamocolumnar junction, which may be on the *ectocervix,* or *external os,* in some adolescents.
- Next collect cervical swabs for chlamydia and gonorrhea, unless collecting urine or a high vaginal swab or nucleic acid amplification test (NAAT) for STI screening.
- Use a moistened cotton-tipped swab or plastic or wooden spatula to collect some vaginal secretions for wet mount and KOH preparations from both the vaginal pool and the vaginal wall, unless there is significant blood present.

Make sure to release the locking mechanism of the speculum before withdrawal to avoid pinching the cervix when closing the speculum bills. Do not force the speculum bills closed, as this may cause the cervix or vaginal walls to be pinched. Testing vaginal pH is a valuable adjunct to the wet mount and KOH prep exams,

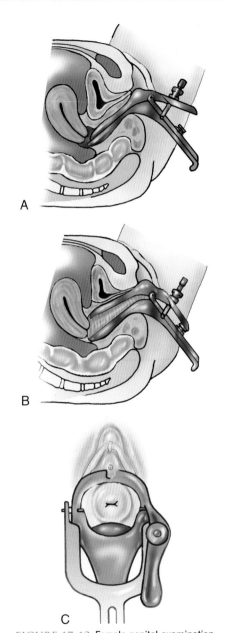

A

B

C

FIGURE 17-13 Female genital examination.

Inspection of the Vagina and Cervix

Inspect the walls of the vagina, and note the presence, color, and consistency of any discharge. Carefully inspect the cervix for color, lesions, and any discharge at the *cervical os.* The *cervical os,* the opening of the cervix

TABLE 17-5 ABNORMAL FINDINGS OF FEMALE GENITALIA ON PELVIC EXAM

Findings	Descriptions
Vulvar and vaginal abnormalities	Imperforate hymen, hematocolpos, vaginal agenesis or signs of a transverse vaginal septum (caused by congenital incomplete fusion of upper and lower vagina), external condyloma, signs of trauma, erythema, and discharge
Cervical abnormalities	Reddened, friable (bleeds with insertion of cotton swab into os), visible condyloma, petechiae ("strawberry spots" rarely seen with trichomoniasis), erosions, double cervix (associated with uterus didelphys), absence of cervix
Pelvic masses	Masses resulting from intrauterine or ectopic pregnancy or from pelvic infection (salpingitis or tuboovarian abscess); adnexal torsion secondary to cyst (which presents with twisting sensation, intermittent bouts of severe pain separated by generalized aching, can be surgical emergency); functional, corpus luteum or dermoid, or other complex ovarian cysts; endometriosis Uterine tumors (such as leiomyomas) are rare in the adolescent; ovarian cancers comprise approximately 1% of all childhood cancers, but they are the most common genital tract cancer in adolescents All adnexal masses should be imaged, first with ultrasound, then (if needed) with computed tomography or magnetic resonance imaging

and vaginal discharge adhering to the speculum bills can be collected for pH testing before the speculum is discarded or placed in cleaning solution. Alternatively, a swab of vaginal secretions can be applied to a pH tape or strip.

The Bimanual Exam

The purpose of the bimanual exam is to assess the cervix, the corpus of the uterus, and the adnexa. The adolescent should be encouraged to relax the abdominal muscles by breathing slowly and steadily, or performing a Valsalva maneuver, which may facilitate insertion of the examiner's fingers. The examiner applies lubricant to the fingers, and then inserts the middle and index fingers of a gloved hand into the vagina, keeping the pressure against the posterior fourchette and the pubococcygeal muscle and away from the delicate anterior structures of the clitoris and urethra (Figure 17-14). In virginal adolescents, it may only be possible to insert one finger. If the need for a bimanual exam is indicated, the examiner should consider the alternative option of a *rectoabdominal exam*

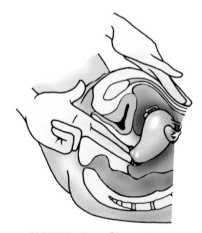

FIGURE 17-14 Bimanual exam.

for adolescents who request to avoid vaginal penetration for cultural or religious reasons.

- **Palpate the cervix:** Note consistency of the cervix, normally firm and shaped like the tip of a nose. Note presence of any bumps on the cervix, such as nabothian cysts, 3- to 8-mm smooth, nontender, firm lumps, which result from blockage of endocervical gland ducts.

- **Palpate the uterus:** Press down on the abdomen with the other hand while supporting the cervix. Assess the size, shape, consistency, mobility, and tenderness of the uterus and any palpable masses. The position of the uterus varies from anteverted, anteflexed, midposition, and retroverted to retroflexed (Figure 17-15). The normal uterus is shaped like an upside-down small pear and is approximately 7.5 cm long and 2.5 cm thick.
- **Assess for cervical motion tenderness:** The examiner wiggles the cervix side-to-side and forward and backward between the palpating fingers. In a normal exam, the movement of the uterus creates an unusual sensation in the pelvis for an adolescent. Ask the adolescent to distinguish between pain and discomfort or an unusual feeling. Tenderness or pain on exam is a symptom of pelvic infection.
- **Assess the adnexae and ovaries:** Place the examining fingers in the vagina first at the right lateral fornix then at the left lateral fornix, posteriorly and high. Begin with the opposite hand on the abdomen just below and medial to the iliac crest and move diagonally toward the symphysis pubis. Apply a firm, steady sweeping motion with the hand on the abdomen as you palpate briefly. Normal ovaries are smooth and almond-shaped, slightly tender to deep palpation, and approximately 3 cm by 1.5 cm by 1 cm. Tenderness or fullness of the adnexae is abnormal and may indicate infection, ectopic pregnancy, or endometriosis.
- **Rectovaginal exams:** This exam is usually omitted in adolescents, unless there is a suspicion of abnormality or an extremely retroflexed uterus, or the hymenal ring is too tight to adequately assess for the cervix and uterus. It is performed with the index finger in the vagina, the middle finger in the rectum and the opposite hand on the abdomen. The *rectovaginal septum* should be thin, pliable, and free of masses. The teen should be reassured that although she may feel the urge to defecate, she will not.
- **Sizing an intrauterine pregnancy:** Recognizing a pregnancy in the adolescent can aid

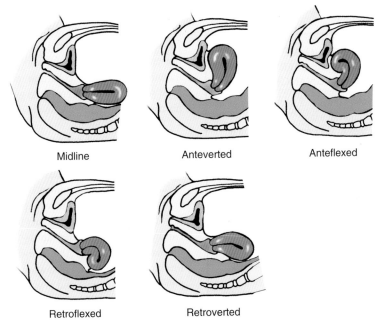

Midline   Anteverted   Anteflexed

Retroflexed   Retroverted

FIGURE 17-15 Various positions of the uterus.

in the swift diagnosis of the cause of complaints ranging from fatigue and nausea to secondary amenorrhea, abdominal fullness, or a mass. The health care provider should maintain a high index of suspicion for pregnancy, even in the youngest adolescents who deny a history of sexual activity. Adolescents may be reluctant to disclose early or unwanted sexual activity. Point of care urine testing for β-hCG is invaluable. The weeks of pregnancy are counted from the first day of the last menstrual period, even though ovulation generally occurs 2 weeks after the beginning of menses (Box 17-1). Fundal height provides a guide for estimating uterine size (Figure 17-16).

Wrapping Up the Examination

The adolescent should be handed some tissues, so she may wipe off the lubricant used. The examiner should stay in the room long enough to ensure that the adolescent does not feel dizzy upon sitting up, and then leave while she dresses. Results of the exam should be given while the teen is dressed, and any abnormalities should be thoroughly explained. To ensure

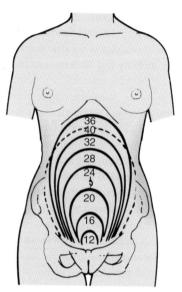

FIGURE 17-16 Fundal height.

confidentiality, present and discuss results with the adolescent alone.

SUSPICION OF SEXUAL ABUSE

In cases of suspected child sexual abuse, the history and behavioral observations are crucial. Any history of abuse disclosed to the health care provider that occurred within the previous 72 hours (up to 120 hours in some states) requires immediate referral for a forensic examination with possible collection of evidence. Most sexually abused prepubertal girls will have normal physical exams because of the following:
- Delays in disclosure
- Rapid healing of genital and anal tissue in prepubertal children
- Predominance in this age-group of sexual abuse involving fondling or oral-genital contact, which does not leave physical signs

It is important to remember that up to 95% of children reporting sexual abuse will have a normal genital exam.[1] The following physical findings in prepubertal girls should raise suspicion of sexual abuse and prompt referral for an exam by specially trained practitioners:
- Hymenal irregularities or absence of hymen including notches, transections, or thin,

---

BOX 17-1	SIZING AN INTRAUTERINE PREGNANCY

Nulliparous uterus: 7.5 × 2.5 cm (size of small lime on bimanual exam)

Eight-week uterus: 9-11 cm × 5 cm (size of orange on bimanual exam)

Twelve-week uterus: 12-14 cm × 7 cm (size of grapefruit, very soft, sometimes difficult to palpate on bimanual exam); just palpable, abdominally at level of symphysis pubis

Sixteen-week uterus: Palpate abdomen, felt halfway between symphysis pubis and umbilicus

Twenty-week uterus: Palpate abdomen, felt at umbilicus

Over twenty-weeks: Measure from symphysis pubis to height of fundus (number of cm — approximate number of weeks)

rounded edges, particularly posterior from the 3 to 9 o'clock position with the child supine; should be confirmed in knee-chest position, because an apparent notch may be a fold in a redundant hymen

- Acute trauma to the hymen or posterior fourchette, or laceration of vaginal mucosa, particularly extending to the rectal mucosa
- Confirmed sexually transmitted infection, including human papillomavirus (HPV) infection in a child ≥2 years old

Other possible findings include increased erythema, irritation, and vaginal discharge, which may be signs of sexual abuse. However, it is essential for health care providers to keep in mind they should not solely rely on physical findings when considering a diagnosis of sexual abuse. The examiner should keep the possibility of sexual abuse in mind whenever other nonvenereal infections, chemical irritation, foreign bodies, and/or poor hygiene are included in the differential diagnosis. Failure or delay of fusion of the median *raphe* between the posterior fourchette and the anus is often mistaken for trauma or sexual abuse.

FEMALE GENITAL CONDITIONS

Table 17-6 presents common conditions and findings of the genitalia in the prepubertal and pubertal female. The prepubertal vagina is hostile to yeast, and vulvovaginal candidiasis is rare except in cases of diabetes mellitus, recent

TABLE 17-6   FEMALE GENITAL CONDITIONS

Condition	Description
Labial adhesions	Adherence of labia minora or majora, primarily seen in girls 3 months to 6 years of age; adhesion may persist until puberty, or may separate spontaneously; treatment is controversial if opening is large enough for normal urinary flow and vaginal drainage
Labial abscesses	Usually caused by *Staphylococcus aureus* and *Streptococcus pyogenes*
Labial lipoma	May be initially mistaken for a hernia
Clitoral lesions	Edema of clitoris, with hypoproteinemia, in conditions such as nephrotic syndrome Hypertrophy of clitoral hood and clitoris, caused by neurofibromatosis, rhabdomyosarcoma, increased androgens Hemorrhages around clitoris caused by lichen sclerosis or trauma (see later)
Urethral prolapse	Presents with bleeding and friable, red-blue doughnutlike annular mass that may be visible in perineum ("hemorrhagic cranberry")
Lichen sclerosis	Uncommon; presents with atrophic, hypopigmented, parchmentlike friable skin around vulva and anus, often in an "hourglass" configuration, with inflammation and subepithelial hemorrhages
Vulvar irritation	Often results from irritants such as bubble bath, poor hygiene, candidal overgrowth caused by antibiotics or diaper occlusion; rarely scratching can occur secondary to pruritus from a pinworm infestation
Vulvovaginitis	Vaginal discharge may be caused by bacteria (e.g., *Streptococcus, Shigella*) or overgrowth of normal flora; foreign body in vagina (typically toilet paper); poor hygiene; sexually transmitted infection (STI)
Straddle injuries to vulva	Straddle injuries (as in playground falls) generally cause trauma to anterior vulvar structures and rarely cause trauma to posterior portion of hymen or posterior fourchette; in addition, injury is usually somewhat asymmetrical and not penetrating in nature

antibiotic usage, compromised immune system, or diaper use in infants or children with special health care needs. Sexually transmitted pathogens, such as *Neisseria gonorrhoeae* and *Chlamydia trachomatis*, infect the columnar epithelium of the vagina rather than the *cervix* in sexually active adolescents. Bacterial infections, such as *Streptococcus* and *Shigella,* can cause purulent or even bloody vaginal discharge in infected individuals.

SUMMARY OF EXAMINATION

- The genital exam in the child and asymptomatic adolescent includes an assessment of the external genitalia only.
- SMR in girls is based on breast development and pubic hair distribution.
- Secondary sexual development must be assessed in the context of overall growth and development.
- The norms for SMR are based on data collected on white children. Children of Asian or Native American descent may not have pubic hair development that matches SMR. Pubic hair development may not correlate well with sexual maturity.
- There are currently few indications for a pelvic exam in an adolescent.
- A pelvic exam is not necessary for recommended STI screening in asymptomatic, sexually active adolescents.
- Ninety-five percent of children reporting sexual abuse will have a normal genital exam.
- Variations in external genitalia may be due to congenital disorders or cultural practices, such as female circumcision.

Charting

Charting on a Sexually Active Female Teen

External Genitalia: Pink, no discharge noted, without lesions. Tanner stage 4 to 5 pubic hair distribution.

Vaginal Exam: Cervix pink without lesions, scant blood at os from menses, scant mucoid discharge in vault.

Bimanual: No pain on deep palpation or with movement of cervix. Uterus midposition. Adnexae nontender, nonthickened.

Rectal: No fissures, lesions, or hemorrhoids; stool brown, guaiac neg.

REFERENCES

1. Adams JA: Medical evaluation of suspected child sexual abuse: 2011. update, *J Child Sex Abus* 20(5):588-605, 2011.
2. Holm I: Ambiguous genitalia in the newborn and disorders of sex development. In Emans SJ and Laufer MR, editors: *Pediatric and adolescent gynecology*, ed 6, Philadelphia, 2012, Lippincott Williams & Wilkins.
3. World Health Organization (WHO): *An update on WHO's work on female genital mutilation (FGM).* Progress report, 2011, WHO (website). Available at www.who.int/reproductivehealth/publications/fgm/rhr_11_18/en/index.html. Accessed April 20, 2013.
4. Simpson, J, Robinson, K, Creighton SM, et al: Female genital mutilation: the role of health professionals in prevention, assessment, and management, *BMJ* 344:e1361, 2012.
5. Strickland JL: Female circumcision/female genital mutilation, *J Pediatr Adolesc Gynecol* 14(3):109-112, 2001.
6. Moyer VA: Screening for cervical cancer: U.S. Preventive Services Task Force recommendation statement, *Ann Intern Med* 156(12):880-91, W312, 2012.
7. Emans SJ: Office evaluation of the child and adolescent. In Emans SJ and Laufer, MR, editors: *Pediatric and adolescent gynecology*, ed 6, Philadelphia, 2012, Lippincott Williams & Wilkins.
8. Hennigen L, Kollar LM, Rosenthal SL: Methods for managing pelvic examination anxiety: individual differences and relaxation techniques, *J Pediatr Health Care* 14(1):9-12, 2000.

CHAPTER 18

MUSCULOSKELETAL SYSTEM

Karen G. Duderstadt; Naomi A. Schapiro

The assessment of the musculoskeletal system is challenging in pediatrics because of the variations in growth and development and the normal range of rotational changes in the extremities in infants and children. Increasing knowledge and comfort in the pediatric health care provider regarding the physical examination of the musculoskeletal system is key to accurate assessment, management, and referral of common orthopedic conditions.

EMBRYOLOGICAL DEVELOPMENT

The rudimentary skeletal system forms as early as the fourth week of gestation when the development of the vertebrae begins and the upper extremities begin as buds on the fetus. As early as the seventh week of gestation, embryonic vascular growth progresses toward the center of the *osteoblasts* in the long bone, which forms cartilage. During the ninth week of gestation, *ossification*, or bone growth, begins in the ossification centers in the lower thoracic and upper lumbar vertebrae, and ossification continues in the femur. The hand pads develop from the extremity buds by days 33 to 36, and the finger rays begin to form on days 41 to 43.[1] It is during this period of gestation that *polydactyly*, the presence of extra digits, or *syndactyly*, the webbing or fusing of the digits, occurs along with other deformities of the extremities. The *calcaneus*, the largest tarsal bone of the foot, ossifies at the sixth month of fetal life. The position of the fetus in utero has the greatest impact on the skeletal system and the most common variants present at birth.

Muscle structures, including the tendons, ligaments, cartilage, and joints, originate from the embryonic *mesoderm*. Muscle fibers are developed by the fourth or fifth month of gestation. They increase in size along with changes in muscle and fat proportions throughout childhood and adolescence.

DEVELOPMENTAL VARIATIONS

At birth, the *epiphyses* of the long bone are composed of hyaline cartilage. Shortly after birth, the secondary ossification centers begin to replace the cartilage along the *epiphyseal plate*. During early periods of rapid growth, ossification occurs in secondary sites throughout the body: the ends of the long bones, the vertebrae, the flat bones in the clavicle, and the skull. The replacement of cartilage by bone is known as *endochondral ossification*. The epiphyseal plate ossifies, becoming the *diaphysis*, the shaft of the long bone; and cartilage at the metaphyseal plate replaces bone cells (Figure 18-1).

Bone growth continues in infants and children along the *epiphysis* as new bone is added to the outer surface of existing bone. Growth along the epiphyseal plate continues until the cells in the growth plate stop dividing in puberty, and closure of the growth plate occurs in young adults when the metaphysis and the epiphysis fuse.

Several factors influence the health of the bones and growth of cells at the epiphyseal plate. Trauma during childhood can cause separation of the epiphysis and the blood vessels to rupture, resulting in cessation of bone growth and a shortened extremity.[1] Nutritional factors such as adequate protein in the diet, the amount of calcium intake, and adequate intake of vitamin D, particularly in breastfed infants, impact bone growth. Vitamin D absorbs

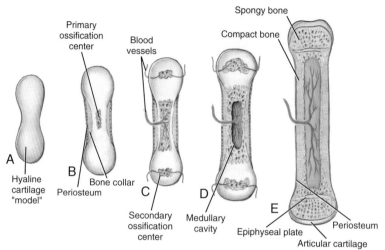

FIGURE 18-1 Growth plates and transition from cartilage to bone at the epiphyseal plate. **A,** Hyaline cartilage "model." **B,** Periosteum and bone collar form. **C,** Blood vessels and osteoblasts infiltrate primary ossification centers. **D,** Osteoclasts form medullary cavity. **E,** Ossification is complete. Hyaline cartilage remains as articular cartilage and in the epiphyseal plate. (From Applegate E: *The anatomy and physiology learning system*, ed 4, St. Louis, 2011, Saunders.)

dietary calcium and phosphorus from the intestines and promotes bone health by maintaining normal levels of these minerals in the blood. Adequate levels of vitamin D in childhood may also have a role in improving muscle and immune function. Parents are often advised to keep infants and children out of the sun due to long-term risks of skin cancer, therefore reducing vitamin D synthesis from the skin. Maintaining adequate levels of vitamin D in infants and children is important to maintaining bone strength. *Rickets* is a deficiency of vitamin D in which the growth plate is impaired by calcification of newly formed bone on the metaphyseal plate. Alterations in thyroid or growth hormones can also impact normal growth.[1] Recent evidence indicates environmental and chemical hazards may be a contributing factor to malformations in the musculoskeletal system.

ANATOMY AND PHYSIOLOGY

Head and Neck

Assessment of the head and neck area is reviewed in Chapter 9.

Upper Extremities and Torso

The *clavicle* lies in a horizontal plane above the first rib and rotates between the sternum and the superior surface of the *scapula* (Figure 18-2). The *scapula*, a large, flat triangular bone, forms the posterior portion of the upper extremity and the superior, lateral angle articulates with the capsule or rounded head of the *humerus,* the large bone in the upper arm. The distal end of the *humerus* forms the *condyle* and is divided into the *medial epicondyle* and the *lateral epicondyle.* The proximal end of the *ulna* attaches at the articulating surface of the humerus and forms one of two long bones in the forearm. The *olecranon* is the outer, rounded distal surface of the *ulna* and forms the major portion of the elbow. The distal end of the ulna is small and articulates with the wrist bones. The *radius* is along the lateral side or thumb side of the forearm, and the distal end of the *radius* forms a large portion of the wrist bones.

The hand consists of eight carpal and five metacarpal bones. Many of the carpal bones are cartilaginous at birth. A radiograph of a child's hand at 2½ years of age illustrates ossification of only the *capitate* and *hamate* bones

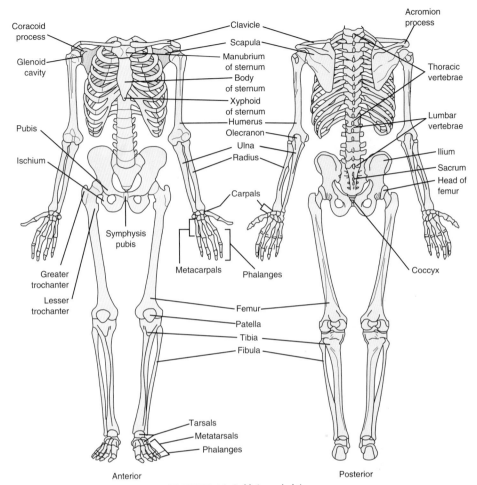

FIGURE 18-2 Mature skeleton.

in the hand. Development and ossification of the hand continues until 11 years of age when all of the carpal bones are ossified except for the small *pisiform* bone, which develops by 12 years of age. Abnormalities of the *phalanges*, or fingers, such as *syndactyly*, webbing, or fusion between adjacent digits of the hands or feet, may be indicative of profound developmental delay (Figure 18-3). *Polydactyly*, the presence of supernumerary digits, is a more common variant and is not usually associated with other congenital anomalies.

Spine

The infant has a C-shaped spinal curve at birth in comparison to the double S curvature that is present in late adolescence. Thoracic and pelvic curves are present at birth, and the secondary cervical curve is present by 3 to 4 months of age when the infant begins to hold up his or her head. The lumbar curvature begins to form as the infant bears weight and begins to walk. The young child often has an exaggerated thoracic-lumbar curvature and a protuberant abdomen until 3 years of age, when gait and balance become more normal (Figure 18-4). The *sacrum* is composed of five separate bones at birth and by 18 to 20 years of age is fused into one large bone. The *coccyx* consists of three or four small bones that begin to ossify between the first and fourth years of life and

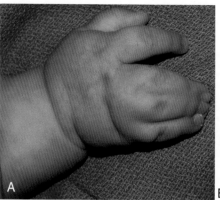
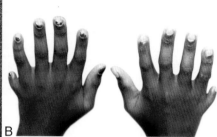

FIGURE 18-3 **A,** Syndactyly. **B,** Polydactyly. (**A,** From Davis P, Cladis F, Motoyana E: *Smith's anesthesia for infants and children,* ed 8, Philadelphia, 2012, Mosby. **B,** From Valiathan A, Sivakumar A, Marianayagam D, et al: Thurston syndrome: report of a new case, *Oral Surg Oral Med Oral Pathol Oral Radiol Endod* 101(6):757-760, 2006.)

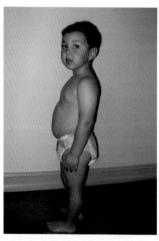

FIGURE 18-4 Protuberant abdomen of the young child. (From Seidel H, Ball J, Dains J, et al: *Mosby's guide to physical examination,* ed 7, St. Louis, 2011, Mosby.)

fuses into one bone by 25 years of age (Figure 18-5).

Pelvis

The hip bone contains three distinct parts in childhood, which are later fused in adulthood. The *ilium* is the superior, broad, flat surface of the hip bone. The *ischium* is the strongest

portion of the hip bone; it contains a portion of the *acetabulum,* which forms the attachment at the hip bone for the femur and the opening or *foramen.* The *pubis* contains the medial portion of the acetabulum and joins medially to form the complete pelvic girdle.

Lower Extremities and Feet

The *femur* is the longest and strongest bone in the body. The head of the femur becomes ossified during the first year of life, but the shaft of the femur does not become completely ossified until 14 years of age. The long bones of the extremities continue to grow at the site of the epiphyseal plate throughout childhood and adolescence; peak bone mass is achieved by young adulthood. In the lower leg, the larger bone is the *tibia,* the proximal end articulates with the femur and the distal end forms the *medial malleolus* of the ankle. The *fibula* is the smaller bone in the lower leg and lateral to the tibia. The distal end of the fibula forms the lateral malleolus of the ankle.

The *patella* is the small triangular bone that forms the kneecap and lies over the junction of the *femur* and the *tibia.* The health of the patella during growth and development depends not only on strong bone growth but also

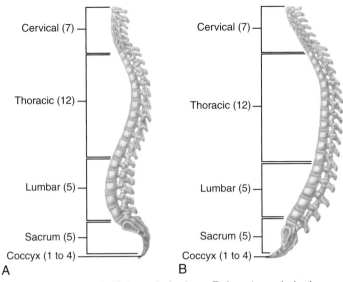

Cervical (7)

Thoracic (12)

Lumbar (5)

Sacrum (5)

Coccyx (1 to 4)

A

Cervical (7)

Thoracic (12)

Lumbar (5)

Sacrum (5)

Coccyx (1 to 4)

B

FIGURE 18-5 **A,** Mature spinal column. **B,** Immature spinal column.

on the strength of the ligaments and tendons supporting the patella.

The seven tarsal bones and five metatarsal bones of the foot undergo dramatic ossification during the first year of life. The ossification of the bones in the foot follows the normal development of the gross motor milestones. The *talus* is ossified by the seventh month of life to form the ankle, and the remaining *metatarsal* bones continue to form during the latter half of the first year of life. The *phalanges* continue the ossification process through adolescence.

The limbs go through a continuous process of rotational change until about 8 years of age. The torsional development is a process that begins in infancy and progresses from sitting position to pulling up, to crawling, then standing, cruising, and finally walking with an exaggerated gait and a wide base of support. The laxity in the ligaments and the torsional forces in the intrauterine environment as well as sitting and sleeping patterns in the early years are responsible for the normal variations in the lower extremities during childhood. Torsional variations

and abnormalities are hereditarily linked and often show a strong family tendency.

Monitoring Growth

During growth, bone has the remarkable capacity to remodel itself. Bone is deposited in areas subjected to stress and reabsorbed in areas where there is little stress. This physiological process explains the ability of children to remodel residual deformity after fractures and explains the biological plasticity in growing bones. The rate of bone growth is greatest in the lower extremities before the onset of puberty; the *distal* extremities reach adult size in early puberty, which is reflected in shoe size in preadolescents. The trunk and *proximal* extremities exhibit the dominant growth during puberty and into young adulthood. Bone growth is completed at age 20 years, and peak bone mass is achieved by age 35 years.

Monitoring the velocity of growth is the key focus of routine well-child visits and when following children with chronic health conditions. For the child with slow growth or delayed onset of puberty, obtaining past growth charts and evaluating the progression of the growth curve along with familial patterns of growth and pubertal development is critical to assessing an abnormal growth pattern.

Muscle Development

The rate of muscle growth and development increases rapidly beginning at age 2 years. Early muscle growth is balanced by a normal decrease in adipose tissue in early childhood.[1] The growth and maturation of the muscles continues with the ossification of the skeletal system (Figure 18-6). *Muscle tone* is the state of normal tension of the muscles, and term infants normally have strong muscle tone at birth. Abnormalities in muscle tone in an infant may be noted shortly after birth when an infant is floppy. Less than normal

muscle tone is described as *hypotonia; rigidity* or increased muscle tone is known as *hypertonia;* and *spasticity* is resistance to flexion and extension and range of motion of the muscles. Normal muscle function requires the normal function of the lower motor neurons (LMNs) in the spinal cord and the normal reflexivity of the muscle fibers. Normal muscle tone requires the normal function of the spinal cord stretch reflex and the balance of the upper motor neurons (UMNs) and LMN function. Lesions on the UMNs result in increased tone and LMN lesions result in decreased tone.

The greatest increase in muscle size occurs during puberty when boys' muscle mass and muscle cell size begins to exceed that in girls.

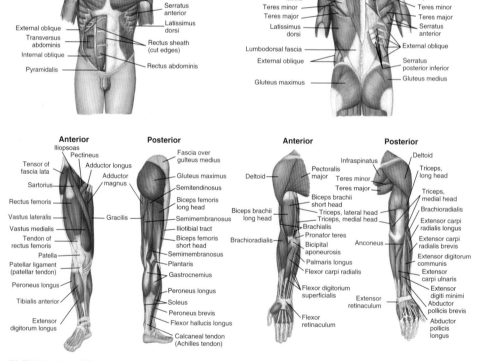

FIGURE 18-6 Muscular system, front and back. (From Mourad LA: *Orthopedic disorders*, St. Louis, 1991, Mosby.)

In early and middle childhood, girls' muscle size increases at a greater rate than in boys up until puberty.

PHYSIOLOGICAL VARIATIONS

Table 18-1 presents physiological and developmental changes in the musculoskeletal system from the newborn through adolescence.

FAMILY, CULTURAL, RACIAL, AND ETHNIC CONSIDERATIONS

African-American infants often have advanced musculoskeletal development and achieve developmental milestones earlier. Asian-American infants often have increased hypotonia at birth due to increased laxity in the ligaments of the muscle, and they may also have an increased abduction of the hips bilaterally on examination in early infancy.

SYSTEM-SPECIFIC HISTORY

Obtaining a complete history or a symptom-related history of the musculoskeletal system is key to accurate assessment in children and adolescents. The Information Gathering table reviews the pertinent areas for each age-group and developmental stage of childhood.

TABLE 18-1 PHYSIOLOGICAL VARIATIONS OF THE MUSCULOSKELETAL SYSTEM AT KEY DEVELOPMENTAL STAGES

Age-Group	Variation
Preterm infant and newborn	Lower extremities in external rotation and flexion at hips; upper femur is anteverted and knees are flexed; tibias are internally rotated; feet are dorsiflexed
Infancy	Tibias gradually rotate externally to about 20 degrees toward midline by 12 months of age; flat feet and bowed legs until walking is firmly established
Early childhood	Stance with wide base of support, hyperflexion of hips and knees with disjointed (toddling) pattern when walking; arms held abducted and elbows extended; in-toeing is common beginning at 15 months; normal arm swing and heel-toe walking generally begin by 18 months of age; longitudinal arch not present in infant but begins to develop by 2½ years of age. At 3 years of age, children exhibit mature pattern of motion and muscle action; resolution of in-toeing and marked torsion of lower extremities normally disappear by school entry
Middle childhood	*Knock-knee* is present until 7 years of age; by 8 to 10 years of age, femur rotates to position of about 14 degrees toward midline from average of 45 degrees at birth
Adolescence	Hormonal changes impact ligaments and tendons; laxity of knees is particularly common in adolescent females, making them vulnerable to injury

INFORMATION GATHERING FOR ASSESSMENT OF THE MUSCULOSKELETAL SYSTEM AT KEY DEVELOPMENTAL STAGES

Age-Group	Questions to Ask
Preterm infant	History of hypoxia in early neonatal period? Intraventricular insult? Any maternal alcohol or substance abuse? When did prenatal care begin?
Newborn	History of maternal infection while in utero? Any trauma sustained at birth? Need for resuscitation or ventilation in immediate newborn period? Presentation at birth? Breech or shoulder? Family history of skeletal deformities or genetic disorders?
Infancy	Family history of bone or joint disorders? Any delay in achieving gross motor milestones? Does infant roll over? Sit without support? Crawl? Stand alone? Walk without support? Any evidence of toe-walking? Any evidence of widening of wrist joints?
Middle childhood	Involved in organized/competitive sports? Any complaint of pain when walking/running or pain that awakens child at night? History of joint stiffness or swelling? Weight of school backpack? History of prolonged steroid use with chronic conditions?
Adolescence	Involved in organized/competitive sports? Any limited range of motion of joints? Is gait normal and erect? History of fractures, sprains, or trauma? Weight of school backpack? Any evidence of habitual slouching? Family history of skeletal deformities? Start of menstrual periods?
Environmental risks	Contact with chemical cleaning agents, hazardous smoke, or chemicals? Exposure to toxic pesticides? History of elevated lead level?

PHYSICAL ASSESSMENT

Preparation for the Examination

For a thorough and complete assessment of the musculoskeletal system, infants must be undressed except for the diaper, and children must be undressed except for underwear. A young child cannot be thoroughly assessed when wearing socks and shoes or when gowned. In preadolescence and adolescence, maintaining modesty while assessing the spine can be challenging, particularly in girls. Maturing females must be in underwear and gown to obtain a thorough examination of the spine. Musculoskeletal terminology is presented in Box 18-1, and skeletal positions are presented in Figure 18-7.

Inspection and Palpation

Initial inspection of the musculoskeletal system in the child from birth to adolescence begins with inspection of skin for color and temperature; inspection of palmar creases; and noting of scars, unusual pigmentation or lesions, swelling, and bruising. Bruising is the most common sign of physical abuse and intentional injury in children. Bruising over bony prominences such as the shins, knees, and forehead are common in children and usually the result of active play. However, bruising seen on the buttocks, neck, face, and earlobes should be considered suspect and require further information gathering and assessment for signs of abuse.[2] Erythema, swelling, tenderness, or temperature changes should also be noted over the joints or extremities.

Observation of posture when standing and sitting, assessing the proportion of upper extremities to lower extremities, and noting any obvious gait abnormalities are part of a complete musculoskeletal assessment. Palpation for bone or joint tenderness, and any unusual

BOX 18-1	MUSCULOSKELETAL TERMINOLOGY
Flexion	A decrease in the angle of the resting joint in the upper or lower extremities
Extension	An increase in the joint angle
Hyperextension	An increase in the angle of the joint beyond the usual arc
Abduction	Movement away from the midline
Adduction	Movement toward the midline
Rotation	Movement around a central axis
Circumduction	Rotation or circular movement of the limbs
Dorsiflexion	Backward rotation
Supine/supination	Lying on back facing upward, palmar surface facing upward
Prone/pronation	Lying face downward/palmar surface facing downward
Inversion	Turning inward/movement towards the body
Subluxation	Partial or incomplete dislocation
Eversion	Turning outward/movement away from body
Varus	Toward midline of body
Valgus	Away from midline of body
Dorsiflexion	Movement of the hands and feet upward

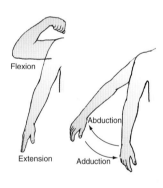

Flexion

Abduction

Extension Adduction

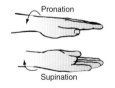

Pronation

Supination

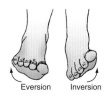

Eversion Inversion

FIGURE 18-7 Skeletal positions.

prominence, thickening, and/or indentations in the bony skeleton as well as muscle tone, muscle strength, and symmetry should be evaluated. Inspection, palpation, and assessment of the mobility of the spine and range of motion of the extremities, including the evaluation of the mobility of the joints, are included in a thorough and complete assessment of the musculoskeletal system.

Joints

Joints in the body have a slightly moveable to freely moveable motion throughout the period of growth and development. The *hinge joint,* between the humerus and the ulna, permits motion in one plane, whereas the *pivotal joint,* between the radial-ulnar joint, allows rotation only. The *condyloid joint* in the wrist allows flexion, extension, adduction, abduction, and circumduction. *Saddle joints,* such as in the thumb, have a similar motion to the condyloid joint in the wrist except that the joint forms a concave-convex fit to achieve motion. The hip and shoulder joints are examples of *ball-and-socket joints.* Finally, the *gliding joints* allow a gliding motion between two flat surfaces, such

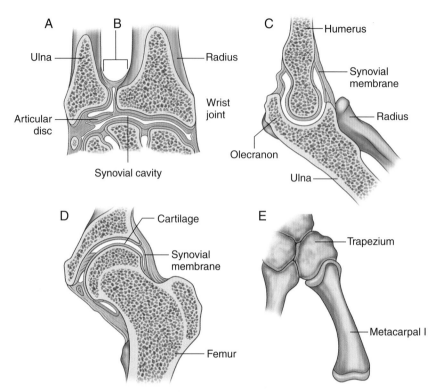

FIGURE 18-8 Skeletal joints. **A,** Condyloid (wrist). **B,** Pivotal (radioulnar). **C,** Hinge or ginglymus (elbow). **D,** Ball and socket (hip). **E,** Saddle (carpometacarpal of thumb). (From Drake R, Vogl AW, Mitchell A: *Gray's anatomy for students*, ed 2, Philadelphia, 2010, Churchill Livingstone.)

as in the vertebrae and carpal joints in the hands and feet (Figure 18-8).

Head and Neck

Assessment of the head and neck is presented in Chapter 9.

Upper Extremities and Clavicle

In the newborn infant, the clavicles should be fully palpated to detect a possible fracture often associated with a traumatic delivery. Localized tenderness at the proximal end of the clavicle shortly after birth often leads to a palpable bony prominence as the fracture heals. A full range of motion of the upper extremities, including the elbows and wrists must be evaluated to determine any trauma that may have affected the clavicles or shoulders during the birth process. In *Erb palsy,* injury to the fifth and sixth cranial nerves, no spontaneous abduction of the shoulder muscles or flexion of the elbow is noted on examination. The arm is adducted and internally rotated, but normal grip in the hand is present.

Range of motion should be passively evaluated in infants and young children and assessed actively when children are cooperative with examination. Any limitation of range of motion in joints and extremities or asymmetrical response should be further investigated. Muscle tone and strength should also be evaluated. In early childhood, the radial-ulnar joint is particularly vulnerable. *Subluxation,* or partial dislocation, of the radius from the humerus, often referred to as *Nursemaid's elbow,* is common in children from 2 to 4 years of age.

Often there is no clear history of trauma, but laxity of the ligaments in the young child predisposes them to injury. In cases of a sub-luxation, the child usually refuses to use the affected arm. Passive range of motion is possible except for *supination* (palm facing upward). Dislocation of the shoulder can also occur in the young child and is marked by swelling, pain, and a limp arm.

Trauma to the upper extremities is common in children and adolescents. Strains, sprains, or fractures can occur with strenuous activity, falls, motor vehicle or pedestrian injuries, or participation in competitive sports. Careful assessment is warranted in the growing child when any history of trauma is obtained. Fractures that are highly suggestive of intentional injury or abuse in children are rib fractures, especially posterior rib fractures, scapular fractures, sternal fractures, fractures of the spinous processes, and metaphyseal lesions.[2] Clavicular fractures and long bone fractures in children older than 1 year of age are common traumatic injuries of childhood.

Lower Extremities and Feet

Assessment of the lower extremities includes evaluating flexion/extension, adduction/abduction, and internal/external rotation. Muscle tone, muscle strength, and symmetry should be evaluated with the child standing and while observing gait. Leg length is evaluated with the infant or child supine, with knee and hip joints extended and legs aligned. A discrepancy in length or asymmetrical appearance may indicate an abnormality in hips, long bones, or knees. In infants, leg length discrepancy may indicate congenital or developmental hip dislocation. Leg length in children can be evaluated by measuring from anterior superior iliac spine to the medial malleolus. Abnormal leg length should be evaluated by bone scan and referred to pediatric orthopedics for further evaluation.

Inspect the *malleoli* to evaluate the presence of torsion in the lower extremities. The medial *malleolus* lies at the distal end of the

tibia, forming the medial ankle, and the lateral *malleolus* forms the lateral ankle at the distal end of the *fibula*. In the infant, the medial and lateral malleoli are parallel when examining the infant supine. A rotation of up to 20 degrees occurs in the lateral malleoli during the normal growth and development of the musculoskeletal system.

At birth, the infant has significant torsion in the lower extremities. Intrauterine positioning may be a contributing factor to the degree of bowleggedness or *genu varum* in the infant and young child. Bowleggedness, or *genu varum,* is a normal condition until 2½ to 3 years of age (Figure 18-9). It is the most common cause of in-toeing in children less than 3 years of age, and normally resolves with growth. Observation of gait, particularly watching the young child walk from the rear view, is important in evaluating the impact of *genu varum* on motor development and performance. Genu varum or bowing after 2½ to 3 years that is severe can be the result of nutritional deficiencies or obesity in young children and may require further evaluation.

To evaluate the young child or school-age child for *tibial torsion,* a curvature or twisting

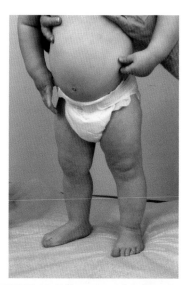

FIGURE 18-9 Genu varum (bowleggedness).

of the tibia also often referred to as *bowleg-gedness*, the child should be examined wearing only underwear and be seated with the legs dangling freely from a chair or exam table (Figure 18-10). The provider places a thumb and forefinger on the lateral and medial malleoli with the knee facing forward to determine the degree of rotation and flexibility of the tibia. The forefoot and hindfoot should be in line with the knees. On inspection, only the anterior edge of the lateral malleolus should be in the midline. Tibial torsion generally resolves with growth and is common until 4 or 5 years of age. Therefore, reassuring the parent is an important component of anticipatory guidance.

Genu valgum, or knock-knee, should be evaluated with the child standing and is present if the medial malleoli are more than an inch apart when the knees are touching. Genu valgum is normal until 7 years of age and resolves in middle childhood with the rotational development of the lower extremities (Figure 18-11). Persistence of genu valgum may be familial or the result of childhood obesity, and if persistent may require further evaluation and referral.

Gower sign is a screening test for muscle weakness in children and is characterized by a child moving from a sitting position to standing by facing prone and the grasping on the legs and hip with the hands until they are

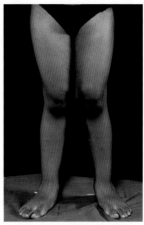

FIGURE 18-11 Genu valgum (knock-knee). (From Chaudhry B, Harvey D: *Mosby's color atlas and text of pediatrics and child health,* St. Louis, 2001, Mosby.)

erect. It is an early sign of a neuromuscular abnormality often associated with *Duchenne muscular dystrophy.*

Assessment of the feet in the infant includes the position and alignment of the forefoot and heels and the range of motion of the ankle and plantar arch. Limited dorsiflexion, or a fixed position of the hindfoot, is abnormal in the newborn, as is adduction of the forefoot and may be diagnostic of *clubfoot.* Decreased range of motion or pain should be noted on exam and referred for further evaluation. With the infant supine and the knees flexed to 90 degrees, inspect the thigh-foot angle and evaluate any adduction of the forefoot past the midline, which may be diagnostic for *metatarsus adductus* (Figure 18-12 and 18-13). A foot that is rigid on range of motion requires further evaluation. A mild deformity with a flexible foot requires passive stretching, which consists of supporting the heel at a right angle to the leg and rotating and stretching the forefoot laterally.

Infants and toddlers do not develop a longitudinal arch until the second or third year of life. Lack of development of a longitudinal arch in the young child may indicate a generalized laxity of the ligaments or flat foot, *pes planus,* and a thorough assessment

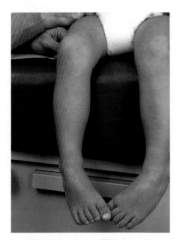

FIGURE 18-10 Tibial torsion.

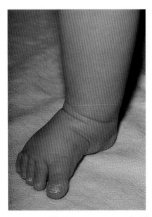

FIGURE 18-12 **Metatarsus varus (adduction of the forefoot).** (From Chaudhry B, Harvey D: *Mosby's color atlas and text of pediatrics and child health,* St. Louis, 2001, Mosby.)

of muscle tone is warranted. Pes planus is hereditary, and use of orthotics and referral is required for further evaluation if symptomatic. Older children may have physiological flat feet due to laxity of the ligaments (Figure 18-14). It is a normal variant and usually improves with age.

Hip

Developmental dysplasia of the hip (DDH) is a congenital or acquired condition involving an improper alignment of the radial head of the femur and the acetabulum. DDH is associated with a range of conditions. In hips that have inadequate formation of the acetabulum, the femoral head may be partially displaced outside the acetabulum. With more severe cases, it can

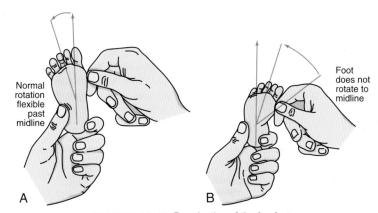

Normal rotation flexible past midline

Foot does not rotate to midline

A   B

FIGURE 18-13 **Examination of the forefoot.**

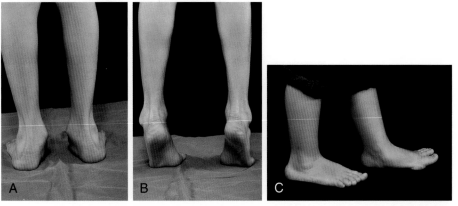

A   B   C

FIGURE 18-14 **A,** Physiological flat feet. **B,** Normal arch on tiptoe. **C,** Pes planus (flat foot). (From Chaudhry B, Harvey D: *Mosby's color atlas and text of pediatrics and child health,* St. Louis, 2001, Mosby.)

be displaced with force by clinical examination, indicating an unstable hip; or the femur may be completely dislocated outside the acetabulum.[3] With misalignment, the hip joint may grow abnormally and lead to premature degenerative joint disease, impaired walking, and pain.[4] Infants born in breech presentation, female infants, infants with a positive family history of DDH, and infants with a positive clinical examination have an increased risk for DDH.[5] The incidence of DDH in infants with risk factors is between 1% and 10%. In the newborn infant, congenital dysplasia of the hip resolves in 60% to 80% of infants with a positive clinical examination by 2 to 8 weeks of age.[4] Screening for DDH leads to earlier detection in affected infants. Proper management of DDH by the pediatric health care provider can limit the impact of DDH in adults. Nine percent of all primary hip replacements and up to 29% of hip replacement in adults up to 60 years of age are related to DDH.[3]

The examination of the hip in the newborn and growing infant is performed with the infant in the supine position with the knees flexed bilaterally and supported by the thumb and forefinger of the examiner, with the pad of the second finger on the bony prominence of the greater trochanter and the thumb near the lesser trochanter (Figure 18-15, *A*). With abduction of the thighs, pressure to the greater trochanter causes the hip to move from an unreduced to a reduced position if it is unstable. *Ortolani sign*, the presence of a *clunk* during the maneuver, is a positive sign for dislocation of the hip (Table 18-2). *Barlow test* also assists in detecting the unstable, dislocatable hip. With the infant supine and the knees flexed, the thigh is grasped and adducted while applying downward pressure (see Figure 18-15, *B*). With pressure on the acetabulum, the hip goes from a reduced position to a dislocated position. A dislocation of the femoral head is a positive Barlow. A *click* can occur during the maneuvers that may radiate from the knee and is often associated with crepitus of the joint, which is a normal finding. With the knees in the infant flexed to 90 degrees,

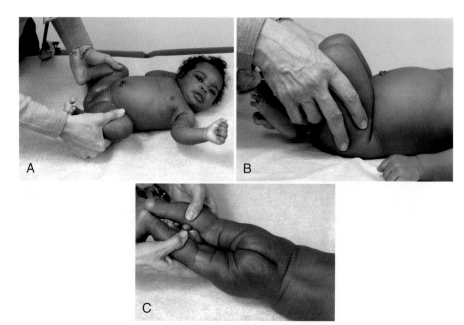

FIGURE 18-15 **A,** Ortolani sign. **B,** Barlow sign. **C,** Inspecting thigh folds.

TABLE 18-2   MUSCULOSKELETAL SCREENING TESTS

Age-Group	Techniques	Referral Criteria
Newborn and early infancy	Ortolani sign Barlow test Galeazzi or Allis sign Foot alignment	Presence of a clunk on abduction of hips Any instability of hip joints Knees when flexed are unequal in height Rigid foot with limited range of motion Rigid in-turning, inability of foot to assume normal angle to leg
Early childhood	Trendelenburg sign	When child bears weight, note any asymmetry in level of iliac crests With leg lifted, iliac crest drops, indicating hip abductor muscles on weight-bearing side are weak
Middle childhood to adolescence	Forward bend test	Asymmetrical elevation of scapula or rib hump; unequal shoulders or iliac crests, uneven waistline A spinal rotation of 5 to 7 degrees should be evaluated
Newborn to adolescence	Flexion of neck Brudzinski sign Kernig sign	Nuchal rigidity—Resistance or pain when neck is flexed when lying supine Involuntary flexion of knees or legs when neck is flexed when lying supine Resistance to or pain on straightening knees or legs from flexed position when lying supine

Data from Chin KR, Price JS, Zimbler S: A guide to early detection of scoliosis, *Contemp Pediatr* 18(9):77-103, 2001.

inspect for symmetry. The knees should be equally aligned. Any asymmetry of the knees is abnormal and may indicate a subluxated or dislocated hip that requires further evaluation. With the infant prone, inspect for the symmetry of the thigh folds (see Figure 18-15, *C*). Asymmetry should be noted, but it is not highly correlated with hip abnormality. Examination of the hips is indicated until an infant is walking independently without support and gait is normal. Box 18-2 presents current recommendations on examination of the hips in infancy.

Examination of the hip in middle childhood and adolescence begins with observation of the standing posture. The height of the iliac crests should be level or equal, and the child should be able to stand on one foot without any tilting of the pelvis.[6] A positive *Trendelenburg sign* is noted when the iliac crest drops, indicating weak hip abductor muscles on the weight-bearing side. The range of motion of the hips should be evaluated with the child or adolescent lying supine. With the hip and knee

BOX 18-2   RECOMMENDATIONS FOR SCREENING FOR DEVELOPMENTAL DYSPLASIA OF HIP IN INFANTS

- All newborns should be routinely screened for DDH by physical examination of hips.
- Ultrasonography of all newborns is not recommended.
- Perform examination of hips until the infant is an established walker.
- Record and document physical findings.
- Assess for changes in physical exam and for signs of DDH.
- If physical findings raise suspicion of DDH or parental concern, refer to a pediatric orthopedic specialist for further evaluation.

fully flexed, rotate the hip joint internally and externally and note any pain or asymmetry in range of motion. Any abnormal findings should be further investigated and referred if indicated.

Predisposing factors for unstable hips:
- Mother is a primipara
- Infant is female
- Positive family history
- Breech presentation
- Other congenital anomalies

Knee

The knee is a common site for both overuse and injury in middle childhood and adolescence. The symmetry and range of motion of the knee should be assessed initially with the child standing. The *patella* should be observed for any abnormal tilt or alignment from the midline. The remainder of the knee examination should be performed with the child lying supine on the exam table. The *patella* should be evaluated while supine for evidence of hypermobility. Joint line tenderness or pain may indicate a *meniscal tear.*[6] Congenital dislocation of the knee, or *patella,* is rare and manifests as limited knee motion in the newborn. Children and youth with a history of knee pain or laxity, as well as those who are unable to fully squat and perform a duck walk require further evaluation and referral. Inspect and palpate knee for any swelling, obvious deformity, incomplete range of motion on medial or lateral rotation, as well as signs of *ligamentous* laxity.

A common complaint of adolescent athletes is medial or anterior patellar pain with exercise or prolonged sitting, and pain or buckling when ascending or descending the stairs. Pain may be elicited on exam; however, findings may also be relatively normal. Sudden traumatic injury of the knee in the young athlete is common, particularly in adolescent females. The following maneuvers may help the pediatric health care provider identify and diagnosis problems with the knee and assist in decision making regarding the need for imaging or referral (Figure 18-16). The maneuvers should be performed bilaterally beginning with the noninjured knee. Some variation in the flexibility and laxity of the joints is normal. Positive findings on knee maneuvers are noted in the following sections.

Lachman Test

- To assess the anterior cruciate ligament (ACL), the knee should be flexed 20 to 30 degrees with the child or adolescent lying supine. With the muscles relaxed, stabilize the femur with one hand while pulling the tibia anteriorly with the dominant hand. Note how far the tibial tubercle moves anteriorly. There should be a firm endpoint. Compare with the unaffected knee.
- **Positive finding:** Excessive movement of the tibial tubercle anteriorly or forward from the neutral position indicates a partial or complete tear of the ACL.[6]

Anterior/Posterior Drawer Test

- To assess the ACL and posterior cruciate ligament (PCL) for efficiency or injury, the hips should be flexed to 45 degrees and the knees flexed to 90 degrees with the child lying supine. The foot should be stabilized on the exam table in a neutral position with the examiner sitting on the child's foot. With the hamstrings relaxed, pull the tibia anteriorly (anterior drawer test) and then move it posteriorly (posterior drawer test) from the neutral position (see Figure 18-16, *A*).
- **Positive finding:** Excessive movement of the tibia anteriorly from the neutral position or lack of a firm endpoint indicates ACL insufficiency. Excessive posterior tibial sag suggests PCL insufficiency.[6] The PCL is normally placed anterior to the femur with the knee flexed to 90 degrees. Significant laxity on exam suggests a tear of the anterior or posterior cruciate ligament.

Varus/Valgus Stress Test

- To assess the stability of the medial collateral ligament (MCL) and lateral collateral

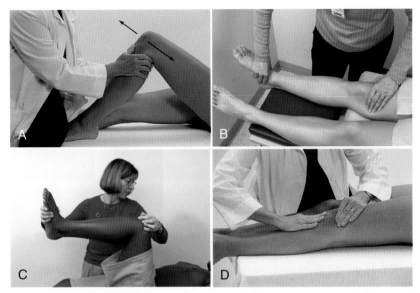

FIGURE 18-16 Examination of the knee. **A,** Drawer test. **B,** Varus/valgus stress test with knee extended. **C,** McMurray test. **D,** Ballottement/bulge test. (**A** and **D,** From Wilson S, Giddens J: *Health assessment for nursing practice,* ed 4, St. Louis, 2009, Mosby.)

ligament (LCL), the knee should be at 0 degrees with the child lying supine and the femur and the ankle stable on the exam table. With the examiner's hand stabilizing the knee joint anteriorly, lift the knee to 20 to 30 degrees and apply varus stress to the tibia. Then move the hand to the posterior side of the knee and apply valgus stress to the knee (see Figure 18-16, *B*).

- Note: For valgus stress, push on the lateral knee, stabilizing at the medial malleolus. For the varus test, push on the medial knee while stabilizing the lateral malleolus.
- **Positive finding**: Lateral knee pain or excessive varus movement of the tibia indicates injury to the LCL. Medial knee pain or increased valgus movement with lack of a firm endpoint indicates injury to the MCL. Laxity or opening in the joint space suggests a tear of the MCL or LCL.

McMurray Test

- Assess the medial and lateral meniscus with the child lying supine, flex the knee

to 90 degrees while supporting the foot and lower leg. Stabilize the medial and lateral joint lines of the knee with thumb and forefinger (see Figure 18-16, *C*). Using the other hand, rotate the tibia medially (valgus force) to test medial meniscus and laterally (varus force) to test the lateral meniscus while extending the knee to 90 degrees.

- **Positive finding:** Any clicking or pain along the medial joint line indicates a medial meniscus tear. A click or pain along the lateral joint indicates a lateral meniscus tear.

Ballottement of Patella Test

- Ballottement sign: With the child lying supine and the knee fully extended, the examiner applies downward pressure on the suprapatellar pouch to force fluid between the patella and the femur and then pushes the patella downward against the femur (see Figure 18-16, *D*).
- **Positive finding:** If patella floats back to the neutral position, fluid is present.

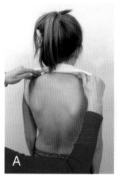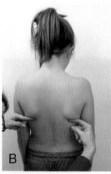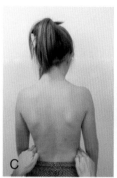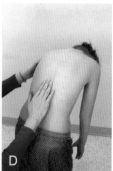

FIGURE 18-17 Assessment of the spine. **A,** Testing shoulder symmetry. **B,** Scapular symmetry. **C,** Iliac crest symmetry. **D,** Beginning Adams forward bend test.

A palpable click of the patella striking the femur on downward pressure is positive for knee joint effusion.

Spine

The spine should be inspected and palpated to note any congenital abnormalities such as hair tufts, dimples, a sacral sinus, or hemangiomas that could indicate spinal abnormalities. Inspection of the spine begins with the child or adolescent standing facing away from the examiner. Assess for the contour of the back, the symmetry of the shoulders, the shape and/or prominence of the scapula and ribs, and the symmetry of the waistline and the iliac crests (Figure 18-17, *A, B,* and *C*). The head should be aligned directly over the sacrum because any deviation from the midline may indicate a spinal deformity. Range of motion of the spine is evaluated by asking the child or adolescent to bend to the side, flex, and extend. An elevated scapula, an uneven waistline, or the presence of a rib hump indicates a positive finding (Figure 18-18) (see Table 18-2). More than five café au lait spots or the presence of axillary freckles suggest *neurofibromatosis.*

Beginning in early childhood, children develop a normal curvature of the spine with *lordosis* of the neck and lumbar region and *kyphosis* of the thorax. An exaggerated *lordosis* is normal in the young child. Viewing the child or adolescent from the side allows the examiner to evaluate normal alignment. Evaluation of SMR or Tanner stage is key to determining skeletal and spinal maturity.

Adams Forward Bend Test

- The child or adolescent should bend forward and touch the toes if possible with hands dangling or in a diving position (see Figure 18-17, *D*). Observe for alignment of spine, any curvature, asymmetry, or rib hump from the rear and sides. A level ruler or *scoliometer* can be used to assess the angle of trunk rotation. Place the scoliometer on the

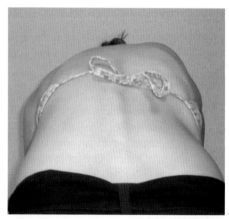

FIGURE 18-18 Positive rib hump. (From Skirven T, Osterman A, Fedorczyk J, et al: *Rehabilitation of the hand and upper extremity,* ed 6, Philadelphia, 2012, Mosby.)

trunk at the peak of the curvature to evaluate alignment.

- **Positive findings:** A rotation of 5 to 7 degrees should be further evaluated.

DIAGNOSTIC PROCEDURES

Concern over the relationship of frequent cumulative exposure to radiological diagnostic procedures and later health effects into adulthood have prompted pediatric health care providers to adopt As Low As Reasonably Achievable (ALARA) and an Image Gently policy in most pediatric health care settings.[7] Computed tomography (CT) has been used more judiciously in the pediatric population as a diagnostic tool following injury or for acute and chronic health conditions in nonurgent situations.

Bone age radiographs of the secondary ossification centers at the end of the long bones are used to assess growth rate in children who lag behind in height velocity compared to the norm or who have delayed onset of puberty. A *bone scan* is used to evaluate unequal leg length.

PREPARTICIPATION SPORTS PHYSICAL

Preparticipation Sports History

The primary purpose of the preparticipation sports physical exam is to exclude or restrict the young athlete with a temporary or permanent contraindication from participation in competitive sports. Additionally, the pediatric health care provider can help match the athlete to the appropriate type and level of sport and can help prevent injury by recommending the appropriate stretching or strengthening exercises. The *preparticipation physical evaluation (PPE)* is often the healthy adolescent's only contact with a pediatric health care provider during an important period of physical and psychosocial growth and development. Therefore the PPE should incorporate routine health maintenance as well as confidential psychosocial screening. It is important to evaluate any risks related to sports participation and use the encounter as an opportunity for anticipatory guidance regarding reproductive health and in encouraging positive health behaviors.

The PPE is also an opportunity for the pediatric health care provider to evaluate risky health practices related to participation in sports, particularly unhealthy weight loss or weight gain (Box 18-3). Sports such as wrestling, boxing, and martial arts are graded by weight class, which creates significant pressure on the young athlete to maximize body strength and bulk. There are equally powerful pressures on dancers and gymnasts to maintain a low weight. By contrast, youth playing positions such as linebacker in football may want to increase weight gain, even if their body mass index (BMI) is over the 95th percentile for age. Information gathering during the PPE should include satisfaction with or concerns about weight. Athletes should also be questioned about such practices as severe food restriction, binging or purging, weight loss, or muscle-enhancing supplements, including medications containing *ephedra, creatine,* and anabolic steroids or their analogs. Tables 18-3 and 18-4 present a review of systems and medical conditions related to participation in competitive sports.

To perform the PPE, the young pubertal female athlete should be examined in gym shorts and sports bra, and young males should be in gym shorts to ensure a thorough assessment of the joints and muscles. A 14-step orthopedic exam is included in the PPE to assess the athlete's musculoskeletal health (Figure 18-19). The components of the 14-point orthopedic examination are as follows:

1. With the young athlete standing, assess for frontal symmetry of trunk, shoulders, and extremities.
2. Assess neck flexion, extension, lateral flexion side to side, and rotation to evaluate range of motion of cervical spine.
3. Assess trapezius strength by having the young athlete shrug shoulders against resistance from the practitioner.
4. Assess deltoid strength by having the young athlete abduct the shoulders against resistance from the practitioner.

BOX 18-3 FOCUSED HISTORY FOR PREPARTICIPATION PHYSICAL EVALUATION FOR THE MIDDLE CHILDHOOD AND ADOLESCENCE

Current Medical History	Past Medical History	Family History	Dietary History
• Sport youth intends to play, including position and weight class if relevant • Any medications used by the youth, including diet supplements, creatine, anabolic steroids and their analogs, *macrolide antibiotics, tricyclic antidepressants, neuroleptics* • Any chronic illnesses, including asthma, how controlled, and any exacerbations during exercise	• Any previous experience in the same or other sports, including previous injuries, especially injuries requiring exclusion for >1 week • Any history of shortness of breath, syncope, or chest pain during exertion • History of seizures, including type, frequency, controlling medication, and past complications • *For young women:* Age of menarche, regularity of menses, and any prior disturbances of menses during sports	• Family history of cerebrovascular accident (CVA) or myocardial infarction (MI) before age 50 years • Any family history of sudden, unexplained death in adolescent or young adult relative • Family history of hypertrophic cardiomyopathy (HCM), prolonged QT syndrome, Marfan syndrome, or other cardiac/circulatory abnormalities	• Are you happy with current weight? Want to gain or lose for sport? • *Weight loss methods:* Ask explicitly: any bingeing, purging, restricting? • Fruits/vegetables daily? Milk or calcium intake? • Fluids for hydration (water, sports drinks, sodas, caffeine intake)? • Supplements, medications for weight loss, weight gain, muscle gain?

5. Assess internal and external rotation of shoulder to evaluate range of motion of the glenohumeral joints.

6. Assess range of motion of the elbows by having young athlete perform flexion and extension of the arms.

7. Assess range of motion of the wrists and elbows by observing pronation and supination of the forearm.

8. Assess range of motion of the hands and fingers by having the young athlete clench the fist and spread the fingers.

9. Assess symmetry from the rear with the young athlete standing.

10. Have the young athlete stand with knees straight and then flex forward and bend backward to assess any discomfort of the lumbar spine.

11. Perform Adams forward bend test by having the young athlete bend forward and touch the toes if possible with hands dangling or in a diving position. Assess for rib hump or asymmetry.

12. To assess for symmetry of leg musculature, have the young athlete stand facing the practitioner with quadriceps flexed.

13. Assess hip, knee, and ankle range of motion, strength, and balance by having the young athlete duck walk four steps.

14. Assess calf strength, symmetry, and balance by having the young athlete stand on heels and then toes.

TABLE 18-3   REVIEW OF SYSTEMS FOR PREPARTICIPATION PHYSICAL
EVALUATION FOR MIDDLE CHILDHOOD AND ADOLESCENCE

System	Disorders
HEENT	Otitis externa, frequent otitis media (OM), allergic rhinitis?
Respiratory	Shortness of breath (SOB), wheezing with exercise?
Cardiovascular	SOB, chest pain, dizziness, syncope with exertion, palpitations with exertion?
Gastrointestinal	Pain or reflux with exercise? Current/chronic problems with diarrhea, constipation?
Genitourinary	*For males:* History or symptoms of hernias, lumps or masses in groin or testicles? *For females:* Menstrual history (menarche, length, regularity of cycles, missed cycles during sports)? Last menstrual period (LMP)?
Musculoskeletal	Instability of any joints (especially shoulder, knee, ankle)? Leg or foot pain with exercise? Swelling of joints? Any weakness?
Neurological	Headaches, dizziness, seizures, recent concussions, recent injuries, weakness, difficulties with sleep, cognitive function, emotional regulation, balance or gait?
Dermatological	*Lesions:* Recent history of herpes, fungal infections, bacterial infections? Extent of acne and usual treatments? Eczema, reaction of skin to perspiration or athletic equipment?

HEENT, Head, eyes, ears, nose, and throat.

TABLE 18-4   MEDICAL CONDITIONS AND LEVEL OF SPORTS PARTICIPATION

Condition	Level of Sports Participation and Rationale
Bleeding disorder	Qualified yes*
Cardiovascular disease	
Carditis (inflammation of the heart)	No May result in sudden death with exertion
Hypertension (high blood pressure)	Qualified yes*
Congenital heart disease (structural heart defects present at birth)	Qualified yes* Those with mild forms may participate fully; those with moderate or severe forms or those who have undergone surgery need evaluation
Dysrhythmia (irregular heart rhythm)	Qualified yes* Those with symptoms (chest pain, syncope, dizziness, shortness of breath) or evidence of mitral valve regurgitation (leaking) need evaluation; all others may participate fully
Heart murmur	Qualified yes* If innocent, full participation is permitted; otherwise, the athlete needs evaluation
Cerebral palsy	Qualified yes*
Diabetes mellitus	Yes Blood glucose concentration should be monitored every 30 minutes during continuous exercise and 15 minutes after completion of exercise
Diarrhea	Qualified no* Unless mild, no participation is permitted, may increase risk of dehydration

Continued

TABLE 18-4   MEDICAL CONDITIONS AND LEVEL OF SPORTS PARTICIPATION—CONT'D

Condition	Level of Sports Participation and Rationale
Eating disorders	
Anorexia nervosa	Qualified yes*
Bulimia nervosa	Qualified yes*
Fever	No
	Increases cardiopulmonary effort, reduces maximum exercise capacity, makes heat illness more likely, and increases orthostatic hypertension during exercise
Hepatitis/HIV	Yes
	All sports may be played that athlete's state of health allows; skin lesions should be covered properly, and universal precautions used when handling blood or body fluids with visible blood
Musculoskeletal disorders	Qualified yes*
Neurological disorders	Qualified yes*
History of serious head or spine trauma, severe or repeated concussions, or craniotomy	Research supports conservative approach to management of concussion, with gradual return to play only when asymptomatic. Athletes with multiple concussions may need an extended time away from sports
Seizure disorder	
Well-controlled	Yes
	Risk of seizure during participation is minimal
Poorly-controlled	Qualified yes*
	Archery, riflery, swimming, weight or power lifting, strength training, or sports involving heights should be avoided because occurrence of a seizure may pose risk to self or others
Obesity	Qualified yes*
Organ transplant recipient	Qualified yes*
Respiratory conditions	
Pulmonary compromise, including cystic fibrosis	Qualified yes*
Asthma	Yes
	Only most severe asthma requires modified participation
Acute upper respiratory infection	Qualified yes*
	Individual assessment required for all but mild disease
Sickle cell disease or trait	Qualified yes*
	Carefully condition, acclimatize, and hydrate to reduce any possible risk
Skin disorders	Qualified yes*
Boils, herpes simplex, impetigo, scabies, molluscum contagiosum	While contagious, participation in gymnastics with mats; martial arts; wrestling; or other collision, contact, or limited-contact sports is not allowed

Adapted from Rice SG: Medical conditions affecting sports participation, *Pediatrics* 121(4):841-848, 2008; Halstead ME, Walter KD: American academy of pediatrics. Clinical report—sport-related concussion in children and adolescents, *Pediatrics* 126(3):597-615, 2010.
*Patient needs evaluation.

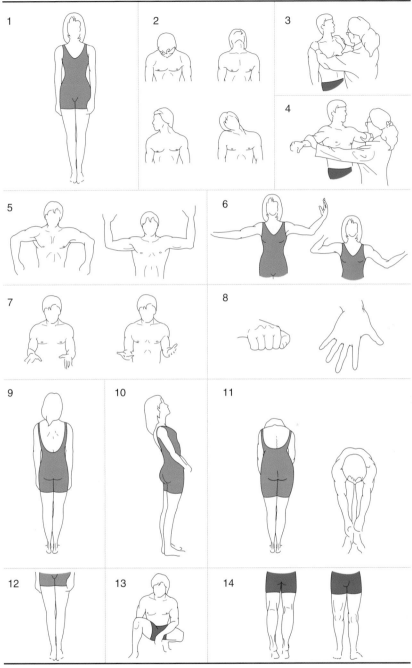

FIGURE 18-19 14-step orthopedic examination. (Adapted from American Academy of Family Physicians, American Academy of Pediatrics, American College of Sports Medicine, American Medical Society for Sports Medicine, American Orthopedic Society for Sports Medicine, American Osteopathic Academy of Sports Medicine: *PPE: preparticipation physical evaluation,* ed 4, Elk Grove, IL, 2010, American Academy of Pediatrics.)

Cardiac Preparticipation Physical Evaluation

The American Heart Association (AHA) recommends the PPE include (1) auscultation for heart murmurs, (2) palpation for femoral pulses to assess for coarctation of the aorta, (3) evaluation for the physical findings of *Marfan syndrome,* and (4) blood pressure evaluation of the brachial artery in sitting position.[6] The AHA also recommends gathering a detailed family history and personal history to identify asymtopmatic young athletes with underlying cardiac disease[6] (Box 18-4).

In young athletes, *hypertrophic cardiomyopathy,* a cardiovascular condition caused by an asymmetrical left ventricular hypertrophy and a nondilated left ventricle with impaired diastolic function, is the leading cause of sudden cardiac death. *Sudden cardiac death* is defined as a nontraumatic death by cardiac arrest within 6 hours of a previous state of good health.[8] The incidence is thought to be 1 in 200,000 high school athletes and 1 in 65,000 college athletes. Generally, no evidence of cardiac disease is present before sudden cardiac death. Other cardiac conditions implicated in sudden cardiac death include anomalous coronary arteries, Marfan syndrome, prolonged QT interval, and cardiac *dysrhythmias.* Any findings on physical examination, which include hypertension, absence of femoral pulses, signs of stigmata of Marfan syndrome, or auscultation of heart murmur, would indicate the need for referral to pediatric cardiovascular specialists.[9]

BOX 18-4   AHA RECOMMENDATIONS FOR PREPARTICIPATION CARDIOVASCULAR SCREENING OF COMPETITIVE ATHLETES*

Personal History
1. Exertional chest pain/discomfort
2. Unexplained syncope/near-syncope[†]
3. Excessive exertional and unexplained dyspnea/fatigue, associated with exercise
4. Prior recognition of a heart murmur
5. Elevated systemic blood pressure

Family History
6. Premature death (sudden and unexpected, or otherwise) before age 50 years due to heart disease, in ≥1 relative
7. Disability from heart disease in a close relative <50 years of age
8. Specific knowledge of certain cardiac conditions in family members: hypertrophic or dilated cardiomyopathy, long-QT syndrome or other ion channelopathies, Marfan syndrome, or clinically important arrhythmias

Physical Examination
9. Heart murmur[‡]
10. Femoral pulses to exclude aortic coarctation
11. Physical stigmata of Marfan syndrome
12. Brachial artery blood pressure (sitting position)[§]

Adapted from Siddiqui S, Patel DR: Cardiovascular screening of adolescent athletes, *Pediatric Clin North Am* 57(3):635-647, 2010.
*Parental verification is recommended for high school and middle school athletes.
[†]Judged not to be neurocardiogenic (vasovagal); of particular concern when related to exertion.
[‡]Auscultation should be performed in both supine and standing positions (or with Valsalva maneuver), specifically to identify murmurs of dynamic left ventricular outflow tract obstruction.
[§]Preferably taken in both arms.

SPORTS INJURIES

Sports injuries can be classified as traumatic *(macrotrauma)*, usually from collision or contact sports such as basketball, football, or soccer, or as overuse *(microtrauma)* (Table 18-5). The pediatric health care provider should assess the level of sports participation, recreational versus competitive sports, that young athletes are involved in when gathering history about injuries. Young athletes who play high-contact sports such as football, basketball, and soccer should be screened for history of previous concussion, fractures, and ligament damage. Athletes who participate in lower-contact sports, such as running or swimming, should be screened for repetitive motion and overuse injuries to the shoulder, knee, elbow, or shin (tibia).

Children who are overweight or obese have a higher number of reported fractures, more musculoskeletal discomfort, and impaired mobility. The incidence of lower extremity malalignment predisposing children and adolescents of injury are also more prevalent in overweight

TABLE 18-5   CLASSIFICATION OF SPORTS BY STRENUOUSNESS*

	A. Low Dynamic	B. Moderate Dynamic	C. High Dynamic
I. Low static	Billiards Bowling Cricket Curling Golf Riflery	Baseball/softball[†] Fencing Table tennis Volleyball	Badminton Cross-country skiing (classic technique) Field hockey[†] Orienteering Race walking Racquetball/squash Running (long distance) Soccer[†] Tennis
II. Moderate static	Archery Auto racing[†‡] Diving[†‡] Equestrian[†‡] Motorcycling[†‡]	Fencing Field events (jumping) Figure skating[†] Football (American)[†] Rodeoing[†‡] Rugby[†] Running (sprint) Surfing[†‡] Synchronized swimming[†]	Basketball[†] Ice hockey[†] Cross-country skiing (skating technique) Lacrosse[†] Running (middle distance) Swimming Team handball
III. High static	Bobsledding/luge[†‡] Field events (throwing) Gymnastics[†‡] Martial arts[†] Sailing Sports climbing Waterskiing[†‡] Weight lifting[†‡] Windsurfing[†‡]	Body building[†‡] Downhill skiing[†] Skateboarding[†‡] Snowboarding[†‡] Wrestling[†]	Boxing[†] Canoeing/kayaking Cycling[†‡] Decathlon Rowing Speed skating[†‡] Triathlon[†‡]

Adapted from Rice SG: Medical conditions affecting sports participation, *Pediatrics* 121(4):841-848, 2008.
*Classification of sports is based on peak dynamic and static components during competition.
[†]Danger of bodily collision.
[‡]Increased risk if syncope occurs.

than nonoverweight children and adolescents.[10] A young athlete's sexual maturity rating (SMR) or Tanner stage is also relevant to injury and the mechanism for injury. Rapid growth during adolescence, particularly during Tanner stage 3 in females and Tanner stage 4 in males, results in decreased strength in the growth plates, leading to greater potential for injury. Young athletes at Tanner stage 3 with relative good muscle strength yet incomplete ossification of the growth plate are predisposed to physeal (growth plate) fractures. Because injuries may recur from season to season, young athletes with a history of repetitive injuries such as frequent ankle sprain should be given strengthening exercises at the time of the PPE to help prevent future injury. For most adolescents, the physical and social benefits of carefully monitored sports participation outweigh the risks, including adolescents with chronic health conditions and special health care needs.

Pediatric Pearls

Ligaments are stronger than bones until adolescence; therefore, injuries to long bones and joints in the preadolescent are more likely to cause fractures rather than sprains.

Sports-Related Concussions

Concussions are common, often unrecognized, and usually do not involve loss of consciousness.[6] *Concussion* is defined as any impact to the brain, face, or neck resulting in rapid onset of neurological symptoms, with or without loss of consciousness, with spontaneous (though often delayed) resolution.[11] There has been an increased focus on the immediate and long-term sequelae of concussion or *traumatic brain injury* (TBI) in the pediatric and adolescent athlete that is due to their increased in participation in high-impact competitive sports. It has been estimated that by the time a young athlete reaches high school, 53% will have reported a history of concussion.[6] Athletes

younger than 18 years take longer to recover from concussion than older athletes. The short sequelae of concussion may include *postconcussion syndrome,* which can last for weeks to months, and *second impact syndrome* if a second head injury occurs during the postconcussion period. The long-term sequelae of concussion include permanent neurological deficits such as decreased cognitive functioning and limiting cognitive potential.[6]

Current guidelines for concussion recommend cognitive rest in addition to exclusion from play until completely asymptomatic with a gradual return to play after symptoms resolve.[11] Information gathered during the PPE should include screening questions related to prior concussions and related symptoms, including any headaches, or cognitive, emotional, or sleep impairment. See Box 18-5 for signs and symptoms of concussion. Appendix H

BOX 18-5   Signs and Symptoms of Concussion

Cognitive Symptoms
- Confusion
- Posttraumatic amnesia
- Disorientation
- Difficulty focusing
- Excessive drowsiness
- Delayed verbal or motor responses
- Slurred or incoherent speech
- Vacant stare
- Loss of consciousness

Physical Symptoms
- Headache
- Fatigue
- Nausea and vomiting
- Visual disturbance
- Phonophobia

Affective Symptoms
- Irritability
- Emotionally labile

Data from Bernhardt DT, Roberts WO: *PPE: Preparticipation physical evaluation*, ed 4, Elk Grove, IL, 2010, American Academy of Pediatrics.

includes the *Sports Concussion Assessment Tool 2 (SCAT2)* for evaluation of young athletes 10 years of age and older following history of head injury or concussion.

The Female Athlete

Female athletes are at higher risk than male athletes for certain musculoskeletal injuries such as noncontact ACL injuries, dislocation of the patella, and idiopathic scoliosis. The lowest intake of vitamin D and calcium are in female adolescents and female young adults. Eating disorders are also more common in female adolescents than male adolescents. Undernutrition in female adolescents can impair skeletal health and impact bone mineral density (BMD) in adulthood. Training intensity can also cause irregular menses and increase the occurrence of stress fractures in young female athletes. *Patellofemoral pain syndrome* is also more common in female athletes, and it often presents as complaints of anterior knee pain radiating from the posterior patella and biomechanical or physical changes in the patellofemoral joint. It is an overuse or overload injury occurring from repeated weight-bearing impact, and may be managed with rest and quadriceps strengthening exercises.

Young women with disordered eating in competitive sports should be screened for *female athlete triad* characterized by anorexia, amenorrhea, and osteopenia or osteoporosis. As many as 20% of female athletes meet one of the criteria for female athlete triad.[12] This triad in young female athletes begins with disordered eating that leads to amenorrhea (absence of menses), and eventually leads to osteoporosis (loss of bone mass), in some cases by the late teens or early 20s. This is a preventable condition and yet it is increasing in frequency because of the lack of understanding on the part of coaches, parents, and athletes regarding the triad symptoms. A strong competitive environment contributes to this serious safety issue. The pediatric health care provider also should be aware that long-distance runners and swimmers may have irregular menses during their sports seasons without necessarily having an eating disorder.

MUSCULOSKELETAL CONDITIONS

Table 18-6 presents the most common abnormal orthopedic conditions seen in infants, children, and adolescents by the pediatric health care practitioner.

TABLE 18-6   MUSCULOSKELETAL CONDITIONS

Condition	Description
Blount disease	Growth disorder of the tibia abnormal ossification of the proximal tibia, also known as *tibia vara*
Clubfoot	Rigidity of foot and inability of foot to right itself from fixed medial position
Talipes equinovarus	Inversion of forefoot, plantar flexion, and heel inversion
Talipes calcaneovalgus	Eversion and dorsiflexion of forefoot
Metatarsus adductus	*Varus* abnormality of forefoot at the tarso-metatarsal junction; ankle and hindfoot are normal; lateral border of foot is curved rather than straight, usually shaped like a "kidney bean;" line drawn medially from heel often intersects third toe
Pes planus (flat feet)	Flattening of longitudinal arch in school-age child when standing erect with full weight bearing on feet bilaterally; flat feet in early childhood are developmentally normal and often are accentuated by fat pad on ventral surface

Continued

TABLE 18-6   MUSCULOSKELETAL CONDITIONS—CONT'D

Condition	Description
Tibial torsion	Inward twisting or bowing of tibia and fibula, often a variation of normal rotational development; intrauterine position may be contributing factor; most common cause of in-toeing children <3 years of age; resolves with normal growth; continued reassurance to parent is important
Slipped femoral capital epiphysis	Proximal femoral epiphysis slips in a posterior and inferior direction over neck of femur; presenting symptoms are limp, knee or hip pain, particularly with strenuous activity; occurs more commonly between 8 and 16 years of age during rapid growth periods
Legg-Calvé-Perthes	Blood supply to femoral capital epiphysis is disturbed and produces avascular necrosis of femoral head; affects children 3 to 12 years of age, with peak incidence in males 4 to 8 years old; children may present with diffuse pain in hip, knee, or the upper thigh; may have history of intermittent limp; early diagnosis and management are key to preventing long-term sequelae
Femoral anteversion	Increased forward rotation of femoral head in relation to knee; may be exacerbated by child sitting in "W" position when playing, watching TV, or sleeping; common cause of in-toeing after 3 years of age; evaluate child when undressed and lying in prone position; note internal rotation of hip; resolution usually occurs after 7 years of age
Osgood-Schlatter syndrome	Inflammation of tibia causing swelling and tenderness at insertion of infrapatellar tendon into tibial tubercle; presents with knee pain after vigorous activity; common finding in adolescent athletes, especially 9 to 15 years of age
Osteogenesis inperfecta	Genetic bone disorder causing defect of connective tissue and deficiency of type I collagen resulting in brittleness of bone, spontaneous fractures, and short, bowed extremities. May result in hearing loss
Developmental dysplasia of the hip	Condition in which femoral head has abnormal relationship to acetabulum: unstable, subluxated, or dislocated; incidence of unstable hip 1/100 and 1 to 1.5/1000 for dislocation, incidence higher in girls; management ranges from observation of unstable hip to reduction and stabilization of dislocated hip with *Pavlik* harness
Idiopathic scoliosis	Lateral bending of spine and associated rotation of vertebral bodies; lateral curvature of >10 degrees indicates scoliosis; scoliometer reading of 7 degrees correlates with 20 degrees radiological curvature; 30% have positive family history

SUMMARY OF EXAMINATION

- Several factors influence the health of the bones such as adequate nutrition and protein in the diet, the amount of calcium intake, and adequate intake of vitamin D.
- Growth along the epiphyseal plate continues until the cells in the growth plate stop dividing in puberty, and closure of the growth plate occurs in young adults.
- Evaluating progression of the height growth curve is critical to assessing normal and abnormal growth patterns along with familial patterns of growth and pubertal development.
- Note any obvious gait abnormalities; observe posture when standing and sitting, assess proportion of upper extremities to lower extremities.

- Evaluate range of motion of joints and assess muscle tone of trunk and extremities.
- Evaluation of the lower extremities includes assessment of flexion/extension, adduction/abduction, and internal/external rotation.
- Observation of gait, particularly watching the young child walk from the rear view, is important in evaluating torsional variations of *genu varum* and *genu valgum.*
- Assessment of the hip in infant is performed in supine position with the knees flexed bilaterally and thumb and forefinger of examiner on the bony prominence of greater trochanter. *Ortolani sign* tests for dislocation of hip and *Barlow test* evaluates stability of hip.
- Knee assessment maneuvers should be performed bilaterally beginning with the noninjured knee. Some variation in the flexibility and laxity of knee joints is normal.
- Assess for contour of back, symmetry of shoulders, shape and/or prominence of scapula and ribs, and symmetry of iliac crests.
- Observe for alignment of spine with child or adolescent in forward bend position. Note any curvature, asymmetry, or rib hump from the rear and sides of the back.
- To perform the *preparticipation physical evaluation* (PPE), a 14-step orthopedic exam is included to assess the athlete's musculoskeletal health.
- The American Heart Association (AHA) recommends the PPE include (1) auscultation for heart murmurs; (2) palpation of femoral pulses; (3) evaluation for *Marfan syndrome;* and (4) blood pressure evaluation.

Charting

A Healthy Young Child

Extremities and Back: nl ROM (range of motion), mild tibial torsion and in-toeing bilaterally R > L, spine straight with mild lordosis.

REFERENCES

1. Porth CM, Matfin G: *Pathophysiology: concepts of altered health status,* Philadelphia, 2010, Wolters Kluwer/Lippincott Williams & Wilkins.
2. Hornor G: Physical abuse: recognition and reporting, *J Pediatr Health Care* 19(1):4-11, 2005.
3. Gelfer P, Kennedy KA: Developmental dysplasia of the hip, *J Pediatr Health Care* 22(5):318-322, 2008.
4. U.S. Preventive Service Task Force: Screening for developmental dysplasia of the hip: recommendation statement, *Pediatrics* 117(3):898-902, 2006.
5. de Hundt M, Vlemmix F, Bais JM, et al: Risk factors for developmental dysplasia of the hip: a meta-analysis, *Eur J Obstet Gynecol Reprod Biol* 165(1):8-17, 2012.
6. Bernhardt DT, Roberts WO: *PPE: preparticipation physical evaluation,* ed 4, Elk Grove Village, Ill., 2010, American Academy of Pediatrics.
7. Frush DP, Frush KS: The ALARA concept in pediatric imaging: building bridges between radiology and emergency medicine: consensus conference on imaging safety and quality for children in the emergency setting, *Pediatr Radiol* 36(2):121-125, 2010.
8. Siddiqui S, Patel DR: Cardiovascular screening of adolescent athletes, *Pediatr Clin North Am* 57(3):635-647, 2010.
9. Maron BJ, Thompson PD, Ackerman MJ, et al: Recommendations and considerations related to preparticipation screening for cardiovascular abnormalities in competitive athletes. American Heart Association Council on Nutrition, Physical Activity, and Metabolism, *Circulation* 115(12):1643-1655, 2007.
10. Taylor ED, Theim KR, Mirch MC, et al: Orthopedic complications of overweight in children and adolescents, *Pediatrics* 117(6):2167-2174, 2006.
11. Halstead ME, Walter KD: American Academy of Pediatrics. Clinical report—sport-related concussion in children and adolescents, *Pediatrics* 126(3):597-615, 2010.
12. Womack J: Give your sports physicals a performance boost, *J Fam Pract* 59(8):437-444, 2010.

CHAPTER 19

NEUROLOGICAL SYSTEM

Karen G. Duderstadt

For the pediatric health care provider, monitoring the development of the nervous system is one of the most important aspects of assessment in infants and children. The nervous system contains the most complex and delicate pathways in the body and is the center of all vital bodily functions. The normal development of these pathways provides the vital motor, sensory, and cognitive functions that sustain human life and comprise human behavior. The challenge is to assess not only the progress of gross motor and fine motor skills in infants and children, but also to assess cognitive development and subtle deficits in attention and information processing that may impact learning behavior.

EMBRYOLOGICAL DEVELOPMENT

The formation of the nervous system begins very early during the third week of embryonic life. The early integral development is essential in influencing the organization and development of the skeleton, skeletal muscles, eyes and ears, and other body systems.[1] The *notochord*, which becomes the spinal column, develops during this period and forms the neural plate and neural folds. Closure of the neural plate is complete by the fourth week of embryonic development and the neural tube is formed. Any fetal insults that occur during this period can result in defects in the brain and spinal cord, such as *spina bifida* defects, which occur in 1 of 1000 live births. During the fifth week of fetal development, the anterior portion of the neural tube enlarges to form the segments of the brain. Brain growth proceeds, with the most rapid brain growth occurring between 15 and 20 weeks of gestation.

By 24 weeks of gestation, the fetus has developed all of the nerve cells, or neurons, needed for the formation of the neural pathways. The *neuron* is the basic unit of the nervous system, and each neuron contains numerous dendrites and one axon (Figure 19-1). Dendrites are the protoplasmic branches of the cell body. Neural impulses enter the cell body through the dendrites and leave through the single axon. They then connect by a series of synapses with another dendrite of the next axon. *Myelin*, a lipoid material surrounding cell fibers, covers only a portion of the axons at birth.

DEVELOPMENTAL VARIATIONS

The development of intelligence in infants depends on the normal progression through the two primary developmental domains—problem solving and language.[2] Brain growth is rapid after birth with 50% of postnatal brain growth achieved by 1 year of age. By 2 to 3 years of age, the brain is 80% of adult size.[1] Head circumference increases sixfold in the first year of life and is the best indication of normal brain growth. *Myelination*, the deposit of the protective fatty substance around the axons, continues in the brain throughout the first 2 years of life, and in the preterm infant continues into the third year of life. Myelination proceeds from head to toe, *cephalocaudal*, beginning with the spinal cord and cranial nerves and then from midline to fingertips, *proximodistal*, following with the brainstem, corticospinal tracts, and sensory pathways. Preterm or very low birth weight (VLBW) infants may develop from toe to head,

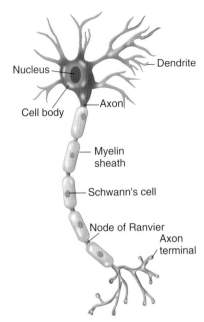

FIGURE 19-1 The neuron.

which is associated with persistent hypertonia in the lower extremities. The control of motor functions in infancy and early childhood is closely associated with the normal myelination of the nerve fibers.[1] Completion of brain growth occurs in early adolescence.

ANATOMY AND PHYSIOLOGY

Central Nervous System

Cerebrum

The outermost part of the brain is the *cerebral cortex,* which is often referred to as the gray matter because the neurons are unmyelinated and give a gray rather than a white appearance. The outer layer of the brain is composed of fissures and grooves, or *sulci,* and the ridge between grooves is the *gyrus.* The young infant has fewer convolutional surfaces, or sulci, in the cerebral cortex and more pliable skull bones. These characteristics decrease the incidence of bruising and tearing of the cerebral cortex in the young infant with minor head trauma. The sulci of the brain deepen throughout childhood

and continue to mature and change into young adulthood.

The *cerebrum* is the largest part of the brain and is covered by the cerebral cortex. The cerebrum is divided into two hemispheres, the left and right hemispheres, with the left hemisphere being dominant in 95% of individuals. The right hemisphere controls the functions of the left side of the body, and the left hemisphere controls the functions of the right side of the body. The hemispheres are connected by a bridge of myelinated axons, the *corpus callosum,* which lies between the fissures of the left and right hemispheres.[1] The corpus callosum controls and integrates motor, sensory, and higher intellectual functions. The right and left hemispheres are divided into four lobes with arbitrary borders named the same as the skull bones that cover them. Each lobe controls particular bodily functions and behaviors (Figure 19-2).

- **Frontal lobe:** Initiates movement control of the flexor muscles of hands and feet. *Broca area* in the frontal lobe controls the ability to articulate speech. Prefrontal area controls thought processes for anticipation and prediction of behavior, and the frontal region is involved in complex learning movement patterns and writing. Damage to the frontal region causes *expressive aphasia.*
- **Parietal lobe:** Controls processing and interpretation of sensory input—visual, auditory,

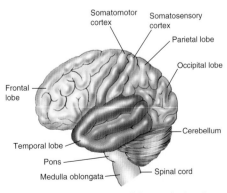

FIGURE 19-2 Regions of the cerebral cortex.

smell, taste, and touch sensations, including pain and temperature. Perceives where a stimulus or pressure is and on which part of the body, and provides *proprioception,* the sense of the position of the limbs of the body. Damage to the parietal region results in *agnosia,* an inability to recognize or perceive the meaningfulness of an object, persons, sounds, shapes, or smells.

- **Temporal lobe:** Primary center for the perception and interpretation of auditory input, auditory association and perception, and memory recall. Wernicke area in the temporal lobe is related to spoken words and language comprehension.
- **Occipital lobe:** Primary visual cortex in the brain and is the center for receiving and interpreting visual data and depth perception.

The *basal ganglia* are masses of myelinated axons that form a subcortical layer of white and gray matter through the central hemispheres. They border the lateral ventricle deep in the brain. The maturation of the basal ganglia occurs in early childhood, and they are involved in movement functions such as arm swinging during walking and running and throwing a ball overhand. Dysfunction of the basal ganglia results in abnormal postural movement patterns as in *cerebral palsy* and *Huntington chorea.*

Cerebellum

The *cerebellum* is located in the posterior cranium and has an outer layer of gray matter overlying white matter. The cerebellum maintains the body's equilibrium and coordinates both voluntary and involuntary movements of the limbs, trunk, head, larynx, and eyes.[1] The motor cortex in the cerebrum relays signals to the cerebellum, which results in the fluid and skilled muscle movements requiring a high level of dexterity. It is the portion of the brain that processes the sensory input from the musculoskeletal system as well as from the visual, auditory, and touch receptors, and it transmits signals to the motor system to direct or correct

muscle activity. Damage to the cerebellum causes *ataxia* (loss of coordination of motor movement, inability to perform rapid alternating movements, a wide-based gait), hypotonia, and nystagmus. In preterm infants, arrested development of the cerebellum can result in deficits in language, visual reception, and social/behavioral function.

Brainstem

The *brainstem* is in the central core of the brain and includes the *pons, medulla oblongata,* and *midbrain* (Figure 19-3). The *pons* acts as the neural transmission center from all parts of the central cortex and supports ascending and descending nerve fibers. It controls basic breathing, eating, and motor functions. Cranial nerve V *(trigeminal nerve)* and cranial nerve VI *(abducens nerve)* arise from the pons. Damage to the peripheral pons causes a loss of sensory functions of the facial and mouth area and a loss of outward or lateral motion of the eye muscles resulting in *strabismus.* The *medulla oblongata,* which lies between the pons and the cerebellum, is a continuation of the spinal cord. The medulla processes impulses from the hypoglossal, vagal, spinal accessory, glossophyarngeal, and the vestibular and acoustic cranial nerves. It also aids in the life functions of respiration and circulation, and controls involuntary reflexes such as coughing, sneezing, and yawning. Damage to the medulla

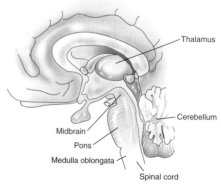

FIGURE 19-3 Brain and brainstem.

causes weakness in the shoulder muscles, affects tongue muscles and salivary function, decreases gastrointestinal motility, alters swallowing and speech functions, causes nerve deafness, and diminishes cardiovascular and respiratory functions.

The *diencephalon* (Figure 19-4) is the extension of the brainstem and lies embedded in the cerebral cortex. It contains the *thalamus, hypothalamus, pituitary gland,* and the *pineal gland* (an endocrine gland that produces melatonin, a hormone that regulates sleep-wake cycle). Parts of the third ventricle and the nuclei of the cranial nerves also arise from the diencephalon. The *midbrain* contains the neural fibers that come from the spinal cord and merge into the thalamus and hypothalamus. The *midbrain* controls the integration of basic bodily functions.

- **Thalamus:** Acts as the brain's relay station and receives input from the sensory and motor systems of the body and dispatches input to the appropriate region of the cerebral cortex.
- **Hypothalamus:** Regulates body temperature, metabolic processes, and involuntary response activity.
- **Pituitary gland:** Responsible for hormonal control of growth, lactation, and metabolism.

The *limbic system* is the group of subcortical structures in the diencephalon including the *hypothalamus* and the *hippocampus.* This system regulates emotion and motivation and organizes memories. Aggression and fear also are regulated by the limbic system. Disruption that occurs during the development of the limbic system causes distorted perceptions and aggressive behavior. Maternal substance abuse early in pregnancy can disrupt the migration of neuron activity in the cerebral cortex, and later prenatal exposure disrupts neuronal synapses. Children exposed to illicit drug use in utero often have disturbances in memory, learning, attention span, and oppositional behavior disorders.

Spinal Cord

The spinal cord is an extension of the medulla oblongata and is composed of gray and white matter extending to the lumbar region. The gray matter runs laterally along the spinal cord and protects the myelinated and unmyelinated fibers of the white matter. *Proprioceptors,* the specialized nerve endings in muscles, tendons, and joints, are located in the white matter and are sensitive to changes in the tension of muscles and tendons. Temperature, pain, touch, and equilibrium are transmitted through the proprioceptors to the brainstem.

The brain and spinal cord are lubricated by *cerebrospinal fluid,* normally a clear liquid that is formed in the ventricles of the brain. It flows from the lateral ventricles to the third and fourth ventricles through a series of foramens. The fourth ventricle, which lies in the medulla, contains three openings that allow the cerebrospinal fluid to pass into the subarachnoid space.

The brain is covered by protective layers that cushion and lubricate the outer surface (Figure 19-5). The *dura mater* lies just beneath the skull bone and periosteum and consists of layers of fibrous connective tissue. Adjacent to the dura mater is the *arachnoid,* the avascular, weblike membrane that cushions the cortex. The dura mater is separated from the arachnoid by the *subdural* space. The *pia mater* is the highly vascular area of the cortex that attaches directly to the gray matter or irregular surface of the brain.

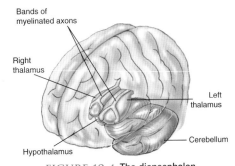

Bands of myelinated axons

Right thalamus

Left thalamus

Cerebellum

Hypothalamus

FIGURE 19-4 **The diencephalon.**

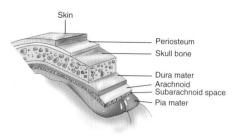

FIGURE 19-5 The meningeal layers.

The subarachnoid area and a cushion of cerebrospinal fluid separate the arachnoid from the pia mater.

Upper and Lower Motor Neurons

Upper motor neurons are located within the central nervous system and convey impulses from the motor areas of the cerebral cortex to the *lower motor neurons* in the spinal cord. They can influence the function of the lower motor neurons as evidenced in conditions such as *cerebral palsy.* The lower motor neurons are located primarily in the peripheral nervous system and provide pathways for nerve fibers to translate movement of the muscles into action. Muscle wasting can be the result of dysfunction in the anterior horn cells of the upper motor neurons. Dysfunction in the lower motor neurons can cause wasting of localized muscle groups and a soft rather than firm tone to the muscle mass. Acquired atrophy of the muscles accompanied by a wide-based gait and muscle weakness when arising from a sitting position is characteristic of *muscular dystrophy,* a developmental muscle wasting condition with onset in early childhood.

Peripheral Nervous System

The *spinal nerves* originate in the spinal cord and exit from the intervertebral spaces. They contain sensory and motor fibers, and with the cranial nerves and visceral fibers of the *autonomic nervous system* compose the pathways of the *peripheral nervous system.* The autonomic nervous system carries impulses to and from the central nervous system. It is divided into the *sympathetic* and *parasympathetic nervous systems* and is made up of unmyelinated nerves. The sympathetic nervous system activates in times of stress and provides increased energy for needed bursts of activity. The parasympathetic nervous system balances the activities of the sympathetic nervous system by restoring stability and maintaining reserve energy for daily bodily functions such as digestion and elimination.

Spinal Nerves

There are 32 pairs of *spinal nerves* that innervate the upper and lower torso, extremities, skin, and muscles (Figure 19-6). The spinal nerves form complex nerve networks called *plexuses.* There are four major plexuses in the peripheral nervous system—the cervical, brachial, lumbar, and sacral plexuses. The body surface that is innervated by the plexus of a spinal nerve is called a *dermatome.* Although dermatomes map specific segments of the body surface, spinal nerve sensation can be transmitted to adjacent dermatomes (see Figure 19-6). The sensory pathways of the spinal nerves carry sensations of touch, temperature, and pain; the motor fibers activate reflexes and impulses that control skeletal muscles and the involuntary muscles of the viscera. The spinal nerves function as part of the lower motor neurons and become dysfunctional in the presence of spinal cord lesions.

Spinal Reflexes

Reflex behavior provides the major assessment of brainstem function. A *reflex* is an expected response between a stimulus and an elicited motor response. The *reflex arc* operates outside the level of conscious control and is the basic defense mechanism of the nervous system. Reflexes help the body maintain appropriate muscle tension and react to painful or harmful stimuli. A stimulus creates an impulse that is transmitted instantaneously outward by the motor neurons of the spinal cord via the spinal nerve and peripheral nervous system to produce a brisk muscle contraction (Figure 19-7).

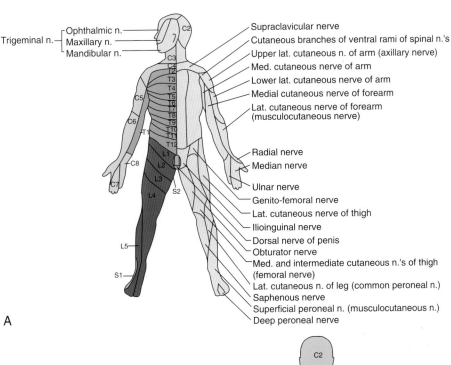

Trigeminal n. — ┌ Ophthalmic n.
                ├ Maxillary n.
                └ Mandibular n.

C2
C3
C4
T1
T2
T3
T4
T5
T6
T7
T8
T9
T10
T11
T12
L1
L2
L3
C5
C6
T1
C8
C7
L4
S2
L5
S1

Supraclavicular nerve
Cutaneous branches of ventral rami of spinal n.'s
Upper lat. cutaneous n. of arm (axillary nerve)
Med. cutaneous nerve of arm
Lower lat. cutaneous nerve of arm
Medial cutaneous nerve of forearm
Lat. cutaneous nerve of forearm
(musculocutaneous nerve)

Radial nerve
Median nerve
Ulnar nerve
Genito-femoral nerve
Lat. cutaneous nerve of thigh
Ilioinguinal nerve
Dorsal nerve of penis
Obturator nerve
Med. and intermediate cutaneous n.'s of thigh
(femoral nerve)
Lat. cutaneous n. of leg (common peroneal n.)
Saphenous nerve
Superficial peroneal n. (musculocutaneous n.)
Deep peroneal nerve

A

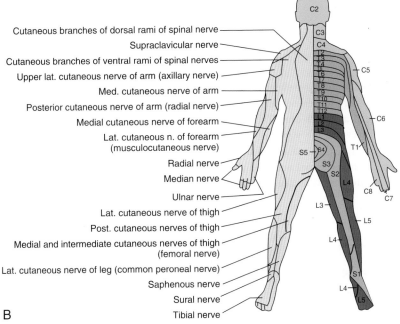

Cutaneous branches of dorsal rami of spinal nerve
Supraclavicular nerve
Cutaneous branches of ventral rami of spinal nerves
Upper lat. cutaneous nerve of arm (axillary nerve)
Med. cutaneous nerve of arm
Posterior cutaneous nerve of arm (radial nerve)
Medial cutaneous nerve of forearm
Lat. cutaneous n. of forearm
(musculocutaneous nerve)
Radial nerve
Median nerve
Ulnar nerve
Lat. cutaneous nerve of thigh
Post. cutaneous nerves of thigh
Medial and intermediate cutaneous nerves of thigh
(femoral nerve)
Lat. cutaneous nerve of leg (common peroneal nerve)
Saphenous nerve
Sural nerve
Tibial nerve

C2
C3
C4
T2
T3
T4
T5
T6
T7
T8
T9
T10
T11
T12
L1
L2
L3
C5
C6
S5
S4
S3
S2
T1
L4
C8
C7
L3
L5
L4
S1
L4
L5

B

FIGURE 19-6 The spinal nerves and dermatomes.

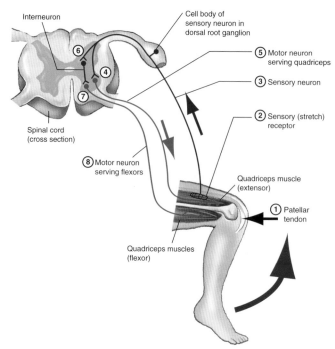

FIGURE 19-7 Reflex arc.

Cranial Nerves

The twelve *cranial nerves* originate in the cranium and supply motor and sensory function primarily to the head and neck area. The exception is cranial nerve X, the *vagus nerve,* which innervates part of the cardiac and abdominal viscera. Both the spinal and cranial nerves are myelinated nerves. The cranial nerves function by way of impulses conveyed from the motor and sensory pathways and the parasympathetic nervous system to the cerebral cortex.

PHYSIOLOGICAL VARIATIONS

Table 19-1 reviews the physical, developmental, and cognitive variations that occur during

TABLE 19-1 PHYSIOLOGICAL VARIATIONS DURING DEVELOPMENT

Age-Group	Physical Variations	Developmental Variations	Cognitive Variations
Preterm infant	Head lag persists for 6 months; myelination of brain continues until 3 years of age	Increased extensor tone in lower extremities; with marked stiffening and toe pointing	Sensorimotor reflexive response to stimulus
Newborn	Brain surface initially smooth at birth; cerebral cortex is half the adult thickness	Exhibits primitive reflexes until 3 to 4 months; requires strong stimulus to elicit response	Innate knowledge of environment, evokes survival response such as sucking

TABLE 19-1 PHYSIOLOGICAL VARIATIONS DURING DEVELOPMENT—CONT'D

Age-Group	Physical Variations	Developmental Variations	Cognitive Variations
Infancy	Head circumference increases sixfold in first year; in term infant, important myelination of brain continues until 2 years of age	*Plagiocephaly,* asymmetrical head, shape, is common; most often related to sleeping position; normally, resolves by 3 months	Develops mental image of hidden object; imitates sounds by 6 months
Early childhood (1 to 3 years of age)	Proprioception, awareness of spatial/body positions begins; increased movement and sphincter control	Develops basic self-control and ability to separate from attachment person; body exploration and realization of sexuality	Parallel play; independence increases; attention span develops
Early childhood (3 to 5 years of age)	Slowed growth, minimal change in head circumference; increased connectivity between neurons to initiate complex thought	Hand preference established; rapid fine motor development; gross motor athletic ability	Egocentric; aggressive behavior; one-dimensional understanding; magical thinking
Middle childhood	Brain reaches 90% of adult size by 5 to 7 years of age; deepening of sulci in brain, increasing complex thought	Transmission of nerve impulses improves, thereby enhancing fine motor and gross motor development	Consequential understanding; concrete operations and objective thought
Adolescence	Neurological development continues into adolescence	Defines self-concept; role diffusion causes conflict	Develops abstract thinking ability

the development and maturation of the nervous system in infancy and childhood.

FAMILY, CULTURAL, RACIAL, AND ETHNIC CONSIDERATIONS

Cultural practices may affect the progress of developmental milestones. Infants who are swaddled on a mother's back for the first year may stand and begin walking at a later age. Increased muscle tone is normally seen in African-American infants, with an equal balance between increased flexor and extensor tone. Decreased tone is common in Asian infants and is usually unbalanced with more extensor tone throughout movement.

SYSTEM-SPECIFIC HISTORY

The Information Gathering table reviews the pertinent areas for the neurological system for each age-group and developmental stage of childhood. Obtaining a complete history of gross motor and fine motor milestones in infancy, assessing speech and language development, and assessing learning ability is key to early identification of insults to the nervous system.

INFORMATION GATHERING FOR NEUROLOGICAL ASSESSMENT AT KEY DEVELOPMENTAL STAGES

Age-Group	Questions to Ask
Preterm infant	History of hypoxia in early neonatal period? Intraventricular insult? Maternal alcohol/substance abuse? Exposure to TORCH viruses?
Newborn	Vaginal or cesarean birth? History of birth injury? Shoulder presentation? Need for resuscitation/ventilation in immediate newborn period? Maternal infection or toxemia? Fetal movement during pregnancy? Age of mother and father at time of infant's birth? Appropriate gestational age? Apgar scores? Jaundice? Neonatal meningitis? Congenital abnormalities? Newborn screening results?
Infancy	Difficulty feeding? Protuberant tongue or tongue thrust? Any delay in achieving gross motor milestones? Does infant roll over? Sit without support? Crawl? Stand alone? Walk without support? Cooing, babbling? Any evidence of toe-walking? Any loss of developmental milestones?
Early childhood	Hand dominance? Feeds self? Any loss of developmental milestones? Any stumbling, limping, poor coordination? History of seizures/spasms, staring spells, daydreaming? Speech development? Attention span? Completion of tasks? Ability to dress independently? Independent toileting achieved?
Middle childhood	Visual and auditory perceptions? Learning difficulties/delays? History of headaches?
Adolescence	Headache history? Sports-related concussions?
Environmental risks	Maternal exposure to potential irritants? Location of housing in relation to hazardous exposures? History of housing and lead exposures? Contact with chemical cleaning agents, hazardous chemicals, smoke? Pesticide exposures?

TORCH, *T*oxoplasmosis, *o*ther (congenital syphilis and viruses), *r*ubella, *c*ytomegalovirus infections, and *h*erpes simplex virus.

PHYSICAL ASSESSMENT

The comprehensive assessment of the pediatric neurological system includes evaluation of mental status, sensory and motor function, and muscle strength and tone; observation of balance, coordination, and gait; and age-appropriate assessment of reflexes, speech and language development, and learning and cognition. An infant or child presenting with a developmental delay or neurological symptoms requires a more focused neurological examination targeted to the appropriate age and developmental stage, performing the most invasive aspect of the examination (e.g., the gag reflex, ophthalmological examination) last. In early childhood, it is important to remember to assess balance, gait, and agility as the child walks, pivots, and turns while holding onto the parent's hand. If the young child is fearful or refuses to walk as requested, gently pick up the child and direct him or her toward the parent and observe the gait with the child undressed except for a diaper. Observing the gait will assist the pediatric health care provider with parental anticipatory guidance about the normal neuromuscular developmental process in early childhood. Box 19-1 presents the basics of the neurological examination in infants and young children.

Evaluation of Motor Function

Muscle tone, the normal degree of tension maintained by muscles while at rest, changes during the first 2 years of life as myelination of the neuronal pathways proceeds and the cerebral cortex begins to control motor functions. The assessment of muscle tone begins in the young infant by observing the resting posture. In the term infant at birth, arms and legs are in a semiflexed position with the hips slightly abducted (Figure 19-8). At the 2-month-old visit, tone in the neck and trunk is evaluated by *gently* pulling the infant upward from the exam table grasping the hands and forearms. Significant head lag or inability of the infant to exhibit strength in the neck and shoulders when pulled

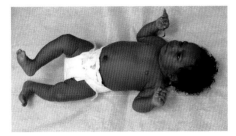

FIGURE 19-8 Normal flexion in term infant.

to sitting may indicate *hypotonia,* a decrease in the normal resting tension in the muscle. In the 4- to 6-month-old, strength in the extremities and trunk is evaluated by *gently* pulling the infant to a sitting position, and is evaluated by pulling the infant from sitting position to standing at the 9-month-old well-child visit.

Abnormal muscle tone and abnormal positioning or posturing of the extremities in the newborn and young infant indicate neurological dysfunction. Hips positioned in external rotation or in a "frog-leg" position in the newborn indicates abnormal muscle tone. *Hypotonia* most commonly presents in the newborn period as a floppy infant. When supine, a floppy infant has limited muscle tone and strength in the extremities, arms are often straight at the infant's side, and hips are abducted with lower extremities abducted on the exam table. When placed in ventral suspension, the infant's head and extremities will hang or drape over the examiner's hand with inability to maintain or move to a horizontal position. Infants with hypotonia can actively move all extremities through normal range of motion, but spontaneous movements may be less frequent than in infants with normal tone.

Hypotonia and muscle weakness may be caused by lesions in the central or peripheral nervous system, as well as neuromuscular disorders, sepsis, organ failure, and metabolic dysfunction.[3] Infants and children with a central nervous system etiology may have a history of neonatal hypoxia or seizures, and prenatal insult including infection, drug exposure, and environmental toxins.

BOX 19-1   **PEDIATRIC NEUROLOGICAL ASSESSMENT CHECKLIST**

- Infant reflexes at <1 year of age
- Fontanels at <18 months
- Level of alertness or consciousness
- Motor and sensory function
- Cranial nerves
- Deep and superficial reflexes
- Coordination
- Balance and gait

Preterm infants may have *hypertonia*, or increased extensor tone in their lower extremities, during their first year of life as well as decreased truncal tone. Infants who have hypotonia initially may later develop spasticity as the cerebral cortex matures. Asymmetry in muscle tone may not be identified early in infancy because of the lack of voluntary control of the musculoskeletal system from the cerebral cortex. Transient hypertonia may be noted in drug-exposed infants in the neonatal period. It generally diminishes during the first year of life and disappears by 2 years of age. If the infant exhibits *opisthotonos*, a persistent arching of the back and extension of the neck, this indicates serious neurological compromise.

Delays in preterm and term infants can occur in any area of development—gross motor, fine motor, language, or cognitive development—but delays are usually first noted in gross motor skills and abilities. Evaluating the primitive and postural reflexes will assist the pediatric health care provider to detect evidence of delayed maturation of sensory and motor function and prompt earlier referral for evaluation and earlier intervention. Table 19-2 presents indicators for delayed cognitive development in an infant with developmental delay.

Primitive Reflexes

The *primitive reflexes* appear as early as 25 weeks' gestation and are involuntary and controlled at birth by the brainstem. Movement is dominated by a primitive grasp reflex at birth.[4] The primitive reflexes should always be symmetrical and are considered abnormal if asymmetrical or absent at birth (Table 19-3; Figures 19-9 through 19-12). In the first 3 months after birth, infants search out objects with their eyes rather than their hands and visually fixate on objects and faces by tracking with their eyes. As the primitive reflexes diminish, infants start to voluntarily grasp with their hands.[4] The primitive reflexes diminish by 3 to 4 months of age as the cerebral cortex matures during the first year of life. They disappear altogether in the normal term

TABLE 19-2	COGNITIVE RED FLAGS
Age	Red Flag
2 months	Lack of fixation
4 months	Lack of visual tracking
6 months	Failure to turn to sound or voice
9 months	Lack of babbling consonant sounds
24 months	Failure to use single words
36 months	Failure to speak in three-word sentences

From Wilks T, Gerber RJ, Erdie-Lalena C: Developmental milestones: cognitive development, *Pediatr Rev* 31(9): 364-367, 2010.

newborn by 4 to 6 months of age, and are considered abnormal if persistent after 6 months of age. The primitive reflexes provide the earliest indication of central nervous system dysfunction. If an infant is very sleepy, irritable, or satiated after feeds, the primitive reflexes will be diminished and should be reevaluated when the infant is alert between feedings.

Postural Reflexes

The appearance of the *postural reflexes* predicts normal development (Table 19-4). The postural reflexes appear between 5 and 6 months in the term infant and progress in a cephalocaudal direction beginning with head control to grasping objects. If postural reflexes do not appear by 8 to 9 months of age, it is considered an abnormal finding. When evaluating tone in early infancy, the infant's head must be kept in the midline position when supine to eliminate eliciting the *asymmetrical tonic neck reflex* (Figure 19-13). When holding the infant firmly suspended prone in the examiner's hand, the infant should lift the head and extend the spine and lower extremities (Figure 19-14). While supporting the trunk, hold the infant just above the examination table and lower the infant to touch the feet gently on the surface of the table to elicit extension of the legs and partial weight bearing (Figure 19-15). The normal development of the postural reflexes makes

TABLE 19-3   PRIMITIVE REFLEXES

Reflex	How Initiated	Response
Asymmetrical tonic neck	With infant on flat surface turn head 90 degrees to surface	Arm and leg extend on same side infant is turned toward, arm and leg on opposite side flex
Moro	Support infant at 30-degree angle above flat surface with examiner's hand; allow head and trunk to drop back to surface supported by examiner's hand; or pull infant up by hands to 30-degree angle above examining table; gently drop infant back to surface quickly and release arms	Arms extend and abduct, hands open, fingers fan out, thumb and forefinger form a C; then arms flex and adduct, knees clench, hips flex, eyes open, infant may cry
Palmar grasp	With infant's head midline, touch palm of infant's hand on ulnar surface with examiner's thumb	Fingers clasp examiner's thumb
Placing	Hold infant upright under arms over edge of table; touch dorsal surface of foot to table edge	Flexion of knees/hips, foot lifts as if stepping up on table
Plantar grasp	Touch infant on plantar surface of foot at base of toes	Toes curl downward
Rooting	Touch or stroke cheek	Infant's head turns toward stimulus and mouth should open
Stepping	Hold infant upright under the arms above exam table; palmar surface of feet should be allowed to just touch table surface	Stepping-like motion with alternate flexion and extension of legs
Sucking	Gently stroke the lips	Infant's mouth opens, sucking begins; gloved finger inserted into mouth evaluates strength of suck reflex
Truncal incurvation or Galant reflex	Hold infant firmly suspended in prone position with examiner's hand supporting chest; with opposite hand, stroke along spine lightly with fingernail just adjacent to vertebrae from shoulders to coccyx	Hips and buttocks curve/turn toward stimulus side

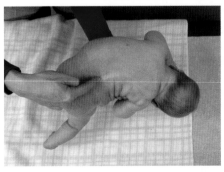

FIGURE 19-9 Truncal incurvation reflex.

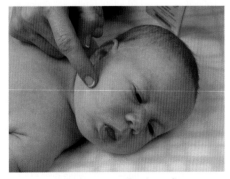

FIGURE 19-10 Rooting reflex.

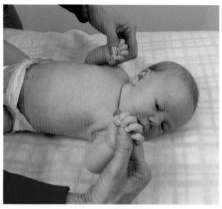

FIGURE 19-11 Palmar grasp reflex.

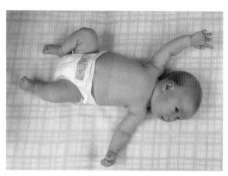

FIGURE 19-13 Asymmetrical tonic neck reflex.

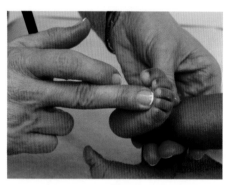

FIGURE 19-12 Plantar grasp reflex.

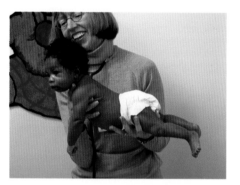

FIGURE 19-14 Landau reflex.

TABLE 19-4   Postural Reflexes

Reflex	How Initiated	Response
Neck righting	Infant's head is turned to the right or left from the midline 90 degrees to the examination table	Rotation of the trunk in the direction in which the head of the supine infant is turned; this reflex is absent or decreased in infants with spasticity
Landau	Hold infant firmly suspended in prone position with examiner's hand supporting abdomen and head; legs should extend over hand	Infant should lift head, extend spine/lower extremities
Lateral parachute	Assessed at 5 to 7 months of age in term infant. Hold infant prone and firmly supported; slowly lower infant toward flat surface	Observe symmetry of hand opening; infant should try to protect self by extending arms/legs
Forward parachute	Assessed at 7 to 9 months of age in term infant. Suspend infant in prone position with arms/legs extended, support with both hands over flat surface	Observe symmetry of hand opening; infant will lift head and extend spine along horizontal plane
Positive support	Hold infant upright and firmly supported under arms while over exam table; touch infant's feet to surface	Infant should extend legs and bear some weight

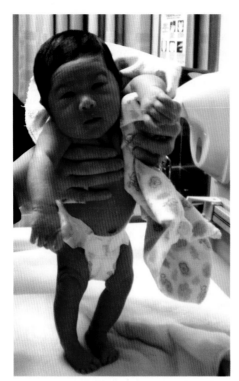

FIGURE 19-15 **Positive support reflex.** (From Gerber RJ, Wilks T, Erdie-Lalena C: Developmental milestones: motor development, *Pediatr Rev* 31(7): 267-277, 2010.)

upper posture possible, and remnants of the postural reflexes persist throughout life.

Involuntary Motor Function

Tremors, coarse repetitive shaking, can be observed intermittently in the term newborn in the first few days after birth and they are generally considered within normal limits. Persistent tremors in the newborn period and beyond are abnormal and require further diagnostic evaluation. *Clonus,* rhythmic tonic-clonic movements of the foot, in the newborn can be normal. Clonus can be elicited by the examiner's firm touch on the sole of the foot with the finger. With sustained clonus beyond the newborn period, the examiner should suspect upper motor neuron dysfunction and consider further diagnostic evaluation. *Tics,* involuntary muscle contractions and/or audible sounds or words, are abnormal neurological signs and can be the result of

emotional upset, severe anxiety in the child related to language or learning difficulties, or the onset of *Tourette syndrome. Chorea* is an involuntary slow, irregular, twisting and writhing movement often seen in *Huntington chorea. Infantile spasms,* or West syndrome, occur in 2 to 3.5 of 10,000 live births.[5] Infantile spasms present as repetitive flexor/extensor movements with head nod, mixed movements, or as myoclonic-tonic spasms or seizures. The peak onset is between 3 and 7 months of age.[5] The spasms may be subtle, brief, and sudden and may be associated with an underlying disorder. Electroencephalography (EEG) is the initial diagnostic for these infants and referral is indicated.

Evaluation of Sensory Function

Touch, deep pressure, pain, temperature, and vibration are all characteristics assessed in sensory function. Tactile sensation can be tested in the verbal child by gently touching different areas of the body with a cotton swab when the eyes are closed. The child should be able to identify the spot by pointing to the area of the body. Pain sensation can be tested similarly in the verbal child by touching the body with the sharp and dull ends of a reflex hammer. Temperature and vibration are sensations not usually elicited in the child. Discrimination sensation can be assessed in the verbal child using the following tests:

- **Stereognosis:** The ability to recognize an object by its feel. With eyes closed, ask the verbal child to identify small familiar objects placed in the palm, such as a key or a coin. If you are not testing expressive language, have the child point to the correct object when eyes are open. Children with cerebral palsy are generally unable to identify the object.
- **Graphesthesia:** The ability to identify shapes traced on the palm. Young verbal children are usually tested with shapes and older children with numbers. May be repeated in each palm to ensure accuracy in testing. Children with spatial and proprioceptive dysfunction will not be able to discriminate shapes or numbers.
- **Two-point discrimination:** A test of spatial discrimination of the body. With the child's

eyes closed, touch lightly on the skin with two points in close proximity on the body, and then follow with touching the child with one point. Ask whether the child felt one or two points. Children under 5 years of age may have difficulty comparing touch points. Loss of sensation can reflect impairment in the peripheral nervous system, spinal column, brainstem, or cerebral cortex. Dysfunction of the lower motor neurons or cognitive processing disorders can cause the verbal child to have image confusion.

Cranial Nerves

Assessment of the cranial nerves is performed as part of a comprehensive physical examination. Cooperative young children and school-age children usually delight in the activity of testing the cranial nerves. Tables 19-5 and 19-6 summarize the assessment of cranial nerves in infancy and early and middle childhood. Cranial nerve testing may be difficult to assess in infants if they are drowsy, crying, or satiated after feeding, and in young children if they are fearful or irritable during the physical examination.

TABLE 19-5 CRANIAL NERVE TESTING IN THE NEWBORN AND INFANT

Cranial Nerve	Test	Response
Cranial nerve I, olfactory	Pass strong-smelling substance (e.g., cloves, peppermint, anise oil) under nose (not often tested in newborns)	Observe for startle response, grimace, sniffing
Cranial nerve II, optic	Light source/ophthalmoscope on medium/large aperture	Pupils constrict in response to light, able to fix on object and follow for 60 to 90 degrees
Cranial nerve III, oculomotor Cranial nerve IV, trochlear Cranial nerve VI, abducens	Elicit pupillary response to test optic nerve by shining pen light toward pupil "Doll's eye" or oculovestibular maneuver—rotate head and body from side to side, observe eyes moving away from direction of rotation	Evaluate shape, size, symmetry, spontaneous movements of pupil Eyes should deviate left when turning head right; if eyes remain fixed or do not track in opposite direction, suspect brainstem dysfunction
Cranial nerve V, trigeminal	Touch infant's cheek area Test jaw muscles by placing gloved finger in infant's mouth	Infant turns cheek toward touch stimulus Infant should bite down on gloved finger and begin sucking
Cranial nerve VII, facial	Observe infant's face for symmetry of facial movements and observe when crying	Asymmetrical nasolabial folds/asymmetrical facial expression may indicate nerve palsy
Cranial nerve VIII, acoustic	With infant lying supine, ring bell sharply within a few inches of infant's ears	Observe for response to sound stimulus, such as mild startle/blink reflex NOTE: Auditory-evoked response required in many states evaluates acoustic nerve function and has replaced rough assessment of acoustic nerve and acoustic blink response to loud clap
Cranial nerve IX, glossopharyngeal	Use tongue blade to apply pressure on midtongue area to overcome tongue thrust	Elicit gag reflex; observe tongue movement, strength

TABLE 19-5 CRANIAL NERVE TESTING IN THE NEWBORN AND INFANT—CONT'D

Cranial Nerve	Test	Response
Cranial nerve X, vagus	Observe infant while crying	Evaluate pitch of cry and assess for hoarseness, stridor; normal cry is loud and angry; shrill, penetrating cry indicates intracranial hemorrhage; whiny, high-pitched cry indicates central nervous system dysfunction
Cranial nerve XI, accessory	With infant lying supine, turn infant's head to one side	Infant should work to bring head to midline
Cranial nerve XII, hypoglossal	Observe infant when feeding	Sucking, swallowing should be efficient, coordinated

Data from Thureen PJ, Deacon J, Hernandez J, et al: *Assessment and care of the well newborn,* ed 2, Philadelphia, 2005, Saunders.

TABLE 19-6 CRANIAL NERVE TESTING IN EARLY TO MIDDLE CHILDHOOD

Cranial Nerve	Test
Cranial nerve II, optic	• Allen vision cards, tumbling E, or Snellen chart for visual acuity testing
Cranial nerve III, oculomotor Cranial nerve IV, trochlear Cranial nerve VI, abducens	• Use ophthalmoscope or light source to test direct and consensual pupillary response to light • With examiner's hand under chin, have child follow toy, light source, or index finger through six cardinal fields of gaze to test eye movement
Cranial nerve V, trigeminal	• Observe child chewing and swallowing to test normal jaw strength • Touch facial area with cotton swab and observe child move away from stimulus
Cranial nerve VII, facial	• Ask child to smile, frown, and puff cheeks, observe for symmetrical facial expressions
Cranial nerve VIII, acoustic	• Perform audiometric testing to evaluate range of hearing
Cranial nerve IX, glosso-pharyngeal, Cranial nerve X, vagus	• Observe tongue strength and movement and elicit gag reflex with tongue blade • Child is able to swallow without difficulty • Voice quality and sound is normal and intact
Cranial nerve XI, accessory Cranial nerve XII, hypoglossal	• Have child stick tongue out and push tongue against tongue blade • Shrug shoulders to assess trapezius muscle strength • Turn head from side to side against resistance

Deep Tendon Reflexes

The reflex arc of the deep tendon reflexes is a complex function of the musculoskeletal and nervous systems and requires an intact sensory neuron, a functional synapse in the spinal cord, an intact motor neuron, a functional neuromuscular junction, and a competent muscle (Table 19-7; Figures 19-16 through 19-22). Reflex testing is useful in young children as it provides information on the normal development and maturation of the neuromuscular system. Assessment of the deep tendon reflexes

TABLE 19-7   DEEP TENDON AND SUPERFICIAL REFLEXES

Reflex	Test	Response
Deep Tendon Reflexes		
Biceps reflex	With examiner's thumb pressed against biceps tendon in antecubital space, support arm with palm prone; tap thumb briskly; tendon should respond by tightening	Flexion of forearm
Triceps reflex	Hold arm in flexed position slightly forward toward chest with forearm dangling downward, tap directly behind elbow on triceps tendon	Contraction of triceps and elbow should extend slightly
Brachioradialis reflex	Support child's forearm with palm resting down; tap briskly on radius about 2 inches above wrist	Flexion of elbow and pronation of forearm
Patellar reflex	Palpate patellar tendon just below patella and tap briskly with leg dangling; having child lock fingers and pull hard in outward direction can help elicit reflex	Contraction of quadriceps and extension of knee
Achilles tendon reflex	Support foot with ankle slightly flexed and leg relaxed, tap above heel; vary degree of flexion of foot to assist in eliciting reflex	Observe plantar flexion
Clonus	In infant, knee should be slightly flexed with infant in supine position; apply pressure to sole of foot to bring ankle into dorsiflexion	In newborn, rapid tonic-clonic movement of 4 to 5 beats is normal response; beyond newborn period, no rhythmic movements are expected
Superficial Reflexes		
Plantar reflex	Stroke sole of foot from heel to ball of foot curving medially with flat object	Movement of toes
Abdominal reflex	Stroke briskly above and below umbilicus	Abdominal muscles contract and umbilicus deviates toward the stimulus
Cremasteric reflex	In male, lightly scratch upper inner thigh	Testicle will elevate slightly on stimulated side
Anal reflex	Gently stroke anal area to test sphincter tone	Quick contraction of sphincter

may help distinguish between upper and lower motor neuron lesions. Abnormally brisk reflexes with clonus may suggest upper motor tract involvement. Absent reflexes are consistent with a neuropathic lesion or severe myopathy.[3] Further discussion of reflexes is presented in Chapter 18. When performing deep tendon reflexes (DTRs) bilaterally, the response is graded as follows:

- 4+: Brisk, markedly hyperactive with clonus
- 3+: Active, brisker than normal
- 2+: Normal response
- 1+: Diminished response, low normal
- 0: Absent or no response

Evaluation of Cerebellar Function

Assessment of cerebellar function evaluates balance, coordination, and cognitive processing. The following simple tests can be performed as an activity during the physical examination, which is fun for the school-age

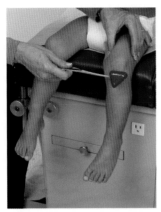

FIGURE 19-16 Patellar reflex.

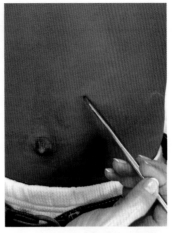

FIGURE 19-19 Abdominal reflex.

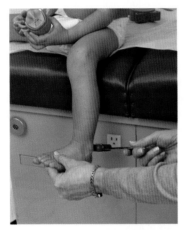

FIGURE 19-17 Achilles tendon reflex.

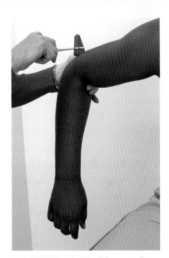

FIGURE 19-20 Triceps reflex.

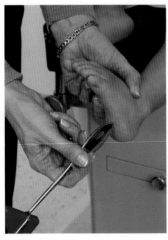

FIGURE 19-18 Plantar reflex.

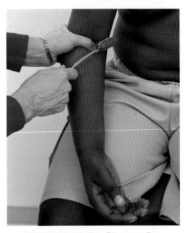

FIGURE 19-21 Biceps reflex.

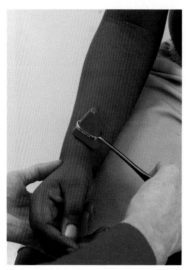

FIGURE 19-22 Brachioradialis reflex.

child and effective in assessing cerebellar function:

- **Romberg test:** Assesses balance and equilibrium. This test can be performed in the cooperative preschool child. Ask the child to stand erect with eyes closed and hands touching the sides. Observe the child's balance for several seconds while monitoring the child closely. Lesions in the cerebellum can cause the child to stagger or fall.
- **Finger-to-thumb test:** Assesses cerebellar function, coordination, and cognitive processing disorders in the school-age child. Ask the child to touch each finger to the thumb in rapid succession. Test may be repeated with one hand at a time.
- **Hopping in place:** Ask the child to alternately hop on one foot and then the other. Tests for balance, cerebellar function, intact motor function, and spatial sense. The child should be able to maintain balance on one leg by 4 years of age.
- **Heel-to-toe walking or tandem walking:** Assesses balance and coordination. Ask the child in the prekindergarten physical exam to walk heel to toe in a straight line. This requires a high level of neuromuscular

coordination and is often not accomplished until 6 years of age.
- **Rapid alternating movements test:** Assesses for cerebellar function, coordination, and cognitive processing disorders in the school-age child. Ask the child to place his or her hands palm down on the thighs. Then demonstrate the rapid, rhythmic movement of the hands back and forth, asking the child to repeat the movement. Next ask the child to perform the rapidly alternating movement with one hand only. Inability to perform the task may indicate cognitive or behavioral dysfunction and requires further evaluation. The child should be able to perform by 8 to 9 years of age.
- **Finger-to-nose test:** Ask the child to close their eyes and then touch their nose with the first finger of one hand and then with first finger of the other hand. Then, with eyes open, have the child touch their nose with first finger and then touch the examiner's finger held about 18 inches in front of the child. Repeat with both hands. Then increase speed of movements with examiner's finger changing position. Consistent failure of child to point at the finger indicates dysfunction in spatial perception and coordination. The child should be able to perform this by 8 to 9 years of age.
- **Heel to shin test:** Assesses coordination and balance in the school-age child. Ask the child to place the right heel on the left shin below the knee, and then slide the heel down the shin to the foot. Repeat with the left leg. Inability to perform the task may indicate decreased motor strength, a cerebellar lesion, or an alteration in proprioception.

PEDIATRIC PEARLS

Findings of *motor overflow,* noted when one hand performs a motor task and the other hand mirrors the movement, or when mirroring movements of the lower extremities occur, indicate a lag in the normal progression of fine motor development, which may impact the child's learning.

Evaluation of Cerebral Function

Assessing general cerebral function in children requires evaluating the level of consciousness, mood and affect, thought, memory, judgment, and communication. In the developing child, cerebral function is more challenging to assess than in adults. In the child with head trauma, the basic components of the initial neurological examination include (1) level of consciousness assessment, (2) sensory function, (3) pupil reactivity, and (4) motor function.

Determining the level of consciousness using an adapted Glasgow Coma Scale (GCS) score is an appropriate assessment in the verbal child (Table 19-8). The adapted GCS assesses three major areas: eye opening, which relates to arousal and alertness; verbal ability, which relates to content and mentation; and motor ability, which reflects mentation as well as the functional integrity of the major central nervous system (CNS) pathways. A modified GCS for infants assesses visual acuity with the

TABLE 19-8   PEDIATRIC ADAPTATION OF THE GLASGOW COMA SCALE

Eye Opening

Birth to 1 Year Old	>1 Year Old		Score
Spontaneously	Spontaneously		4
To loud noise	To verbal command		3
To pain	To pain		2
No response	No response		1

Motor Response

Birth to 1 Year Old	>1 Year Old		Score
Spontaneous responses	Obeys		6
Localizes pain	Localizes pain		5
Withdrawal to pain	Withdrawal to pain		4
Involuntary flexion	Involuntary flexion		3
Involuntary extension	Involuntary extension		2
No response	No response		1

Verbal Response

Birth to 2 Years Old	2 to 5 Years Old	>5 Years Old	Score
Cries as response, vocalizes	Purposeful words	Oriented and responds	5
Cries	Incoherent words	Disoriented and converses	4
Inappropriate crying	Cries or screams	Inappropriate words	3
Grunts	Grunts	Incomprehensible words	2
No response	No response	No response	1

Severity of Injury*

Mild head injury	**13-15**	
Moderate head injury	**9-12**	
Severe head injury	**<8**	

Modified from Barkin RM, Rosen P: *Emergency pediatrics: a guide to ambulatory care,* ed 6, St. Louis, 2003, Mosby.
*Calculate total score for age by assessing eye opening, best motor response, and verbal response and assigning a score for each area. Total Glasgow Coma Scale score indicates severity of the head injury.

ability to open the eye spontaneously (response to speech, to pain, or no response), verbal cues (coos and babbles appropriately, irritable cries inconsolable, cries or screams persistently to pain, grunts or moans to pain, or no response), and motor function (normal spontaneous movements, withdraws to touch, withdraws to pain, abnormal flexion, abnormal extension, or no response).

DIAGNOSTIC PROCEDURES

Computerized tomography (CT) is the most common diagnostic tool for evaluation of possible cranial lesions. Magnetic resonance imaging (MRI) is more often used to evaluate neurological injury or a cerebral abnormality related to developmental delay. Evidence on CT versus MRI in a clinical setting may influence provider choice as well as access to timely imaging and need for conscious sedation. Electroencephalography (EEG) is used to diagnose infants or children presenting with spasms or seizures. Ultrasound may be used in evaluating neonates for hydrocephalus or intraventricular hemorrhages. Pediatric health care providers in most pediatric health care settings have adopted an As Low As Reasonably Achievable (ALARA) and an Image Gently policy to limit frequent cumulative exposure to radiological diagnostic procedures.[6]

NEUROLOGICAL CONDITIONS

Table 19-9 presents the most common neurological conditions occurring in infants, children, and adolescents. Traumatic brain injury and concussion are addressed in Chapter 18.

Cerebral Palsy

Cerebral palsy (CP) is a static, nonprogressive disorder of posture and movement caused by a defect, or a brain insult or injury to the central nervous system during the prenatal, perinatal, or postnatal period. It is the major developmental disability affecting function in children.[7] It is often referred to as *static encephalopathy* with a delayed developmental presentation. Although CP is a motor disorder, it can also be associated with additional developmental disabilities and cognitive impairment depending on the degree of brain injury. There are numerous risk factors for the development of CP including vascular and

TABLE 19-9   NEUROLOGICAL CONDITIONS IN INFANTS, CHILDREN, AND ADOLESCENTS

Condition	Description
Abusive head trauma	Characterized by severe trauma or shaking in small infants causing acceleration and deceleration of the delicate brain tissue within the periosteum, resulting in retinal hemorrhages and subarachnoid and subdural hematomas. *Shaken baby syndrome* can also result in epidural hematoma. Severe trauma can be fatal.
Prader-Willi syndrome	A rare chromosomal disorder characterized by hypotonia, insatiable appetite, obesity and uncontrolled appetite, hypogonadism, incomplete sexual development, and developmental delay.
Neurofibromatosis	Characterized by six or more café au lait macules over 5 mm in diameter, axillary or inguinal freckling noted in infancy or early childhood.
Migraine headache in children	Characterized by pulsating pain and high pain intensity. May be associated with chronic daily headaches in up to 53% of children presenting with migraine headaches.[8]
Tension-type headaches in children	Characterized by pressing, mild pain and described as less intense than migraine headaches.

intraventricular insults, but the most common risk factors for CP are perinatal hypoxia and neonatal asphyxia. CP may be classified as a *pyramidal* (spastic) or an *extrapyramidal* (nonspastic) disorder, indicating the area of the brain that has been affected and the predominant disability.[7] It is important for the pediatric health care provider to serially assess cognitive and intellectual function and gross and fine motor skills in children with CP to ensure early interventions that foster the child's full developmental potential.[9]

Down Syndrome

Down syndrome, or *trisomy 21,* occurs is 1.1 out of 1000 live births. Common characteristics of Down syndrome include facies with upward slanting palpebral fissures and inner epicanthal folds, flattened nasal area, brachydactyly or abnormal shortening of fingers and toes with wide-spaced first and second toes, simian crease, hypotonia, macroglossia, and mental retardation. Infants and children with Down syndrome are at increased risk for congenital cardiac defects, duodenal atresia, leukemia, thyroid dysfunction, visual and hearing defects, obesity, atlanto-occipital joint instability that impacts extension and flexion movements, and delayed sexual development. Strabismus and refractive errors are also common. Approximately 5% to 10% of children with Down syndrome have autism spectrum disorder. Careful assessment of cognitive and intellectual function by the pediatric health care provider as well as developmental milestones is important to assist the child in developing to his or her full potential.

SUMMARY OF EXAMINATION

- Assessment of muscle tone and strength is a key component of evaluating the development of the neurological system. Evaluate tone and strength in the young infant by observing the resting posture and assessing movement of extremities.
- Assess balance, gait, and agility as the older infant walks, pivots, and turns while holding on to the parent's hand.
- Development delays in preterm and term infants can occur in any area of gross motor, fine motor, language, or cognitive skills, but delays are usually first noted in gross motor skills and abilities.

- Evaluating primitive and postural reflexes assesses sensory and motor function in the young infant.
- Cranial nerve testing and deep tendon reflex testing is useful in young children to assess normal development and maturation of the neuromuscular system.
- Cerebellar function in a child presenting with head trauma is assessed by evaluating level of consciousness, pupil reactivity, motor and function with a modified Glasgow Coma Scale.

Charting

18-Month-Old

Neurological: Alert, active, follows simple directions; gait, balance, and coordination normal for age, DTRs intact +2 bilaterally, muscle strength equal and symmetrical, cranial nerves II-XII grossly intact, ASQ normal for age.

DTR, Deep tendon reflex.

REFERENCES

1. Porth CM, Matfin G: *Pathophysiology: concepts of altered health status*, Philadelphia, 2010, Wolters Kluwer/Lippincott Williams & Wilkins.
2. Wilks T, Gerber RJ, Erdie-Lalena C: Developmental milestones: cognitive development, *Pediatr Rev* 31(9):364-367, 2010.
3. Bodamer OA, Miller G: *UpToDate*, Waltham, Ma., 2012, UpToDate.
4. Gerber RJ, Wilks T, Erdie-Lalena C: Developmental milestones: motor development, *Pediatr Rev* 31(7): 267-277, 2010.
5. Wheless JW, Gibson PA, Rosbeck KL, et al: Infantile spasms (West syndrome): update and resources for pediatricians and providers to share with parents, *BMC Pediatrics* 12:108, 2012.
6. Frush DP, Frush KS: The ALARA concept in pediatric imaging: building bridges between radiology and emergency medicine: consensus conference on imaging safety and quality for children in the emergency setting, *Pedatr Radiol* 36(2):121-125, 2010.
7. Jones MW, Morgan E, Shelton JE, et al: Cerebral palsy: introduction and diagnosis (part I), *J Pediatr Health Care* 21(3):146-152, 2007.
8. Wager J, Hirschfeld G, Zernikow B: Tension-type headache or migraine? Adolescents' pain descriptions are of little help, *Headache* 53(2):322-332, 2013.
9. Jones MW, Morgan E, Shelton JE: Primary care of the child with cerebral palsy: a review of systems (part II), *J Pediatr Health Care* 21(4):226-237, 2007.

UNIT III CHARTING PEDIATRIC HEALTH CARE VISITS

CHAPTER 20

CHARTING PEDIATRIC COMPREHENSIVE AND SYMPTOM-FOCUSED HEALTH CARE VISITS

Karen G. Duderstadt

CHARTING THE HEALTH CARE VISIT

Comprehensive assessment of the infant, child, and adolescent and accurate charting in the health record are the hallmarks of quality professional practice for the pediatric health care provider. Documentation of the thorough physical examination in the health record is as important to the pediatric health visit as the comprehensive assessment, and it is the legal responsibility of every pediatric health care provider to accurately record all aspects of the health care visit. Included in this chapter are templates for the comprehensive well-child visit, the continuity well-child visit, the symptom-focused visit, and the preparticipation physical evaluation to assist the pediatric health care provider. A sample electronic health record (EHR) is also provided.

COMPREHENSIVE WELL-CHILD VISIT

The initial comprehensive well-child visit is composed of subjective data, which includes all components of the health history, objective data from the physical examination including vital signs and laboratory screening, assessment and/or list of health conditions, anticipatory guidance for activities of daily living, a plan for each health condition, and follow-up with the child and family. Figure 20-1 presents a sample form for charting the comprehensive well-child visit. Figure 20-2 presents a form for a continuity well-child visit.

SYMPTOM-FOCUSED VISIT

The components of the symptom-focused visit are the same as the initial comprehensive well-child visit—subjective, objective, assessment, plan, and follow-up. However, the pediatric health care provider gathers information most relevant to the presenting problem, chief complaint, or the particular acute or chronic health condition and conducts a focused physical examination. Figure 20-3 presents a sample form for charting the symptom-focused visit.

PREPARTICIPATION SPORTS PHYSICAL VISIT

The preparticipation physical evaluation (PPE) visit is the opportunity for the pediatric health care provider to conduct a comprehensive physical assessment of the growing and developing child and adolescent. The focus of the PPE is to identify any health conditions that may impact sports participation and to identify any risks participation in a particular sport

SUBJECTIVE DATA

Demographics
Informant: _____ Relationship to patient: _____

Verify family contact information
Address: _____
Daytime/evening phone: (___)_____ Cell phone: (___)_____

Child Profile
Birth date: __/__/__ Age: _____ Birthplace: _____
Date of last well child visit: __/__/__
Previous health care provider: _____ Phone: (___)_____
Previous medical records available: _____ Requested: _____
Allergies: _____

History of Present Illness (HPI)
Chief complaint or concern(s): _____
_____
_____

Past Medical History
Prenatal history: _____
Birth history: _____
Neonatal course: _____
Prenatal labs/newborn screening: _____
Hospitalizations: _____
Injuries (intentional and unintentional): _____
Chronic health conditions: _____

Current medications: _____
Immunizations: _____

Activities of Daily Living
Nutrition/feeding: _____
    Servings of fruits and vegetables daily: _____
    Calcium intake daily: _____
    Juice/sugary drinks and water intake: _____
Elimination/stools: _____
Sleep: _____
Screen time daily: _____

Oral Health
Brushing teeth twice daily: _____
Dental home: _____ Date of last dental visit:_____

School/Childcare
Childcare/daycare:_____
School/grade: _____
School performance/GPA: _____
After-school programs: _____
Bullying/friends at school: _____
Sports/Interests/Activities: _____
_____

Developmental Surveillance
Meets milestones below:
    Personal-social: _____
    Communication/language: _____
    Fine motor: _____
    Gross motor: _____
    Parent concerned about:_____
Behavior: _____
Discipline method used: _____
Temperament: _____
Home Safety/smoke alarm: _____
Car seat/booster seat/seat belt: _____ **Bicycle/scooter/skateboard helmet:** _____

FIGURE 20-1 Comprehensive well-child visit—initial visit form.

SUBJECTIVE DATA (cont.)

Family Health History
Age and health status of immediate family members: _____
Familial health conditions: _____
Current health risks (HTN*, diabetes, obesity): _____

Family Situation/Social History
Who lives in home? _____
Home environment: _____
Parental employment: _____
Support system: _____
Firearms in home/ammunition/locked: _____
Tobacco use/substance abuse: _____
Cultural/religious practices: _____
Environmental exposure history: _____
        Lead exposure? _____
        Use of pesticides in home? _____

Adolescent History
Menstrual history: _____
        Menarche: _____
        Monthly periods: _____
        Irregular periods: _____
        Concerns: _____

SSHADESS* Assessment (review confidentiality and limitations of information)
Strengths: _____
School: _____
Home: _____
Activities: _____
Drugs/alcohol/tobacco: _____
Emotion/depression: _____
Sexuality: _____
Safety: _____

Review of Systems: _____
_____

FIGURE 20-1, CONT'D Comprehensive well-child visit—initial visit form.   *Continued*

OBJECTIVE DATA

Physical Examination

Height: _____ Weight: _____ H.C.: _____ BMI*: _____

Temperature: _____ Respiration: _____ Heart Rate: _____ Blood Pressure: _____

General Appearance: _____

Skin: _____ Head: _____

Eyes: _____ Ears: _____

Nose: _____ Mouth/Throat: _____

Neck/lymphatics: _____ Chest and Lungs: _____

Breast: _____ Heart: _____

Abdomen: _____ Genitalia: _____

Sexual maturity rating/Tanner stage: _____ Rectum/Anus: _____

Musculoskeletal: _____ Neurological (CNs,* DTRs*): _____

Parent-child interaction: _____

Developmental and Emotional/Behavioral Screening Tests

MCHAT: _____

ASQ: _____

PEDS: _____

PHQ-2 or PHQ-9 Depression Scale: _____

Laboratory Tests: _____

ASSESSMENT

Plan

#1 Health Maintenance

Immunization: _____

Nutrition: _____

Growth & Development: _____

Safety: _____

Follow-up: _____

Problem #2: _____

Diagnostic/Consultation: _____

Therapeutic: _____

Patient Education: _____

Follow-up: _____

Problem #3: _____

Diagnostic/Consultation: _____

Therapeutic: _____

Patient Education: _____

Follow-up: _____

Provider Signature: _____ Date: _____

*BMI, body mass index; CNs, cranial nerves; DTRs, deep tendon reflexes; HC, head circumference; HTN, hypertension; SSHADESS, strengths, school, home, activities, drugs/alcohol/tobacco, emotion/depression, sexuality, safety.

FIGURE 20-1, CONT'D **Comprehensive well-child visit—initial visit form.**

SUBJECTIVE DATA

Demographics
Informant: _____ Relationship to patient: _____

Verify family contact information
Address: _____
Daytime/evening phone: (___)_____ Cell phone: (___)_____

HEALTH HISTORY
History of Present Illness (HPI)
Chief complaint or concern(s): _____

Past Medical History
Illness or injury since last visit: _____
Current medications: _____
Allergies noted: _____
Immunizations: _____
Lab tests—lead/hgb/hct/cholesterol/STI* screen: _____

Activities of Daily Living
Nutrition/feeding: _____
    Servings of fruits and vegetables daily: _____
    Calcium intake daily: _____
    Juice/sugary drinks and water intake: _____
Elimination/stools: _____
Sleep: _____
Screen time daily: _____

Oral Health
Brushing teeth twice daily: _____
Dental home: _____Date of last dental visit: _____

School/Childcare
Childcare/daycare: _____
School/grade: _____
School performance/GPA: _____
After-school programs: _____
Bullying/friends at school: _____
Sports/Interests/Activities: _____

Developmental Surveillance
Meets milestones below:
    Personal-social: _____
    Communication/language: _____
    Fine motor: _____
    Gross motor: _____
    Parent concerned about: _____
Behavior: _____
Discipline method used: _____
Temperament: _____
Home safety/smoke alarm:_____
Car seat/booster seat/seat belt: _____ **Bicycle/scooter/skateboard helmet:**_____

Family Profile/Social History (since last visit)
Parental employment: _____
Home situation: _____
Support system: _____

FIGURE 20-2 Continuity well-child visit form. *Continued*

OBJECTIVE DATA

Physical Examination
Height: _____ Weight: _____ H.C.:_____ BMI*:_____
Temperature:_____ Respiration: _____ Heart Rate: _____ Blood Pressure:_____
General Appearance: _____
Skin: _____ Head: _____
Eyes: _____ Ears: _____
Nose:_____ Mouth/Throat: _____
Neck/lymphatics: _____ Chest and Lungs: _____
Breast: _____ Heart: _____
Abdomen: _____ Genitalia: _____
Sexual maturity rating/Tanner stage: _____ Rectum/Anus: _____
Musculoskeletal: _____ Neurological (CNs,* DTRs*): _____
Parent-child interaction: _____

Developmental and Emotional/Behavioral Screening Tests
MCHAT: _____
ASQ: _____
PEDS: _____
PHQ-2 or PHQ-9 Depression Scale: _____

Laboratory Tests: _____

ASSESSMENT

Plan
  #1 Health Maintenance
    Immunization: _____
    Nutrition: _____
    Growth & Development: _____
    Safety: _____
    Follow-up: _____
  Problem #2: _____
    Diagnostic/Consultation:_____
    Therapeutic: _____
    Patient Education: _____
    Follow-up: _____
  *Problem #3:*_____
    Diagnostic/Consultation: _____
    Therapeutic: _____
    Patient Education: _____
    Follow-up: _____

Provider Signature: _____ Date: _____

*BMI, body mass index; CNs, cranial nerves; DTRs, deep tendon reflexes; HC, head circumference; STIs, sexually transmitted infections.

FIGURE 20-2, CONT'D Continuity well-child visit form.

may pose for a young athlete. The PPE is often the healthy adolescent's only regular contact with the pediatric health care provider, and the visit should include regular health maintenance, a confidential psychosocial screening, and a thorough physical examination, including cardiac and musculoskeletal evaluation. Complete documentation of the PPE health history and physical examination and notation of any restrictions to play provides important health information for school athletic programs and coaches, and may provide protection from injury for the young athlete.

Figure 20-4 is the form recommended by the American Academy of Family Physicians and the American Academy of Pediatrics for PPE.

SUBJECTIVE DATA

Informant: _____ **Relationship to patient:** self / parent / other (Circle one)
Verify child's age: _____
Verify phone: Daytime Tel: (___)_____ Evening Tel: (___)_____ Cell Tel: (___)_____

I. HEALTH HISTORY
   A. Present Concern(s):_____
   _____
   _____

   B. History of Present Illness
      Home management/medications (dosage, time, date):_____
      Exposures: _____
      Pertinent family medical history: _____
   C. Relevant Past Medical History: _____
   D. Relevant Review of Systems: _____

OBJECTIVE DATA

II. PHYSICAL EXAMINATION
      Height: _____ Weight: _____ Temperature:_____ Respiration: _____
      Heart Rate: _____ Blood Pressure:_____
      General Appearance and Parent-Child Interaction
         Skin: _____   Face: _____
         Head: _____   Eyes: _____
         Ears: _____   Nose:_____
         Mouth/Throat: _____   Neck: _____
         Chest and Lungs: _____   Breast: _____
         Heart: _____   Abdomen: _____
         Genitalia: _____   Rectum/Anus: _____
         Musculoskeletal: _____   Neurological (CNs,* DTRs*): _____
         Lab Tests: _____

III. ASSESSMENT: _____

IV. Plan *#1 Health Maintenance*
      Next well child visit: _____
      Immunization update: _____
   Problem list
   Problem #2: _____
      Diagnostic/Consultation:_____
      Therapeutic: _____
      Patient Education: _____
      Follow-up: _____
   Problem #3:_____
      Diagnostic/Consultation: _____
      Therapeutic: _____
      Patient Education: _____
      Follow-up: _____

Provider Signature: _____ Date: _____

*CNs, Cranial nerves; *DTRs*, deep tendon reflexes.

FIGURE 20-3 Symptom-focused visit form.

■ PREPARTICIPATION PHYSICAL EVALUATION

HISTORY FORM

(Note: This form is to be filled out by the patient and parent prior to seeing the physician. The physician should keep this form in the chart.)

Date of Exam _____

Name _____ Date of birth _____

Sex _____ Age _____ Grade _____ School _____ Sport(s) _____

Medicines and Allergies: Please list all of the prescription and over-the-counter medicines and supplements (herbal and nutritional) that you are currently taking

_____

_____

Do you have any allergies? ☐ Yes ☐ No If yes, please identify specific allergy below.
☐ Medicines   ☐ Pollens   ☐ Food   ☐ Stinging Insects

Explain "Yes" answers below. Circle questions you don't know the answers to.

GENERAL QUESTIONS	Yes	No
1. Has a doctor ever denied or restricted your participation in sports for any reason?		
2. Do you have any ongoing medical conditions? If so, please identify below: ☐ Asthma ☐ Anemia ☐ Diabetes ☐ Infections Other: _____		
3. Have you ever spent the night in the hospital?		
4. Have you ever had surgery?		

HEART HEALTH QUESTIONS ABOUT YOU	Yes	No
5. Have you ever passed out or nearly passed out DURING or AFTER exercise?		
6. Have you ever had discomfort, pain, tightness, or pressure in your chest during exercise?		
7. Does your heart ever race or skip beats (irregular beats) during exercise?		
8. Has a doctor ever told you that you have any heart problems? If so, check all that apply: ☐ High blood pressure ☐ A heart murmur ☐ High cholesterol ☐ A heart infection ☐ Kawasaki disease Other: _____		
9. Has a doctor ever ordered a test for your heart? (For example, ECG/EKG, echocardiogram)		
10. Do you get lightheaded or feel more short of breath than expected during exercise?		
11. Have you ever had an unexplained seizure?		
12. Do you get more tired or short of breath more quickly than your friends during exercise?		

HEART HEALTH QUESTIONS ABOUT YOUR FAMILY	Yes	No
13. Has any family member or relative died of heart problems or had an unexpected or unexplained sudden death before age 50 (including drowning, unexplained car accident, or sudden infant death syndrome)?		
14. Does anyone in your family have hypertrophic cardiomyopathy, Marfan syndrome, arrhythmogenic right ventricular cardiomyopathy, long QT syndrome, short QT syndrome, Brugada syndrome, or catecholaminergic polymorphic ventricular tachycardia?		
15. Does anyone in your family have a heart problem, pacemaker, or implanted defibrillator?		
16. Has anyone in your family had unexplained fainting, unexplained seizures, or near drowning?		

BONE AND JOINT QUESTIONS	Yes	No
17. Have you ever had an injury to a bone, muscle, ligament, or tendon that caused you to miss a practice or a game?		
18. Have you ever had any broken or fractured bones or dislocated joints?		
19. Have you ever had an injury that required x-rays, MRI, CT scan, injections, therapy, a brace, a cast, or crutches?		
20. Have you ever had a stress fracture?		
21. Have you ever been told that you have or have you had an x-ray for neck instability or atlantoaxial instability? (Down syndrome or dwarfism)		
22. Do you regularly use a brace, orthotics, or other assistive device?		
23. Do you have a bone, muscle, or joint injury that bothers you?		
24. Do any of your joints become painful, swollen, feel warm, or look red?		
25. Do you have any history of juvenile arthritis or connective tissue disease?		

MEDICAL QUESTIONS	Yes	No
26. Do you cough, wheeze, or have difficulty breathing during or after exercise?		
27. Have you ever used an inhaler or taken asthma medicine?		
28. Is there anyone in your family who has asthma?		
29. Were you born without or are you missing a kidney, an eye, a testicle (males), your spleen, or any other organ?		
30. Do you have groin pain or a painful bulge or hernia in the groin area?		
31. Have you had infectious mononucleosis (mono) within the last month?		
32. Do you have any rashes, pressure sores, or other skin problems?		
33. Have you had a herpes or MRSA skin infection?		
34. Have you ever had a head injury or concussion?		
35. Have you ever had a hit or blow to the head that caused confusion, prolonged headache, or memory problems?		
36. Do you have a history of seizure disorder?		
37. Do you have headaches with exercise?		
38. Have you ever had numbness, tingling, or weakness in your arms or legs after being hit or falling?		
39. Have you ever been unable to move your arms or legs after being hit or falling?		
40. Have you ever become ill while exercising in the heat?		
41. Do you get frequent muscle cramps when exercising?		
42. Do you or someone in your family have sickle cell trait or disease?		
43. Have you had any problems with your eyes or vision?		
44. Have you had any eye injuries?		
45. Do you wear glasses or contact lenses?		
46. Do you wear protective eyewear, such as goggles or a face shield?		
47. Do you worry about your weight?		
48. Are you trying to or has anyone recommended that you gain or lose weight?		
49. Are you on a special diet or do you avoid certain types of foods?		
50. Have you ever had an eating disorder?		
51. Do you have any concerns that you would like to discuss with a doctor?		

FEMALES ONLY		
52. Have you ever had a menstrual period?		
53. How old were you when you had your first menstrual period?		
54. How many periods have you had in the last 12 months?		

Explain "yes" answers here

_____

_____

_____

_____

_____

_____

I hereby state that, to the best of my knowledge, my answers to the above questions are complete and correct.

Signature of athlete _____ Signature of parent/guardian _____ Date _____

FIGURE 20-4 Preparticipation physical evaluation form. (Copyright 2010, American Academy of Family Physicians, American Academy of Pediatrics, American College of Sports Medicine, American Medical Society for Sports Medicine, American Orthopaedic Society for Sports Medicine, and American Osteopathic Academy of Sports Medicine. Used with permission.)

■ PREPARTICIPATION PHYSICAL EVALUATION

THE ATHLETE WITH SPECIAL NEEDS: SUPPLEMENTAL HISTORY FORM

Date of Exam _____

Name _____ Date of birth _____

Sex _____ Age _____ Grade _____ School _____ Sport(s) _____

	Yes	No
1. Type of disability		
2. Date of disability		
3. Classification (if available)		
4. Cause of disability (birth, disease, accident/trauma, other)		
5. List the sports you are interested in playing		
6. Do you regularly use a brace, assistive device, or prosthetic?		
7. Do you use any special brace or assistive device for sports?		
8. Do you have any rashes, pressure sores, or any other skin problems?		
9. Do you have a hearing loss? Do you use a hearing aid?		
10. Do you have a visual impairment?		
11. Do you use any special devices for bowel or bladder function?		
12. Do you have burning or discomfort when urinating?		
13. Have you had autonomic dysreflexia?		
14. Have you ever been diagnosed with a heat-related (hyperthermia) or cold-related (hypothermia) illness?		
15. Do you have muscle spasticity?		
16. Do you have frequent seizures that cannot be controlled by medication?		

Explain "yes" answers here

_____
_____
_____
_____

Please indicate if you have ever had any of the following.

	Yes	No
Atlantoaxial instability		
X-ray evaluation for atlantoaxial instability		
Dislocated joints (more than one)		
Easy bleeding		
Enlarged spleen		
Hepatitis		
Osteopenia or osteoporosis		
Difficulty controlling bowel		
Difficulty controlling bladder		
Numbness or tingling in arms or hands		
Numbness or tingling in legs or feet		
Weakness in arms or hands		
Weakness in legs or feet		
Recent change in coordination		
Recent change in ability to walk		
Spina bifida		
Latex allergy		

Explain "yes" answers here

_____
_____
_____
_____
_____

I hereby state that, to the best of my knowledge, my answers to the above questions are complete and correct.

Signature of athlete _____ Signature of parent/guardian _____ Date _____

FIGURE 20-4, CONT'D Preparticipation physical evaluation form.   *Continued*

■ PREPARTICIPATION PHYSICAL EVALUATION

PHYSICAL EXAMINATION FORM

Name _____   Date of birth _____

PHYSICIAN REMINDERS
1. Consider additional questions on more sensitive issues
   - Do you feel stressed out or under a lot of pressure?
   - Do you ever feel sad, hopeless, depressed, or anxious?
   - Do you feel safe at your home or residence?
   - Have you ever tried cigarettes, chewing tobacco, snuff, or dip?
   - During the past 30 days, did you use chewing tobacco, snuff, or dip?
   - Do you drink alcohol or use any other drugs?
   - Have you ever taken anabolic steroids or used any other performance supplement?
   - Have you ever taken any supplements to help you gain or lose weight or improve your performance?
   - Do you wear a seat belt, use a helmet, and use condoms?
2. Consider reviewing questions on cardiovascular symptoms (questions 5–14).

EXAMINATION						
Height		Weight		☐ Male ☐ Female		
BP / (/) Pulse			Vision R 20/	L 20/		Corrected ☐ Y ☐ N

MEDICAL	NORMAL	ABNORMAL FINDINGS
Appearance • Marfan stigmata (kyphoscoliosis, high-arched palate, pectus excavatum, arachnodactyly, arm span > height, hyperlaxity, myopia, MVP, aortic insufficiency)		
Eyes/ears/nose/throat • Pupils equal • Hearing		
Lymph nodes		
Heart[a] • Murmurs (auscultation standing, supine, +/- Valsalva) • Location of point of maximal impulse (PMI)		
Pulses • Simultaneous femoral and radial pulses		
Lungs		
Abdomen		
Genitourinary (males only)[b]		
Skin • HSV, lesions suggestive of MRSA, tinea corporis		
Neurologic[c]		
MUSCULOSKELETAL		
Neck		
Back		
Shoulder/arm		
Elbow/forearm		
Wrist/hand/fingers		
Hip/thigh		
Knee		
Leg/ankle		
Foot/toes		
Functional • Duck-walk, single leg hop		

[a]Consider ECG, echocardiogram, and referral to cardiology for abnormal cardiac history or exam.
[b]Consider GU exam if in private setting. Having third party present is recommended.
[c]Consider cognitive evaluation or baseline neuropsychiatric testing if a history of significant concussion.

☐ Cleared for all sports without restriction

☐ Cleared for all sports without restriction with recommendations for further evaluation or treatment for _____

_____

☐ Not cleared

     ☐ Pending further evaluation

     ☐ For any sports

     ☐ For certain sports _____

     Reason _____

Recommendations _____

_____

I have examined the above-named student and completed the preparticipation physical evaluation. The athlete does not present apparent clinical contraindications to practice and participate in the sport(s) as outlined above. A copy of the physical exam is on record in my office and can be made available to the school at the request of the parents. If conditions arise after the athlete has been cleared for participation, the physician may rescind the clearance until the problem is resolved and the potential consequences are completely explained to the athlete (and parents/guardians).

Name of physician (print/type) _____   Date _____

Address _____   Phone _____

Signature of physician _____ , MD or DO

9-2681/0410

FIGURE 20-4, CONT'D **Preparticipation physical evaluation form.**

■ PREPARTICIPATION PHYSICAL EVALUATION

CLEARANCE FORM

Name _____ Sex ☐ M ☐ F   Age _____   Date of birth _____

☐ Cleared for all sports without restriction

☐ Cleared for all sports without restriction with recommendations for further evaluation or treatment for _____

_____

☐ Not cleared

    ☐ Pending further evaluation

    ☐ For any sports

    ☐ For certain sports _____

    Reason _____

Recommendations _____

_____

_____

_____

_____

_____

I have examined the above-named student and completed the preparticipation physical evaluation. The athlete does not present apparent clinical contraindications to practice and participate in the sport(s) as outlined above. A copy of the physical exam is on record in my office and can be made available to the school at the request of the parents. If conditions arise after the athlete has been cleared for participation, the physician may rescind the clearance until the problem is resolved and the potential consequences are completely explained to the athlete (and parents/guardians).

Name of physician (print/type) _____ Date _____

Address _____ Phone _____

Signature of physician _____, MD or DO

EMERGENCY INFORMATION

Allergies _____

_____

_____

_____

_____

Other information _____

_____

_____

_____

_____

_____

_____

_____

FIGURE 20-4, CONT'D Preparticipation physical evaluation form.

ELECTRONIC HEALTH RECORD

Electronic health records (EHRs) are now used in many pediatric health care settings and guide the provider in all aspects of the history and physical examination. Often, the EHR is developed for providers working in health care settings with adults. However, most EHR programs can be effectively modified for use with children and adolescents across clinical settings. Figure 20-5 is an example of an EHR that is specifically for use in the pediatric health care setting.

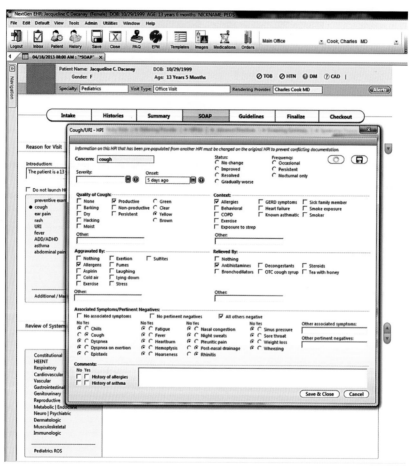

FIGURE 20-5 Electronic health record (EHR) template example. (Copyright 2013, NextGen Healthcare. Used with permission.)

APPENDICES

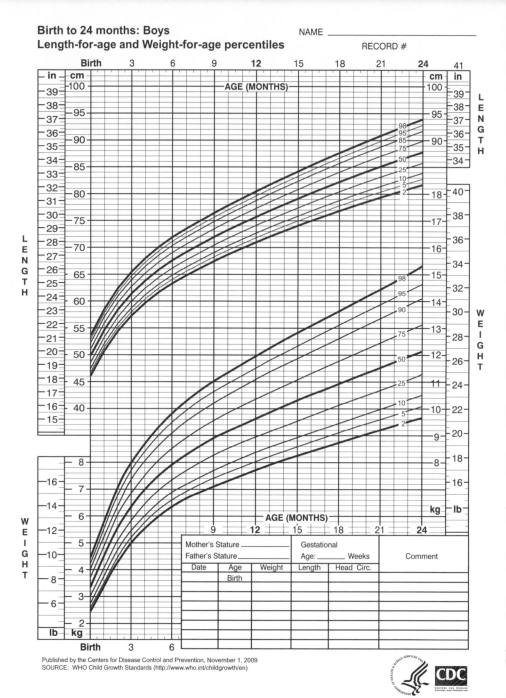

FIGURE A-1 Birth to 24 months: boys' length-for-age and weight-for-age percentiles. (From the National Center for Health Statistics in collaboration with the National Center for Chronic Disease Prevention and Health Promotion, 2000.)

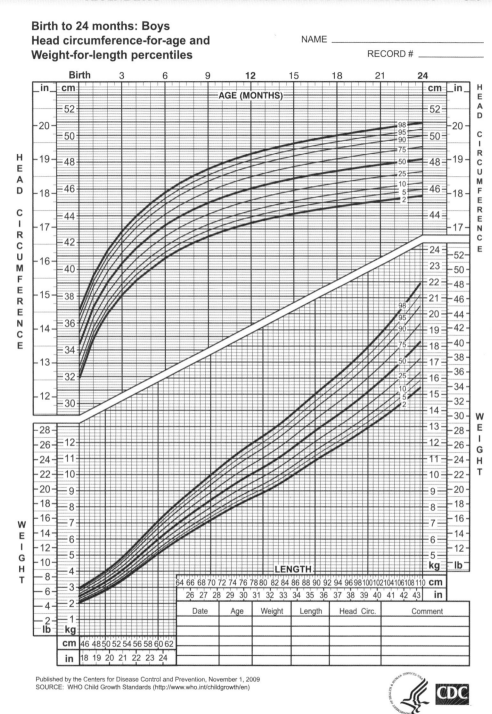

Published by the Centers for Disease Control and Prevention, November 1, 2009
SOURCE: WHO Child Growth Standards (http://www.who.int/childgrowth/en)

FIGURE A-2 Birth to 24 months: boys' head circumference-for-age and weight-for-age percentiles. (From the National Center for Health Statistics in collaboration with the National Center for Chronic Disease Prevention and Health Promotion, 2000.)

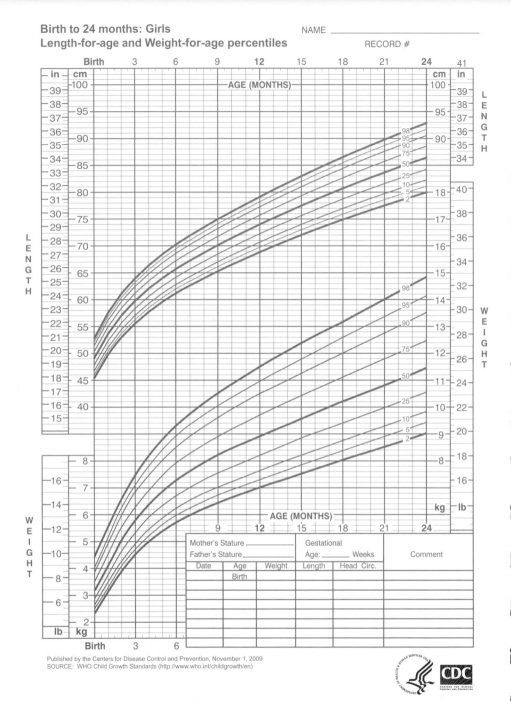

FIGURE A-3 Birth to 24 months: girls' length-for-age and weight-for-age percentiles. (From the National Center for Health Statistics in collaboration with the National Center for Chronic Disease Prevention and Health Promotion, 2000.)

Birth to 24 months: Girls
Head circumference-for-age and
Weight-for-length percentiles

NAME _____

RECORD # _____

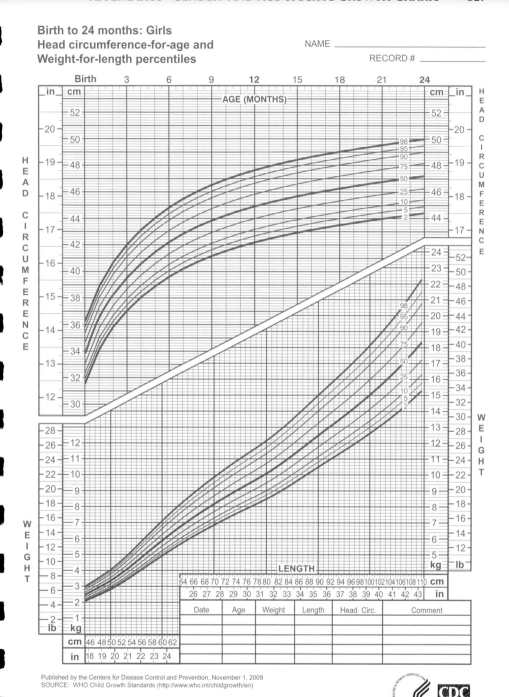

Published by the Centers for Disease Control and Prevention, November 1, 2009
SOURCE: WHO Child Growth Standards (http://www.who.int/childgrowth/en)

FIGURE A-4 Birth to 24 months: girls' head circumference-for-age and weight-for-age percentiles. (From the National Center for Health Statistics in collaboration with the National Center for Chronic Disease Prevention and Health Promotion, 2000.)

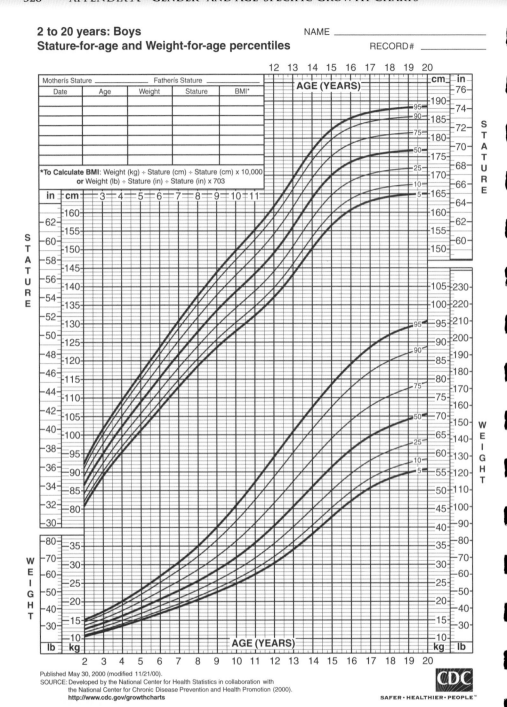

2 to 20 years: Boys
Stature-for-age and Weight-for-age percentiles

Published May 30, 2000 (modified 11/21/00).
SOURCE: Developed by the National Center for Health Statistics in collaboration with
the National Center for Chronic Disease Prevention and Health Promotion (2000).
http://www.cdc.gov/growthcharts

FIGURE A-5 2 to 20 years old: boys' stature-for-age and weight-for-age percentiles. (From the National Center for Health Statistics in collaboration with the National Center for Chronic Disease Prevention and Health Promotion, 2000.)

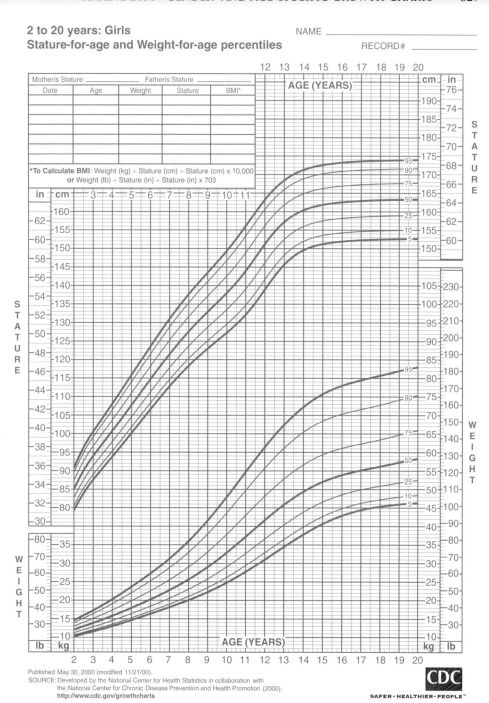

FIGURE A-6 2 to 20 years old: girls' stature-for-age and weight-for-age percentiles. (From the National Center for Health Statistics in collaboration with the National Center for Chronic Disease Prevention and Health Promotion, 2000.)

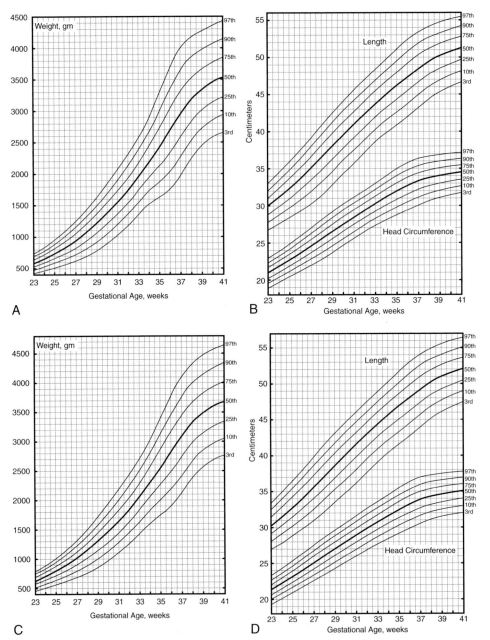

FIGURE A-7 Preterm growth curves. New gender-specific intrauterine growth curves for girls' weight-for-age (A), girls' length- and HC-for-age (B), boys' weight-for-age (C), and boys' length- and HC-for-age (D). Of note, 3rd and 97th percentiles on all curves for 23 weeks should be interpreted cautiously given the small sample size; for boys' HC curve at 24 weeks, all percentiles should be interpreted cautiously because the distribution of data is skewed left. (From Olsen IE, Groveman SA, Lawson ML, et al: New intrauterine growth curves based on United States data, *Pediatrics* 125[2]:e214-224, 2010.)

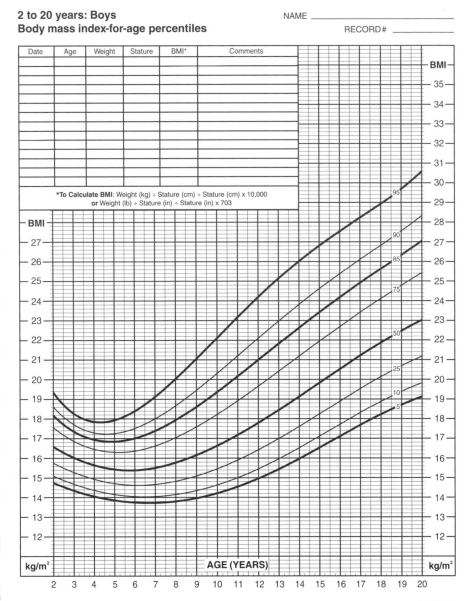

FIGURE B-1 2 to 20 years old: boys' body mass index–for–age percentiles. (From the National Center for Health Statistics in collaboration with the National Center for Chronic Disease Prevention and Health Promotion, 2000.)

2 to 20 years: Girls
Body mass index-for-age percentiles

NAME _____

RECORD# _____

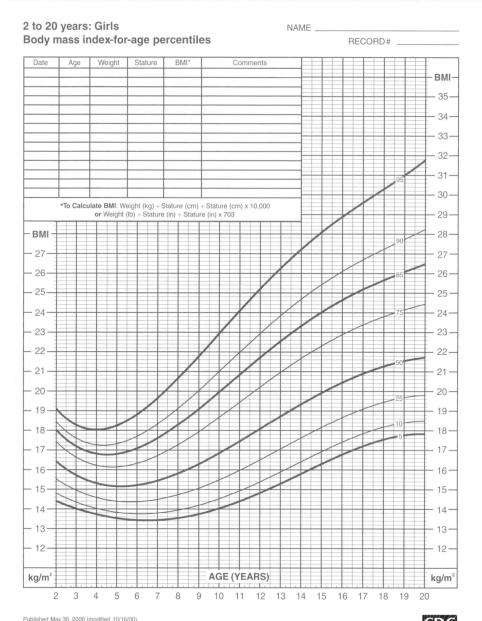

*To Calculate BMI: Weight (kg) ÷ Stature (cm) ÷ Stature (cm) x 10,000
or Weight (lb) ÷ Stature (in) ÷ Stature (in) x 703

Published May 30, 2000 (modified 10/16/00).
SOURCE: Developed by the National Center for Health Statistics in collaboration with
the National Center for Chronic Disease Prevention and Health Promotion (2000).
http://www.cdc.gov/growthcharts

CDC
SAFER · HEALTHIER · PEOPLE™

FIGURE B-2 **2 to 20 years old: girls' body mass index–for-age percentiles. (From the National Center for Health Statistics in collaboration with the National Center for Chronic Disease Prevention and Health Promotion, 2000.)**

Instructions and Permissions for Use of the M-CHAT

The Modified Checklist for Autism in Toddlers (M-CHAT; Robins, Fein, & Barton, 1999) is available for free download for clinical, research, and educational purposes. There are two authorized websites: the M-CHAT and supplemental materials can be downloaded from **www.firstsigns.org** or from Dr. Robins' website, at **http://www.mchatscreen.com**

Users should be aware that the M-CHAT continues to be studied, and may be revised in the future. Any revisions will be posted to the two websites noted above.

Furthermore, the M-CHAT is a copyrighted instrument, and use of the M-CHAT must follow these guidelines:

(1) Reprints/reproductions of the M-CHAT must include the copyright at the bottom (© 1999 Robins, Fein, & Barton). No modifications can be made to items, instructions, or item order without permission from the authors.

(2) The M-CHAT must be used in its entirety. There is no evidence that using a subset of items will be valid.

(3) Parties interested in reproducing the M-CHAT in print (e.g., a book or journal article) or electronically for use by others (e.g., as part of digital medical record or other software packages) must contact Diana Robins to request permission (**drobins@gsu.edu**).

(4) If you are part of a medical practice, and you want to incorporate the M-CHAT into your own practice's electronic medical record (EMR), you are welcome to do so. However, if you ever want to distribute your EMR page outside of your practice, please contact Diana Robins to request permission.

Instructions for Use

The M-CHAT is validated for screening toddlers between 16 and 30 months of age, to assess risk for autism spectrum disorders (ASD). The M-CHAT can be administered and scored as part of a well-child check-up, and also can be used by specialists or other professionals to assess risk for ASD. The primary goal of the M-CHAT was to maximize sensitivity, meaning to detect as many cases of ASD as possible. Therefore, there is a high false positive rate, meaning that not all children who score at risk for ASD will be diagnosed with ASD. To address this, we have developed a structured follow-up interview for use in conjunction with the M-CHAT; it is available at the two websites listed above. Users should be aware that even with the follow-up questions, a significant number of the children who fail the M-CHAT will not be diagnosed with an ASD; however, these children are at risk for other developmental disorders or delays, and therefore, evaluation is warranted for any child who fails the screening.

The M-CHAT can be scored in less than two minutes. Scoring instructions can be downloaded from **http://www2.gsu.edu/~wwwpsy/faculty/robins.htm or www.firstsigns.org**. We also have developed a scoring template, which is available on these websites; when printed on an overhead transparency and laid over the completed M-CHAT, it facilitates scoring. Please note that minor differences in printers may cause your scoring template not to line up exactly with the printed M-CHAT.

Children who fail 3 or more items total or 2 or more critical items (particularly if these scores remain elevated after the M-CHAT Follow-up Interview) should be referred for diagnostic evaluation by a specialist trained to evaluate ASD in very young children. In addition, children for whom there are physician, parent, or other professional's concerns about ASD should be referred for evaluation, given that it is unlikely for any screening instrument to have 100% sensitivity.

FIGURE C-1 Modified Checklist for Autism in Toddlers (M-CHAT). (Copyright Diana Robins, Deborah Fein, and Marianne Barton, 1999. Used with permission.)   *Continued*

M-CHAT

Please fill out the following about how your child usually is. Please try to answer every question. If the behavior is rare (e.g., you've seen it once or twice), please answer as if the child does not do it.

1.	Does your child enjoy being swung, bounced on your knee, etc.?	Yes No
2.	Does your child take an interest in other children?	Yes No
3.	Does your child like climbing on things, such as up stairs?	Yes No
4.	Does your child enjoy playing peek-a-boo/hide-and-seek?	Yes No
5.	Does your child ever pretend, for example, to talk on the phone or take care of a doll or pretend other things?	Yes No
6.	Does your child ever use his/her index finger to point, to ask for something?	Yes No
7.	Does your child ever use his/her index finger to point, to indicate interest in something?	Yes No
8.	Can your child play properly with small toys (e.g., cars or blocks) without just mouthing, fiddling, or dropping them?	Yes No
9.	Does your child ever bring objects over to you (parent) to show you something?	Yes No
10.	Does your child look you in the eye for more than a second or two?	Yes No
11.	Does your child ever seem oversensitive to noise? (e.g., plugging ears)	Yes No
12.	Does your child smile in response to your face or your smile?	Yes No
13.	Does your child imitate you? (e.g., you make a face-will your child imitate it?)	Yes No
14.	Does your child respond to his/her name when you call?	Yes No
15.	If you point at a toy across the room, does your child look at it?	Yes No
16.	Does your child walk?	Yes No
17.	Does your child look at things you are looking at?	Yes No
18.	Does your child make unusual finger movements near his/her face?	Yes No
19.	Does your child try to attract your attention to his/her own activity?	Yes No
20.	Have you ever wondered if your child is deaf?	Yes No
21.	Does your child understand what people say?	Yes No
22.	Does your child sometimes stare at nothing or wander with no purpose?	Yes No
23.	Does your child look at your face to check your reaction when faced with something unfamiliar?	Yes No

© 1999 Diana Robins, Deborah Fein, & Marianne Barton

FIGURE C-1, CONT'D

Child's Name _____   Record Number _____
Today's Date _____   Filled out by _____
Date of Birth _____

Pediatric Symptom Checklist

Emotional and physical health go together in children. Because parents are often the first to notice a problem with their child's behavior, emotions or learning, you may help your child get the best care possible by answering these questions. Please mark under the heading that best fits your child.

			Never (0)	Sometimes (1)	Often (2)
1.	Complains of aches/pains	1	____	____	____
2.	Spends more time alone	2	____	____	____
3.	Tires easily, has little energy	3	____	____	____
4.	Fidgety, unable to sit still	4	____	____	____
5.	Has trouble with a teacher	5	____	____	____
6.	Less interested in school	6	____	____	____
7.	Acts as if driven by a motor	7	____	____	____
8.	Daydreams too much	8	____	____	____
9.	Distracted easily	9	____	____	____
10.	Is afraid of new situations	10	____	____	____
11.	Feels sad, unhappy	11	____	____	____
12.	Is irritable, angry	12	____	____	____
13.	Feels hopeless	13	____	____	____
14.	Has trouble concentrating	14	____	____	____
15.	Less interest in friends	15	____	____	____
16.	Fights with others	16	____	____	____
17.	Absent from school	17	____	____	____
18.	School grades dropping	18	____	____	____
19.	Is down on him or herself	19	____	____	____
20.	Visits doctor with doctor finding nothing wrong	20	____	____	____
21.	Has trouble sleeping	21	____	____	____
22.	Worries a lot	22	____	____	____
23.	Wants to be with you more than before	23	____	____	____
24.	Feels he or she is bad	24	____	____	____
25.	Takes unnecessary risks	25	____	____	____
26.	Gets hurt frequently	26	____	____	____
27.	Seems to be having less fun	27	____	____	____
28.	Acts younger than children his or her age	28	____	____	____
29.	Does not listen to rules	29	____	____	____
30.	Does not show feelings	30	____	____	____
31.	Does not understand other people's feelings	31	____	____	____
32.	Teases others	32	____	____	____
33.	Blames others for his or her troubles	33	____	____	____
34.	Takes things that do not belong to him or her	34	____	____	____
35.	Refuses to share	35	____	____	____

Total score _____

Does your child have any emotional or behavioral problems for which she/he needs help?   ( ) N   ( ) Y
Are there any services that you would like your child to receive for these problems?   ( ) N   ( ) Y

If yes, what services? _____

FIGURE D-1 Pediatric Symptom Checklist. (Copyright M.S. Jellinek and J.M. Murphy, 1988. Used with permission.)

Children with Special Health Care Needs (CSHCN) Screener©
(mail or telephone)

1. Does your child currently need or use **medicine prescribed by a doctor** (other than vitamins)?
   - ☐ Yes → Go to Question 1a
   - ☐ No   → Go to Question 2

   1a. Is this because of ANY medical, behavioral or other health condition?
   - ☐ Yes → Go to Question 1b
   - ☐ No   → Go to Question 2

   1b. Is this a condition that has lasted or is expected to last for *at least* 12 months?
   - ☐ Yes
   - ☐ No

2. Does your child need or use more **medical care, mental health or educational services** than is usual for most children of the same age?
   - ☐ Yes → Go to Question 2a
   - ☐ No   → Go to Question 3

   2a. Is this because of ANY medical, behavioral or other health condition?
   - ☐ Yes → Go to Question 2b
   - ☐ No → Go to Question 3

   2b. Is this a condition that has lasted or is expected to last for *at least* 12 months?
   - ☐ Yes
   - ☐ No

3. Is your child **limited or prevented** in any way in his or her ability to do the things most children of the same age can do?
   - ☐ Yes → Go to Question 3a
   - ☐ No   → Go to Question 4

   3a. Is this because of ANY medical, behavioral or other health condition?
   - ☐ Yes → Go to Question 3b
   - ☐ No   → Go to Question 4

   3b. Is this a condition that has lasted or is expected to last for *at least* 12 months?
   - ☐ Yes
   - ☐ No

4. Does your child need or get **special therapy**, such as physical, occupational or speech therapy?
   - ☐ Yes → Go to Question 4a
   - ☐ No   → Go to Question 5

   4a. Is this because of ANY medical, behavioral or other health condition?
   - ☐ Yes → Go to Question 4b
   - ☐ No   → Go to Question 5

   4b. Is this a condition that has lasted or is expected to last for *at least* 12 months?
   - ☐ Yes
   - ☐ No

5. Does your child have any kind of emotional, developmental or behavioral problem for which he or she needs or gets **treatment or counseling**?
   - ☐ Yes → Go to Question 5a
   - ☐ No

   5a. Has this problem lasted or is it expected to last for *at least* 12 months?
   - ☐ Yes
   - ☐ No

FIGURE E-1 Children with Special Health Care Needs (CSHCN) Screener. (Copyright The Child and Adolescent Health Measurement Initiative. Used with permission.)

Scoring the Children with Special Health Care Needs (CSHCN) Screener©

The CSHCN Screener© uses consequences-based criteria to screen for children with chronic or special health care needs. To qualify as having chronic or special health care needs, the following criteria must be met:

a)   The child currently experiences a specific consequence.
b)   The consequence is due to a medical or other health condition.
c)   The duration or expected duration of the condition is 12 months or longer.

The first part of each screener question asks whether a child experiences one of five different health consequences:

1)   Use or need of prescription medication.
2)   Above average use or need of medical, mental health or educational services.
3)   Functional limitations compared with others of same age.
4)   Use or need of specialized therapies (OT, PT, speech, etc.).
5)   Treatment or counseling for emotional or developmental problems.

The second and third parts* of each screener question ask those responding "yes" to the first part of the question whether the consequence is due to any kind of health condition and if so, whether that condition has lasted or is expected to last for at least 12 months.

*NOTE: CSHCN screener question 5 is a two-part question. Both parts must be answered "yes" to qualify.

All three parts of at least one screener question (or in the case of question 5, the two parts) must be answered "yes" in order for a child to meet CSHCN Screener© criteria for having a chronic condition or special health care need.

The CSHCN Screener© has three "definitional domains:"

1)   Dependency on prescription medications.
2)   Service use above that considered usual or routine.
3)   Functional limitations.

The definitional domains are not mutually exclusive categories. A child identified by the CSHCN Screener© can qualify on one or more definitional domains (see diagram).

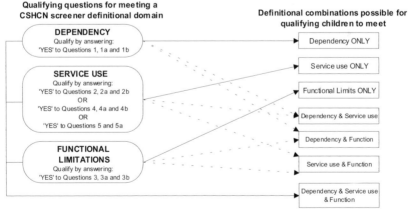

FIGURE E-1, CONT'D

Pediatric Environmental History (0-18 Years of Age)
The Screening Environmental History

For all of the questions below, most are often asked about the child's primary residence. Although some questions may specify certain locations, one should always consider all places where the child spends time, such as daycare centers, schools, and relative's houses.

Where does your child live and spend most of his/her time?	_____
What are the age, condition, and location of your home?	_____
Does anyone in the family smoke?	❑ Yes ❑ No ❑ Not sure
Do you have a carbon monoxide detector?	❑ Yes ❑ No ❑ Not sure
Do you have any indoor furry pets?	❑ Yes ❑ No ❑ Not sure
What type of heating/air system does your home have? ❑ Radiator ❑ Forced air ❑ Gas stove ❑ Wood stove ❑ Other_____	
What is the source of your drinking water? ❑ Well water ❑ City water ❑ Bottled water	
Is your child protected from excessive sun exposure?	❑ Yes ❑ No ❑ Not sure
Is your child exposed to any toxic chemicals of which you are aware?	❑ Yes ❑ No ❑ Not sure
What are the occupations of all adults in the household?	_____
Have you tested your home for radon?	❑ Yes ❑ No ❑ Not sure
Does your child watch TV, or use a computer or video game system more than two hours a day?	❑ Yes ❑ No ❑ Not sure
How many times a week does your child have unstructured, free play outside for at least 60 minutes?	_____
Do you have any other questions or concerns about your child's home environment or symptoms that may be a result of his or her environment?	_____

Follow up/ Notes

_____

_____

The Screening Environmental History is taken in part from the following sources:

▪ American Academy of Pediatrics Committee on Environmental Health. Pediatric Environmental Health 2nd ed. Etzel RA, Balk SJ, Eds. Elk Grove Village, IL: American Academy of Pediatrics; 2003. Chapter 4: How to Take an Environmental History.

▪ Balk SJ. The environmental history: asking the right questions. *Contemp Pediatr.* 1996;13:19-36.

▪ Frank A, Balk S, Carter W, et al. Case Studies in Environmental Medicine. Agency for Toxic Substances and Disease Registry, Atlanta GA. 1992, rev. 2000. Taking an Exposure History.

> This screening environmental history is designed to capture most of the common environmental exposures to children. The screening history can be administered regularly during well-child exams as well as to assess whether an environmental exposure plays a role in a child's symptoms. If a positive response is given to one or more of the screening questions, the primary care provider can consider asking questions on the topic provided in the Additional Categories and Questions to Supplement the Screening Environmental History, accessible at www.neefusa.org/pdf/PEHIhistory.pdf.

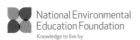

National Environmental
Education Foundation
Knowledge to live by

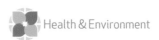

Health & Environment

Additional resources and Spanish language materials available at www.neefusa.org/health
health@neefusa.org

FIGURE F-1 Pediatric Environmental History. (Copyright National Environmental Education Foundation. Used with permission.)

Pediatric Environmental History (0-18 Years of Age)

Additional Categories and Questions to Supplement
The Screening Environmental History

For all of the questions below, most are often asked about the child's primary residence. Although some questions may specify certain locations, one should always consider all places where the child spends time, such as daycare centers, schools, and relative's houses.

General Housing Characteristics (For lead poisoning, refer to Table 3.2 in CDC Managing Elevated Blood Lead Levels Among Young Children 1.usa.gov/KAL9Yc)

Do you own or rent your home? _____

What year was your home built? (Or: Was your home built before 1978? 1950?) _____

Has your child been tested for lead? ☐ Yes ☐ No ☐ Not sure

Is there a family member or playmate with an elevated blood lead level? ☐ Yes ☐ No ☐ Not sure

Does your child spend significant time at another location? (e.g. baby sitters, school, daycare?) _____

Indoor home environment (For asthma, refer to Environmental History Form for Pediatric Asthma Patient)

If a family member smokes, does this person want to quit smoking? ☐ Yes ☐ No ☐ Not sure

Is your child exposed to smoke at the baby sitters, school, or daycare center? ☐ Yes ☐ No ☐ Not sure

Do regular visitors to your home smoke? ☐ Yes ☐ No ☐ Not sure

Have there been renovations or new carpet or furniture in the home during the past year? ☐ Yes ☐ No ☐ Not sure

Does your home have carpet? ☐ Yes ☐ No ☐ Not sure

Is the room where your child sleeps carpeted? ☐ Yes ☐ No ☐ Not sure

Do you use a wood stove or fire place? ☐ Yes ☐ No ☐ Not sure

Have you had water damage, leaks, or a flood in your home? ☐ Yes ☐ No ☐ Not sure

Do you see cockroaches in your home daily or weekly? ☐ Yes ☐ No ☐ Not sure

Do you see rats and/or mice in your home weekly? ☐ Yes ☐ No ☐ Not sure

Do you have smoke detectors in your home? ☐ Yes ☐ No ☐ Not sure

Air Pollution/Outdoor Environment (For asthma, refer to Environmental History Form for Pediatric Asthma Patient)

Is your home near an industrial site, hazardous waste site, or landfill? ☐ Yes ☐ No ☐ Not sure

Is your home near major highways or other high traffic roads? ☐ Yes ☐ No ☐ Not sure

Are you aware of Air Quality Alerts in your community? ☐ Yes ☐ No ☐ Not sure

Do you change your child's activity when an Air Quality Alert is issued? ☐ Yes ☐ No ☐ Not sure

Do you live on or near a farm where pesticides are used frequently? ☐ Yes ☐ No ☐ Not sure

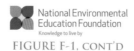

National Environmental
Education Foundation
Knowledge to live by

FIGURE F-1. CONT'D

Food and Water Contamination

If you use well water for drinking, when was the last time the water was tested?
Coliform bacteria_____ Other microbials_____ Nitrites/nitrates_____ Arsenic_____ Pesticides_____

For all types of water sources:

Have you tested your water for lead?	❑ Yes ❑ No ❑ Not sure
Do you mix infant formula with tap water?	❑ Yes ❑ No ❑ Not sure

Which types of seafood do you normally eat? _____

How many times per month do you eat that particular fish or shellfish? _____

How many times a week do you eat any of the following types of fish?
Shark_____ Swordfish_____ Tile fish_____ King mackerel_____ Albacore tuna_____ Other_____

How often do you wash fruits and vegetables before giving them to your child? _____

What type of produce do you buy? ❑ Organic ❑ Local ❑ Grocery store ❑ Other

Toxic Chemical Exposures (Also refer to Taking an Environmental History and Environmental and Occupational History in Recognition and Management of Pesticide Poisonings)

Consider this set of questions for patients with seizures, frequent headaches, or other unusual or chronic symptoms

How often are pesticides applied inside your home?	_____
How often are pesticides applied outside your home?	_____
Where do you store chemicals/pesticides?	_____
Do you often use solvents or other cleaning or disinfectant chemicals?	
Do you have a deck or play structure made from pressure treated wood?	❑ Yes ❑ No ❑ Not sure
Have you applied a sealant to the wood in the past year?	❑ Yes ❑ No ❑ Not sure
What do you use to prevent mosquito bites to your children?	_____
How often do you apply that product?	_____

Occupations and Hobbies

What type of work does your child/teenager do?	_____
Do any adults work around toxic chemicals?	❑ Yes ❑ No ❑ Not sure
If so, do they shower and change clothes before returning home from work?	❑ Yes ❑ No ❑ Not sure
Does the child or any family member have arts, crafts, ceramics, stained glass work or similar hobbies?	❑ Yes ❑ No ❑ Not sure

Health Related Questions

Have you ever relocated due to concerns about an environmental exposure?	❑ Yes ❑ No ❑ Not sure
Do symptoms seem to occur at the same time of day?	❑ Yes ❑ No ❑ Not sure
Do symptoms seem to occur after being at the same place every day?	❑ Yes ❑ No ❑ Not sure
Do symptoms seem to occur during a certain season?	❑ Yes ❑ No ❑ Not sure
Are family members/neighbors/co-workers experiencing similar symptoms?	❑ Yes ❑ No ❑ Not sure
Are there environmental concerns in your neighborhood, child's school, or day care?	❑ Yes ❑ No ❑ Not sure

Has any family member had a diagnosis of any of the following?
❑ Asthma ❑ Autism ❑ Cancer ❑ Learning disability

Does your child suffer from any of the following recurrent symptoms?
❑ Cough ❑ Headaches ❑ Fatigue ❑ Unexplained pain_____

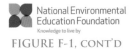

National Environmental
Education Foundation
Knowledge to live by

FIGURE F-1, CONT'D

References

- Agency for Toxic Substances and Disease Registry. Case Studies in Environmental Medicine: Pediatric Environmental Health. 2002. http://www.atsdr.cdc.gov/HEC/CSEM/pediatric/. pp 62-68, 72-73.
- Agency for Toxic Substances and Disease Registry. Case Studies in Environmental Medicine: Taking an Exposure History. 2000. http://www.atsdr.cdc.gov/HEC/CSEM/exphistory/. pp 26-29.
- Agency for Toxic Substances and Disease Registry. Environmental Exposure History (I PREPARE). http://www.atsdr.cdc.gov/Asbestos/medical_community/working_with_patients/_downloads/IPrepareCard.pdf.
- Association of Occupational and Environmental Clinics. Pediatric Environmental Health History (Goldman R., Shannon M., Woolf A). 1999. http://www.aoec.org/resources.htm.
- Centers for Disease Control and Prevention. Managing Elevated Blood Lead Levels Among Young Children: Recommendations from the Advisory Committee on Childhood Lead Poisoning Prevention. Atlanta: CDC; 2002. http://www.cdc.gov/nceh/lead/CaseManagement/caseManage_main.htm.
- Centers for Disease Control and Prevention/ National Center for Environmental Health. Key Clinical Activities for Quality Asthma Care. 2003. http://www.cdc.gov/mmwr/preview/mmwrhtml/rr5206a1.htm. pp 5-6.
- Children's Environmental Health Network. Environmental History-Taking (Balk S., Walton-Brown S., Pope A). 1999. http://www.cehn.org/cehn/trainingmanual/pdf/manual-envhist.pdf.
- Dunn AM, Burns C, Sattler B. Environmental Health of Children. Journal of Pediatric Health Care. Sept-Oct 2003;17(5); 223-23. p. 225.
- Environmental Protection Agency. Asthma Home Environment Checklist. February 2004. http://www.epa.gov/asthma/pdfs/home_environment_checklist.pdf.
- Environmental Protection Agency. Recognition and Management of Pesticide Poisonings. March 1999. http://www.epa.gov/oppfead1/safety/healthcare/handbook/handbook.htm. pp 20-21.
- Environmental Protection Agency. Tips to Protect Children from Environmental Risks. November 2004. http://yosemite.epa.gov/ochp/ochpweb.nsf/content/tips.htm.
- Institute of Medicine. Nursing, Health, and the Environment. http://www.nap.edu/books/030905298X/html/. pp 263-270.
- Pope AM, Snyder MA, Mood LH, eds. Nursing, Health, and the Environment, Institute of Medicine Report. Washington, DC: National Academy Press; 1995.
- Roberts JR, Landers KM, Fargason CA. An unusual source of lead poisoning. Clinical Pediatrics 1998;37:377-9.
- Roberts JR, Reigart JR. Environmental Health Education in the medical school curriculum. Ambulatory Pediatrics 2001;1:108-111.
- The National Environmental Education Foundation. Environmental History Form for Pediatric Asthma Patient. http://www.neefusa.org/health/asthma/asthmahistoryform.htm.
- The National Environmental Education Foundation. National Pesticide Competency Guidelines for Medical & Nursing Education. http://www.neefusa.org/health/pesticidesguidelinepublications/education.htm. pp 35-36.
- The National Environmental Education Foundation. National Pesticide Practice Skills Guidelines for Medical & Nursing Practice. http://www.neefusa.org/health/pesticidesguidelinepublications/practice.htm. pp.30-32.
- The National Environmental Education Foundation. Taking an Environmental History. http://www.neefusa.org/pdf/EnvhistoryNEETF.pdf.
- University of Connecticut Health Center and US Environmental Protection Agency. Guidance for Clinicians on the Recognition and Management of Health Effects Related to Mold Exposure and Moisture Indoors. http://www.oehc.uchc.edu/clinser/MOLD%20GUIDE.pdf. pp 38-39, 41.
- University of Maryland. Developing a Pesticide Exposure History. 2002. http://www.entmclasses.umd.edu/Leaflets/pil25.pdf. pp 3-10.
- University of Maryland School of Nursing. Environmental Health Assessment Guide for a Home and Family. http://www.envirn.umaryland.edu/kellogg/HPDPFamilyAssessment.pdf.

Advisory Committee

Funded in part by The New York Community Trust

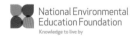

National Environmental
Education Foundation
Knowledge to live by

4301 Connecticut Avenue, Suite 160 • Washington, DC 20008 • Tel. (202) 261-6475 • health@neefusa.org • www.neefusa.org/health

FIGURE F-1, CONT'D

SCAT2

Sport Concussion Assessment Tool 2

Name _____

Sport/team _____

Date/time of injury _____

Date/time of assessment _____

Age _____ Gender ☐ M ☐ F

Years of education completed _____

Examiner _____

What is the SCAT2?[1]

This tool represents a standardized method of evaluating injured athletes for concussion and can be used in athletes aged from 10 years and older. It supersedes the original SCAT published in 2005[2]. This tool also enables the calculation of the Standardized Assessment of Concussion (SAC)[3,4] score and the Maddocks questions[5] for sideline concussion assessment.

Instructions for using the SCAT2

The SCAT2 is designed for the use of medical and health professionals. Preseason baseline testing with the SCAT2 can be helpful for interpreting post-injury test scores. Words in Italics throughout the SCAT2 are the instructions given to the athlete by the tester.

This tool may be freely copied for distribition to individuals, teams, groups and organizations.

What is a concussion?

A concussion is a disturbance in brain function caused by a direct or indirect force to the head. It results in a variety of non-specific symptoms (like those listed below) and often does not involve loss of consciousness. Concussion should be suspected in the presence of **any one or more** of the following:

- Symptoms (such as headache), or
- Physical signs (such as unsteadiness), or
- Impaired brain function (e.g. confusion) or
- Abnormal behaviour.

Any athlete with a suspected concussion should be REMOVED FROM PLAY, medically assessed, monitored for deterioration (i.e., should not be left alone) and should not drive a motor vehicle.

Symptom Evaluation

How do you feel?

You should score yourself on the following symptoms, based on how you feel now.

	none	mild		moderate		severe	
Headache	0	1	2	3	4	5	6
"Pressure in head"	0	1	2	3	4	5	6
Neck Pain	0	1	2	3	4	5	6
Nausea or vomiting	0	1	2	3	4	5	6
Dizziness	0	1	2	3	4	5	6
Blurred vision	0	1	2	3	4	5	6
Balance problems	0	1	2	3	4	5	6
Sensitivity to light	0	1	2	3	4	5	6
Sensitivity to noise	0	1	2	3	4	5	6
Feeling slowed down	0	1	2	3	4	5	6
Feeling like "in a fog"	0	1	2	3	4	5	6
"Don't feel right"	0	1	2	3	4	5	6
Difficulty concentrating	0	1	2	3	4	5	6
Difficulty remembering	0	1	2	3	4	5	6
Fatigue or low energy	0	1	2	3	4	5	6
Confusion	0	1	2	3	4	5	6
Drowsiness	0	1	2	3	4	5	6
Trouble falling asleep (if applicable)	0	1	2	3	4	5	6
More emotional	0	1	2	3	4	5	6
Irritability	0	1	2	3	4	5	6
Sadness	0	1	2	3	4	5	6
Nervous or Anxious	0	1	2	3	4	5	6

Total number of symptoms (Maximum possible 22)

Symptom severity score
(Add all scores in table, maximum possible: 22 x 6 = 132)

Do the symptoms get worse with physical activity?   ☐ Y   ☐ N
Do the symptoms get worse with mental activity?   ☐ Y   ☐ N

Overall rating

If you know the athlete well prior to the injury, how different is the athlete acting compared to his / her usual self? Please circle one response.

no different	very different	unsure

FIGURE G-1   Sports Concussion Assessment Tool 2 (SCAT 2). (From *Br J Sports Med* 43(Suppl 1): i85-i88, 2009.)

Cognitive & Physical Evaluation

1 Symptom score (from page 1)

22 **minus** number of symptoms   of 22

2 Physical signs score

Was there loss of consciousness or unresponsiveness?   Y   N
If yes, how long? _____ minutes
Was there a balance problem/unsteadiness?   Y   N

Physical signs score (1 point for each negative response)   of 2

3 Glasgow coma scale (GCS)

Best eye response (E)

No eye opening	1
Eye opening in response to pain	2
Eye opening to speech	3
Eyes opening spontaneously	4

Best verbal response (V)

No verbal response	1
Incomprehensible sounds	2
Inappropriate words	3
Confused	4
Oriented	5

Best motor response (M)

No motor response	1
Extension to pain	2
Abnormal flexion to pain	3
Flexion/Withdrawal to pain	4
Localizes to pain	5
Obeys commands	6

Glasgow Coma score (E + V + M)   of 15

GCS should be recorded for all athletes in case of subsequent deterioration.

4 Sideline Assessment – Maddocks Score

"I am going to ask you a few questions, please listen carefully and give your best effort."

Modified Maddocks questions (1 point for each correct answer)

At what venue are we at today?	0	1
Which half is it now?	0	1
Who scored last in this match?	0	1
What team did you play last week/game?	0	1
Did your team win the last game?	0	1

Maddocks score   of 5

Maddocks score is validated for sideline diagnosis of concussion only and is not included in SCAT 2 summary score for serial testing.

5 Cognitive assessment
Standardized Assessment of Concussion (SAC)

Orientation (1 point for each correct answer)

What month is it?	0	1
What is the date today?	0	1
What is the day of the week?	0	1
What year is it?	0	1
What time is it right now? (within 1 hour)	0	1

Orientation score   of 5

Immediate memory
"I am going to test your memory. I will read you a list of words and when I am done, repeat back as many words as you can remember, in any order."

Trials 2 & 3:
"I am going to repeat the same list again. Repeat back as many words as you can remember in any order, even if you said the word before."

Complete all 3 trials regardless of score on trial 1 & 2. Read the words at a rate of one per second. Score 1 pt. for each correct response. Total score equals sum across all 3 trials. Do not inform the athlete that delayed recall will be tested.

List	Trial 1	Trial 2	Trial 3	Alternative word list		
elbow	0 1	0 1	0 1	candle	baby	finger
apple	0 1	0 1	0 1	paper	monkey	penny
carpet	0 1	0 1	0 1	sugar	perfume	blanket
saddle	0 1	0 1	0 1	sandwich	sunset	lemon
bubble	0 1	0 1	0 1	wagon	iron	insect
Total						

Immediate memory score   of 15

Concentration
Digits Backward:
"I am going to read you a string of numbers and when I am done, you repeat them back to me backwards, in reverse order of how I read them to you. For example, if I say 7-1-9, you would say 9-1-7."

If correct, go to next string length. If incorrect, read trial 2. One point possible for each string length. Stop after incorrect on both trials. The digits should be read at the rate of one per second.

		Alternative digit lists		
4-9-3	0 1	6-2-9	5-2-6	4-1-5
3-8-1-4	0 1	3-2-7-9	1-7-9-5	4-9-6-8
6-2-9-7-1	0 1	1-5-2-8-6	3-8-5-2-7	6-1-8-4-3
7-1-8-4-6-2	0 1	5-3-9-1-4-8	8-3-1-9-6-4	7-2-4-8-5-6

Months in Reverse Order:
"Now tell me the months of the year in reverse order. Start with the last month and go backward. So you'll say December, November ... Go ahead"

1 pt. for entire sequence correct

Dec-Nov-Oct-Sept-Aug-Jul-Jun-May-Apr-Mar-Feb-Jan	0	1

Concentration score   of 5

[1] This tool has been developed by a group of international experts at the 3rd International Consensus meeting on Concussion in Sport held in Zurich, Switzerland in November 2008. The full details of the conference outcomes and the authors of the tool are published in British Journal of Sports Medicine, 2009, volume 43, supplement 1.
The outcome paper will also be simultaneously co-published in the May 2009 issues of Clinical Journal of Sports Medicine, Physical Medicine & Rehabilitation, Journal of Athletic Training, Journal of Clinical Neuroscience, Journal of Science & Medicine in Sport, Neurosurgery, Scandinavian Journal of Science & Medicine in Sport and the Journal of Clinical Sports Medicine.

[2] McCrory P et al. Summary and agreement statement of the 2nd International Conference on Concussion in Sport, Prague 2004. British Journal of Sports Medicine. 2005; 39: 196-204

[3] McCrea M. Standardized mental status testing of acute concussion. Clinical Journal of Sports Medicine. 2001; 11: 176-181

[4] McCrea M, Randolph C, Kelly J. Standardized Assessment of Concussion: Manual for administration, scoring and interpretation. Waukesha, Wisconsin, USA.

[5] Maddocks, DL; Dicker, GD; Saling, MM. The assessment of orientation following concussion in athletes. Clin J Sport Med. 1995;5(1):32–3

[6] Guskiewicz KM. Assessment of postural stability following sport-related concussion. Current Sports Medicine Reports. 2003; 2: 24-30

FIGURE G-1, CONT'D

6 Balance examination

This balance testing is based on a modified version of the Balance Error Scoring System (BESS)[a]. A stopwatch or watch with a second hand is required for this testing.

Balance testing

"I am now going to test your balance. Please take your shoes off, roll up your pant legs above ankle (if applicable), and remove any ankle taping (if applicable). This test will consist of three twenty second tests with different stances."

(a) Double leg stance:
"The first stance is standing with your feet together with your hands on your hips and with your eyes closed. You should try to maintain stability in that position for 20 seconds. I will be counting the number of times you move out of this position. I will start timing when you are set and have closed your eyes."

(b) Single leg stance:
"If you were to kick a ball, which foot would you use? [This will be the dominant foot] Now stand on your non-dominant foot. The dominant leg should be held in approximately 30 degrees of hip flexion and 45 degrees of knee flexion. Again, you should try to maintain stability for 20 seconds with your hands on your hips and your eyes closed. I will be counting the number of times you move out of this position. If you stumble out of this position, open your eyes and return to the start position and continue balancing. I will start timing when you are set and have closed your eyes."

(c) Tandem stance:
*"Now stand heel-to-toe with your **non-dominant foot** in back. Your weight should be evenly distributed across both feet. Again, you should try to maintain stability for 20 seconds with your hands on your hips and your eyes closed. I will be counting the number of times you move out of this position. If you stumble out of this position, open your eyes and return to the start position and continue balancing. I will start timing when you are set and have closed your eyes."*

Balance testing – types of errors
1. Hands lifted off iliac crest
2. Opening eyes
3. Step, stumble, or fall
4. Moving hip into > 30 degrees abduction
5. Lifting forefoot or heel
6. Remaining out of test position > 5 sec

Each of the 20-second trials is scored by counting the errors, or deviations from the proper stance, accumulated by the athlete. The examiner will begin counting errors only after the individual has assumed the proper start position. **The modified BESS is calculated by adding one error point for each error during the three 20-second tests. The maximum total number of errors for any single condition is 10.** If a athlete commits multiple errors simultaneously, only one error is recorded but the athlete should quickly return to the testing position, and counting should resume once subject is set. Subjects that are unable to maintain the testing procedure for a minimum of **five seconds** at the start are assigned the highest possible score, ten, for that testing condition.

Which foot was tested: Left   Right
(i.e. which is the **non-dominant** foot)

Condition	Total errors
Double Leg Stance (feet together)	of 10
Single leg stance (non-dominant foot)	of 10
Tandem stance (non-dominant foot at back)	of 10
Balance examination score (30 **minus** total errors)	of 30

7 Coordination examination

Upper limb coordination

Finger-to-nose (FTN) task: *"I am going to test your coordination now. Please sit comfortably on the chair with your eyes open and your arm (either right or left) outstretched (shoulder flexed to 90 degrees and elbow and fingers extended). When I give a start signal, I would like you to perform five successive finger to nose repetitions using your index finger to touch the tip of the nose as quickly and as accurately as possible."*

Which arm was tested: Left   Right

Scoring: 5 correct repetitions in < 4 seconds = 1

Note for testers: Athletes fail the test if they do not touch their nose, do not fully extend their elbow or do not perform five repetitions. Failure should be scored as 0.

Coordination score   of 1

8 Cognitive assessment

Standardized Assessment of Concussion (SAC)

Delayed recall
"Do you remember that list of words I read a few times earlier? Tell me as many words from the list as you can remember in any order."

Circle each word correctly recalled. Total score equals number of words recalled.

List		Alternative word list	
elbow	candle	baby	finger
apple	paper	monkey	penny
carpet	sugar	perfume	blanket
saddle	sandwich	sunset	lemon
bubble	wagon	iron	insect

Delayed recall score   of 5

Test domain	Score
Symptom score	of 22
Physical signs score	of 2
Glasgow Coma score (E + V + M)	of 15
Balance examination score	of 30
Coordination score	of 1
Subtotal	**of 70**
Orientation score	of 5
Immediate memory score	of 5
Concentration score	of 15
Delayed recall score	of 5
SAC subtotal	**of 30**
SCAT2 total	**of 100**
Maddocks Score	**of 5**

Definitive normative data for a SCAT2 "cut-off" score is not available at this time and will be developed in prospective studies. Embedded within the SCAT2 is the SAC score that can be utilized separately in concussion management. The scoring system also takes on particular clinical significance during serial assessment where it can be used to document either a decline or an improvement in neurological functioning.

Scoring data from the SCAT2 or SAC should not be used as a stand alone method to diagnose concussion, measure recovery or make decisions about an athlete's readiness to return to competition after concussion.

FIGURE G-1, CONT'D

Athlete Information

Any athlete suspected of having a concussion should be removed from play, and then seek medical evaluation.

Signs to watch for

Problems could arise over the first 24-48 hours. You should not be left alone and must go to a hospital at once if you:
- Have a headache that gets worse
- Are very drowsy or can't be awakened (woken up)
- Can't recognize people or places
- Have repeated vomiting
- Behave unusually or seem confused; are very irritable
- Have seizures (arms and legs jerk uncontrollably)
- Have weak or numb arms or legs
- Are unsteady on your feet; have slurred speech

Remember, it is better to be safe.
Consult your doctor after a suspected concussion.

Return to play

Athletes should not be returned to play the same day of injury. When returning athletes to play, they should follow a stepwise symptom-limited program, with stages of progression. For example:
1. rest until asymptomatic (physical and mental rest)
2. light aerobic exercise (e.g. stationary cycle)
3. sport-specific exercise
4. non-contact training drills (start light resistance training)
5. full contact training after medical clearance
6. return to competition (game play)

There should be approximately 24 hours (or longer) for each stage and the athlete should return to stage 1 if symptoms recur. Resistance training should only be added in the later stages.
Medical clearance should be given before return to play.

Tool	Test domain	Time	Score			
		Date tested				
		Days post injury				
	Symptom score					
	Physical signs score					
	Glasgow Coma score (E + V + M)					
SCAT2	Balance examination score					
	Coordination score					
	Orientation score					
	Immediate memory score					
SAC	Concentration score					
	Delayed recall score					
	SAC Score					
Total	SCAT2					
Symptom severity score (max possible 132)						
Return to play			Y N	Y N	Y N	Y N

Additional comments

Concussion injury advice (To be given to concussed athlete)

This patient has received an injury to the head. A careful medical examination has been carried out and no sign of any serious complications has been found. It is expected that recovery will be rapid, but the patient will need monitoring for a further period by a responsible adult. Your treating physician will provide guidance as to this timeframe.

If you notice any change in behaviour, vomiting, dizziness, worsening headache, double vision or excessive drowsiness, please telephone the clinic or the nearest hospital emergency department immediately.

Other important points:
- Rest and avoid strenuous activity for at least 24 hours
- No alcohol
- No sleeping tablets
- Use paracetamol or codeine for headache. Do not use aspirin or anti-inflammatory medication
- Do not drive until medically cleared
- Do not train or play sport until medically cleared

Clinic phone number

Patient's name

Date/time of injury

Date/time of medical review

Treating physician

Contact details or stamp

FIGURE G-1, CONT'D

INDEX

Note: Page numbers followed by "f" indicate figures, "t" indicate tables, and "b" indicate boxes.